Pediatric Retinal Vascular Diseases

Ulrich Spandau • Sang Jin Kim

Pediatric Retinal Vascular Diseases

From Angiography to Vitrectomy

Springer

Ulrich Spandau
Ophthalmology
University of Uppsala Ophthalmology
Uppsala
Sweden

Sang Jin Kim
Department of Ophthalmology
Samsung Medical Center
Sungkyunkwan University
Seoul
South Korea

Additional material to this book can be downloaded from http://extras.springer.com.

ISBN 978-3-030-13703-8 ISBN 978-3-030-13701-4 (eBook)
https://doi.org/10.1007/978-3-030-13701-4

Library of Congress Control Number: 2019935808

This Springer imprint is published by the registered company Springer Nature Switzerland AG.
The registered company address is: Gewerbestrasse 11, 6330 Cham, Switzerland

Preface

Dear reader,

This book provides comprehensive and up-to-date information on diagnosis, medical, and surgical treatments for pediatric retinal vascular conditions, which are leading causes of childhood blindness throughout the world. Experienced ophthalmologists in this field discuss basic knowledge about these diseases, practical aspects of management such as exam under anesthesia, up-to-date diagnostic approaches including spectral-domain handheld optical coherence tomography (OCT), and OCT angiography. A high emphasis is placed on recent advances in medical and surgical treatments for pediatric retinal vascular diseases. Step-by-step instructions are given for the surgical treatment with anti-VEGF treatment, laser photocoagulation, and vitrectomy. Both the general ophthalmologist who cares for children with retinal diseases and the specialist (pediatric ophthalmologists and vitreoretinal surgeon) will find this book to be an informative resource in providing best care for children with pediatric retinal vascular conditions.

The book includes many videos, which demonstrate the surgeries step-by-step. All videos are listed in the Video list and can be accessed under http://extras.springer.com/Search. Enter the ISBN number of your book and download the videos.

Alternatively, the online version of every chapter contains the videos. Note the following footmark at the beginning of every chapter:

"**Electronic Supplementary Material** The online version of this chapter (https://doi.org/10.1007/978-3-030-13701-4_16) contains supplementary material, which is available to authorized users." Copy and paste the https address in your browser and you can access the videos.

Uppsala, Sweden — Ulrich Spandau
Seoul, South Korea — Sang Jin Kim

Acknowledgments

I want to thank my family and especially my wife Katrin for her never-ending patience with a husband who spends so much time with his books.

Ulrich Spandau

Contents

Abbreviations

FA	fluorescein angiography
FEVR	familial exudative vitreoretinopathy
GA	gestational age
LE	left eye
LIO	laser indirect ophthalmoscopy
PHPV	persistent hyperplastic primary vitreous
PMA	postmenstrual age
RE	right eye
ROP	retinopathy of prematurity

List of Videos

The videos can be accessed under http://extras.springer.com/Search. Enter the ISBN number of your book and download the videos.

Part I
Pediatric Retinal Diseases

Chapter 1
Coats Disease

1.1 Diagnosis of Coats Disease

1.1.1 Introduction

Coats disease is an idiopathic retinal vascular disorder characterized by retinal telangiectasia, exudation, and exudative retinal detachment. In 1908, George Coats first described case series with retinal telangiectasia and massive exudation [1]. Coats disease occurs most commonly in males in the first or second decades, but it can be diagnosed at any age. The majority of cases are unilateral, but recent studies using wide-field fluorescein angiography revealed that subclinical abnormalities such as peripheral nonperfusion are common in contralateral eyes [2, 3]. The clinical manifestations of Coats disease are highly variable, ranging from telangiectasia only to phthisis bulbi.

1.1.2 Pathogenesis

1.1.2.1 Histopathology

A histologic study on enucleated eyes with Coats disease revealed macrophage infiltration and cholesteric clefts in the subretinal space [4]. Retinal vascular abnormalities were also demonstrated including dilated vessels with hyalinized vessel walls [4]. Immunoreactivity for VEGF was observed in the detached retina, dilated vessel, and macrophages infiltrating the subretinal proliferative tissue [4]. VEGFR-2 immunoreactivity was also observed in endothelial cells located in abnormal retinal vessels and inner layer of the detached retina, but not in macrophages infiltrating the subretinal space [4].

U. Spandau, S. J. Kim, *Pediatric Retinal Vascular Diseases*,
https://doi.org/10.1007/978-3-030-13701-4_1

1.1.3 *Genetics*

Previous studies reported mutations in several genes including *NDP* [5], *CRB1* [6], *TINF2* [7], *PANK2* [8], and *ABCA4* [9] in patients with Coats disease or Coats-like retinal phenotype. However, the exact molecular mechanisms remain to be elucidated.

1.1.4 *Clinical Characteristics*

1.1.4.1 **Fundus Findings** [10–12]

Retinal vascular telangiectasis (Figs. 1.1 and 1.2) develop most commonly in the inferior and temporal quadrants between the equator and the ora serrata [12]. Affected vessels show irregular and aneurysmal dilations. Vascular leakage from

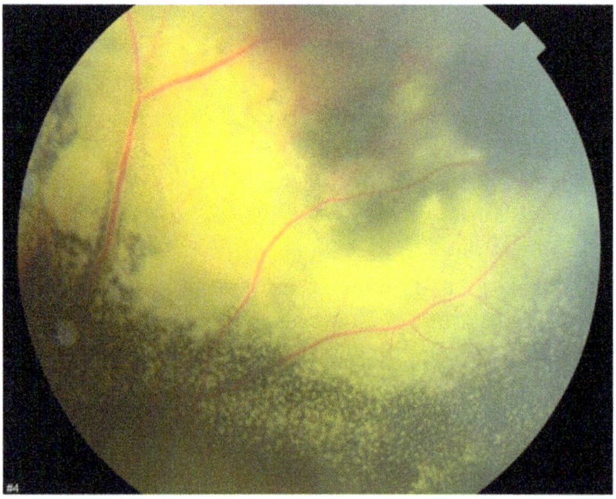

Fig. 1.1 Peripheral telangiectatic vessels with massive exudation and retinal detachment

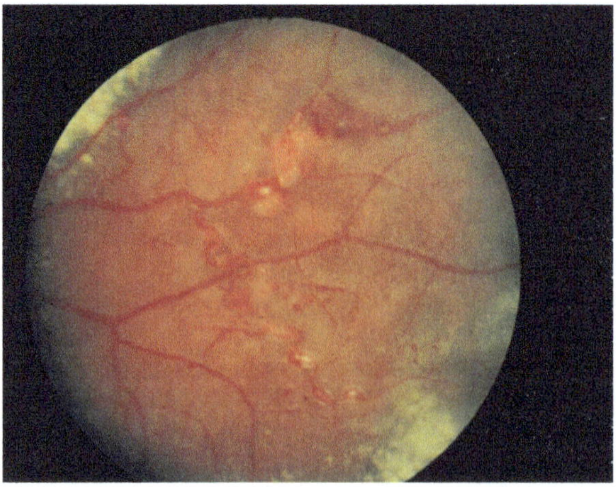

Fig. 1.2 Typical area of retinal telangiectasia without associated exudation. (Reprinted from Shields et al. [12]. Copyright (2001), with permission from Elsevier)

the abnormal vessels result in lipid-rich exudation (Figs. 1.3 and 1.4) and progressive fluid accumulation with subsequent serous retinal detachment (Figs. 1.5, 1.6, and 1.7) [11]. Macular edema or subretinal fluid is a common cause of visual symptom.

Retinal pigment epithelial cells that proliferate and migrate into the subretinal space may develop subretinal fibrous proliferation [11].

The vitreous usually remains clear [11]. Vitreoretinal traction, fibrosis, or proliferative vitreoretinopathy are not common but epiretinal membrane may develop [11].

In a large-scale case series (n = 150 patients) study by Shields et al. in 2001 [10], median age at the diagnosis was 5 years. Among the 150 patients, 114 (76%) were males and 142 (95%) showed unilateral involvement [10]. The most common referral diagnoses were Coats disease in 64 (41%) followed by retinoblastoma in 43 (27%) patients [10]. Visual acuity at presentation was 20/200 or worse in 121 eyes (76%) [10]. The retinal telangiectasia involved the midperipheral or peripheral

Fig. 1.3 Exudates at posterior pole in an 8-year old boy with Coats disease

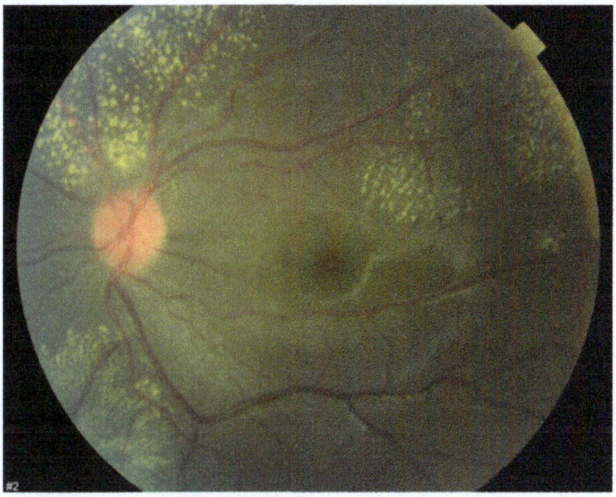

Fig. 1.4 Long-standing exudates at posterior pole in Coats disease

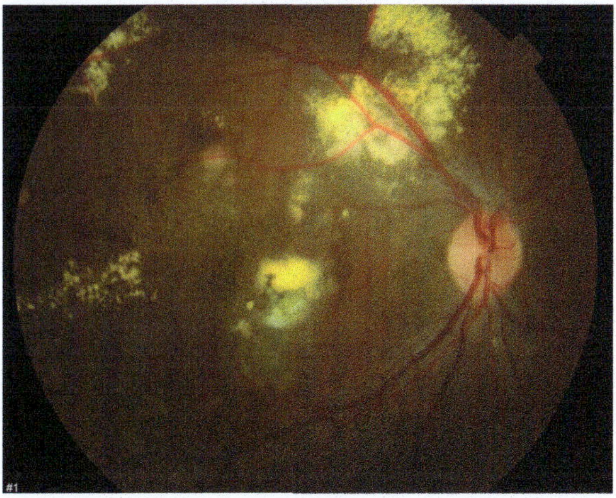

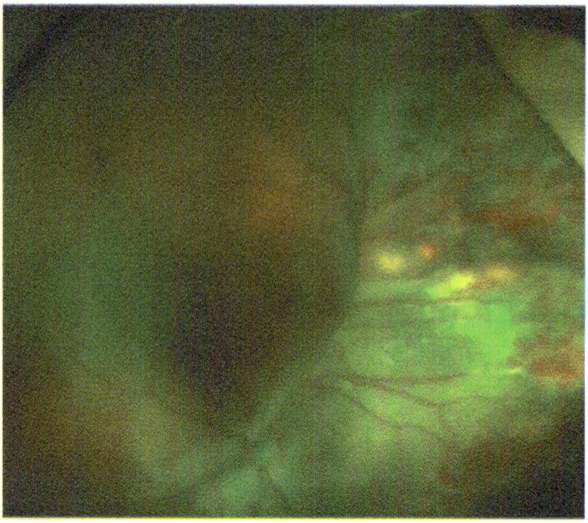

Fig. 1.5 Total retinal detachment in Coats disease

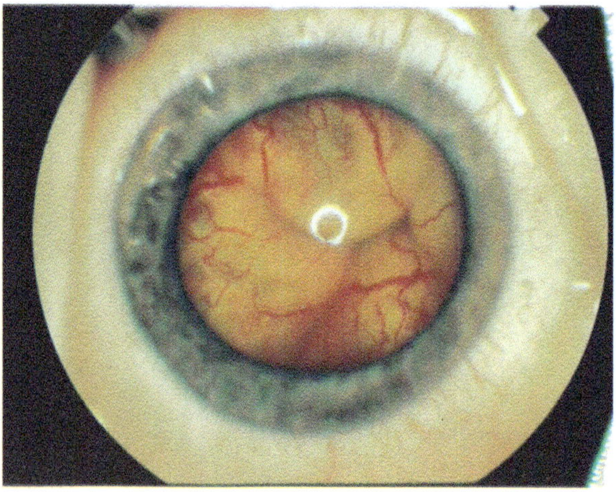

Fig. 1.6 Total retinal detachment in a patient with Coats disease. (Reprinted from Shields et al. [12]. Copyright (2001), with permission from Elsevier)

fundus in 98% of eyes [10]. Retinal exudation was present in six or more clock hours in 115 eyes (73%) [10]. Total retinal detachment was seen in 74 eyes (47%) and neovascular glaucoma in 12 eyes (8%) [10].

1.1.5 Fluorescein Angiography

Wide-field angiography systems such as RetCam (Natus) or Ultra-widefield™ retinal imaging systems (Optos) are essential in diagnosis and management of Coats disease. The angiographic features of Coats disease include areas of nonperfusion, peripheral telangiectatic capillaries and "light bulb" aneurysms, vascular leakage,

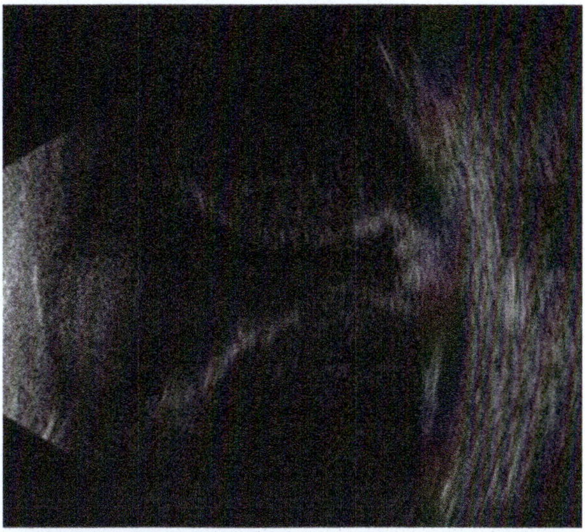

Fig. 1.7 B-scan ultrasonography of total retinal detachment in a 12-year-old boy

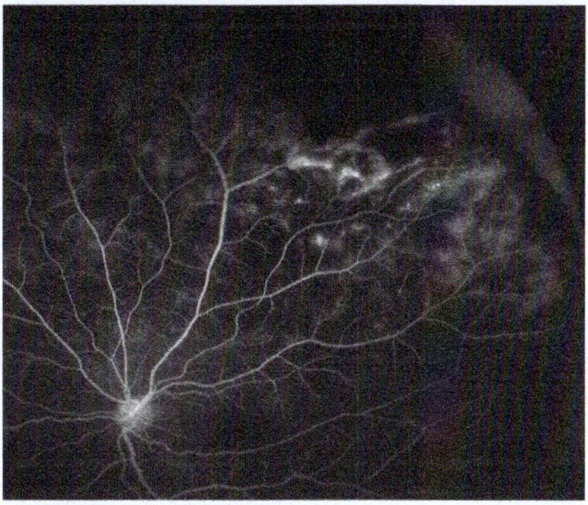

Fig. 1.8 Ultra-wide field fluorescein angiography showing dilated peripheral vessels with leakage in a patient with Coats disease

and blocked fluorescence from exudates (Figs. 1.8, 1.9, 1.10, and 1.11) [11]. Fluorescein angiography is essential in early detection of vascular abnormalities especially in eyes with telangiectasia only.

1.1.6 Optical Coherence Tomography (OCT)

In Coats disease, OCT is useful in identifying macular edema and subretinal fluid and to evaluate response to treatment. Subretinal fluid and exudate may be visible with OCT in patients with Coats disease (Figs. 1.12 and 1.13). It should be noted

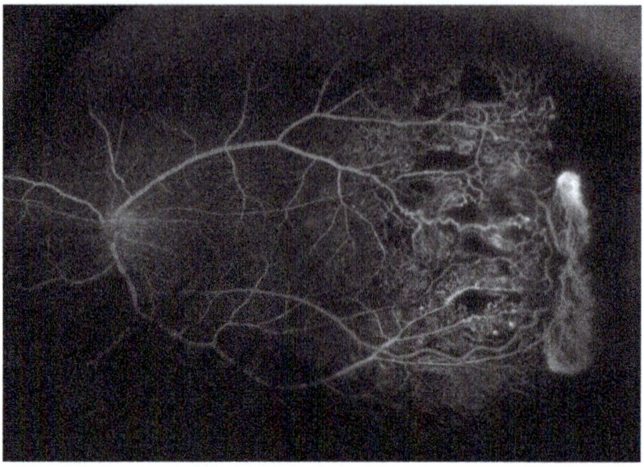

Fig. 1.9 Ultra-wide field fluorescein angiography showing dilated peripheral vessels and nonperfusion in a patient with Coats disease

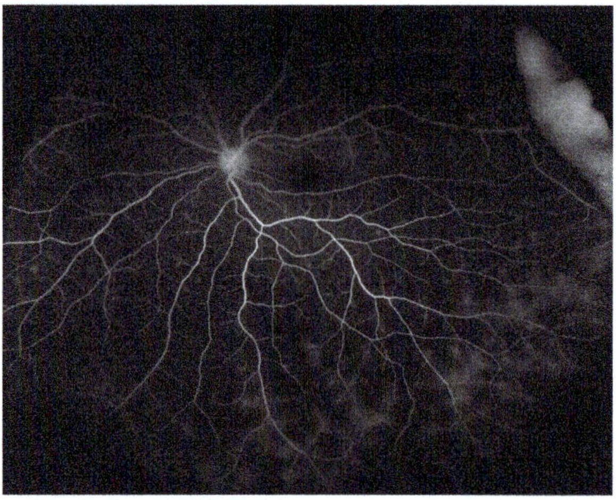

Fig. 1.10 Mild late leakage in normal-looking vessels in the inferior periphery in a patient with Coats disease

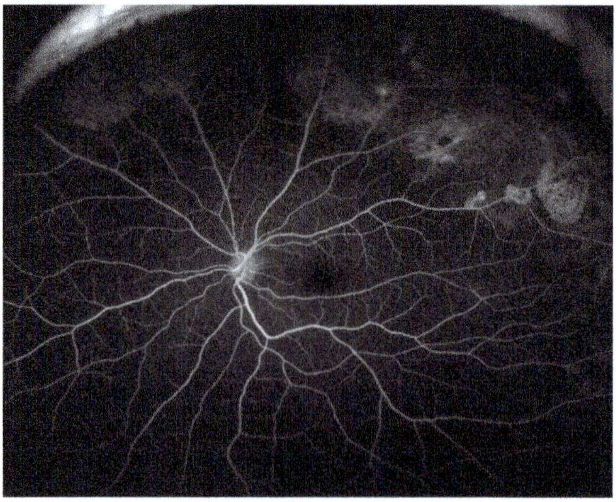

Fig. 1.11 Decreased leakage after cryotherapy in a patient with Coats disease

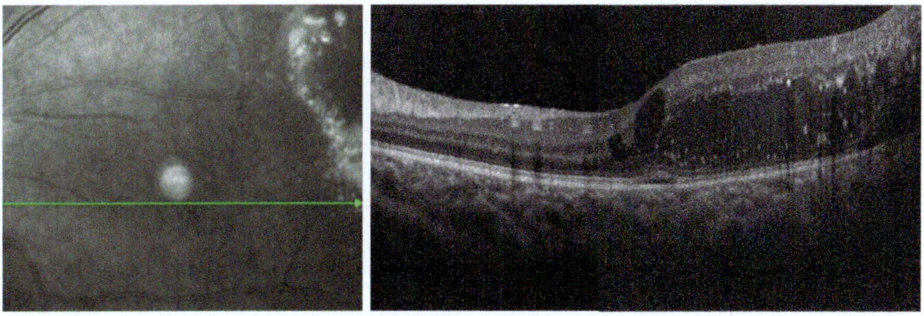

Fig. 1.12 SD-OCT showing macular edema and exudates in a patient with Coats disease

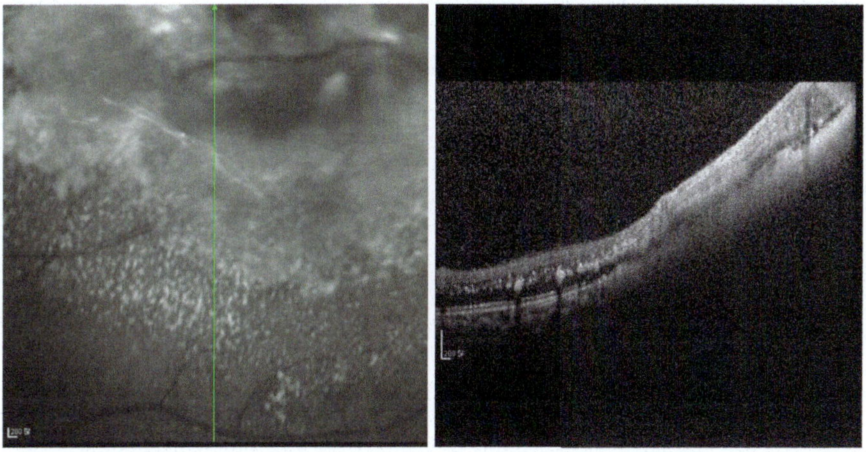

Fig. 1.13 SD-OCT showing intraretinal lipid deposits in a patient with Coats disease

that in eyes with large amount of subretinal fluid, the amount of subretinal fluid seen on OCT scans taken in a sitting position may be different from that in a supine position due to fluid shifting.

1.2 Classification of Coats Disease

1.2.1 A Classification System

Shields et al. proposed a classification system of Coats disease based on their clinical observations in 150 consecutive patients in 2001 [10]. Their proposed classification system is now being widely-used and very helpful for selecting treatment methods and predicting the visual outcomes (Table 1.1 and Fig. 1.14).

Table 1.1 Staging classification of Coats disease [10]

Stage	Findings
1	Retinal telangiectasia only
2	Telangiectasia and exudation
A	Extrafoveal exudation
B	Foveal exudation
3	Exudative retinal detachment
A	Subtotal detachment 1. Extrafoveal 2. Foveal
B	Total detachment
4	Total retinal detachment; glaucoma
5	Advanced end-stage disease

Eyes with stage 1 disease can be managed by either regular follow-up exams or laser photocoagulation [10]. In stage 1 disease, there is high probability that the eye can be salvaged and the visual prognosis is usually favorable [10]. However, stage 1 disease is rare in a real clinical practice probably due to no symptoms.

Eyes with stage 2 disease can be managed by laser photocoagulation or cryotherapy, depending on the extent and location of the disease [10]. In stage 2A, the visual prognosis is generally good [10]. Eyes with stage 2B are usually salvaged and the visual prognosis is fairly good [10]. Visual prognosis of eyes with a dense yellow gray nodule by the foveal exudation is usually worse [10].

Eyes with stage 3A disease can generally be managed by photocoagulation or cryotherapy [10]. Some of the patients with stage 3A1 disease (extrafoveal subtotal retinal detachment) in a sitting position can reveal subfoveal fluid in a supine position (thus stage 3A2). Even if the retinal detachment involves the fovea, it will resolve when the telangiectasias are treated [10]. Laser photocoagulation is less effective in areas of retinal detachment, and cryotherapy is often preferable in such instances [10]. However, Levinson and Hubbard reported good anatomical outcome of 577 nm yellow laser photocoagulation in 16 patients including 5 patients with stage 3B disease [13]. Patients with stage 3B with bullous detachment may require surgical treatment (e.g. external subretinal fluid drainage).

Patients who present with stage 4 disease are often best managed by enucleation to relieve the severe ocular pain [10]. Patients with stage 5 disease generally have a blind, but comfortable eye and require no aggressive treatment [10].

1.2.2 *Stage and Visual Outcome*

The staging system of Coats disease is helpful for selecting treatment and predicting the ocular and visual outcomes. In a case series study including 150 patients from 1975 to 1999, the visual outcome was generally poor [10]. The proportion of

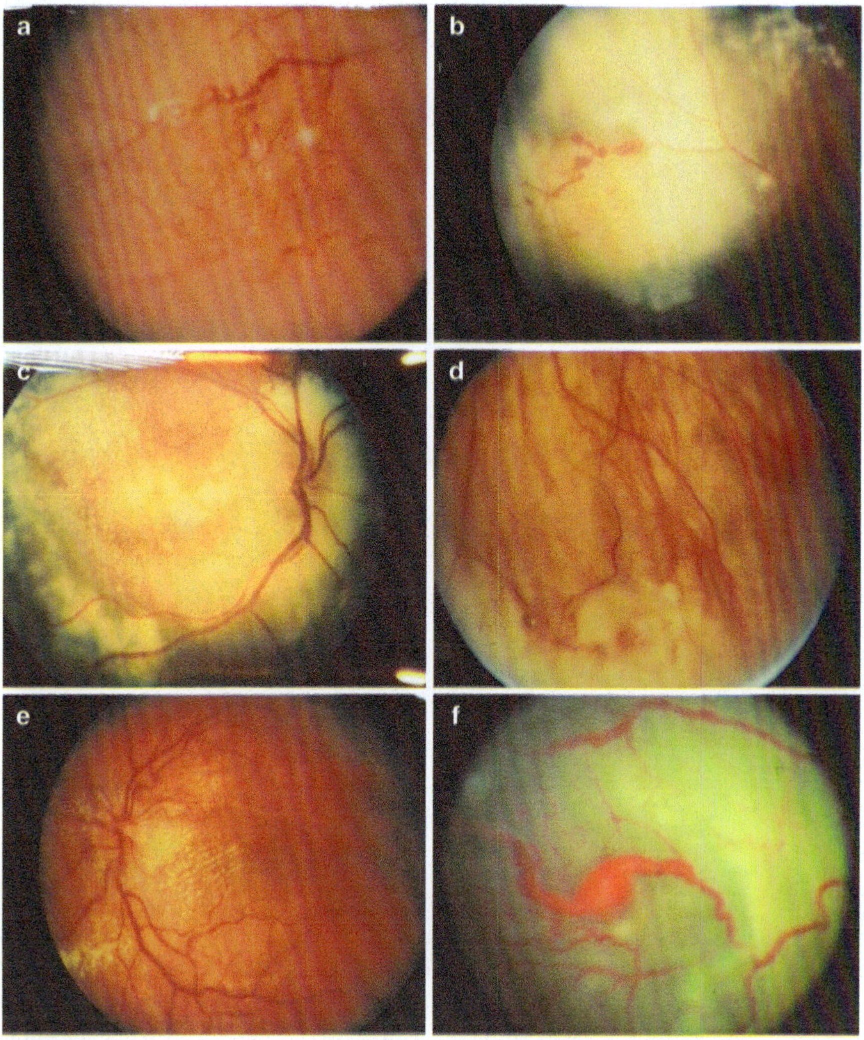

Fig. 1.14 Examples of stages of Coats disease. (**a**) Stage 1, retinal telangiectasia only. (**b**) Stage 2A, telangiectasia and extrafoveal exudation. (**c**) Stage 2B, foveal exudation. (**d**) Stage 3A1, subtotal retinal detachment inferiorly, sparing the fovea. (**e**) Stage 3A2, subtotal retinal detachment extending beneath the fovea. (**f**) Stage 3B, total exudative retinal detachment. (**g**) Stage 4, total exudative retinal detachment behind the lens in eye with secondary glaucoma. (**h**) Stage 5, advanced end stage disease with chronic inflammation, posterior synechia and cataract, secondary to longstanding retinal detachment. (Reprinted from Shields et al. [12]. Copyright (2001), with permission from Elsevier)

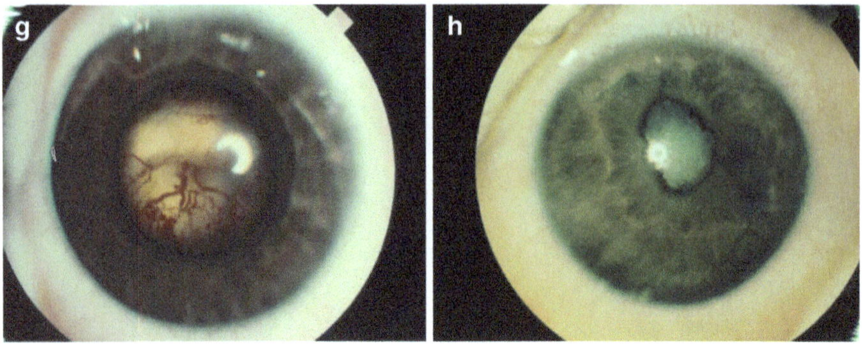

Fig. 1.14 (continued)

Table 1.2 Visual outcome according to the stage of Coats Disease

	Shields et al. [10]		Ong et al. [14] 1995–2005		2006–2015	
Stage	% poor visual outcome[a]	Number of eyes	% poor visual outcome[a]	Number of eyes	% poor visual outcome[a]	Number of eyes
1	0	1				
2A	30	10	50	2	0	1
2B	86	7	67	3	33	3
3A1	70	25	80	5	70	10
3A2	70	23				
3B	94	37	100	5	100	3
4	100	18	100	1		0
5	100	3		0		0

[a]Poor visual outcome was defined as BCVA of 20/200 or worse

poor visual outcome (20/200 or worse) was high in eyes with stage 2B through 5 (Table 1.2). Recently, Ong et al. [14] compared visual outcome between two time periods (decade 1, 1995–2005 and decade 2, 2006–2015), and showed that (1) there was a trend for the mean initial presenting VA for decade 1 eyes to be worse than for decade 2 eyes; (2) from initial to final follow-up visit, mean VA also worsened for decade 1 eyes, but remained stable for decade 2 eyes; (3) at the end of follow-up, there was a trend for mean VA for decade 1 eyes to be worse than for decade 2 eyes; and (4) decade 2 eyes had a higher average number of procedures per eye compared with decade 1 eyes (Table 1.2). In conclusion, this study showed that the earlier presentation of disease in decade 2 suggests improvements in disease detection over time, and there was a trend for eyes to have better final VA in decade 2.

References

1. Coats G. Forms of retinal diseases with massive exudation. Graefes Arhiv für Ophthalmologie. 1912;17:440–525.
2. Blair MP, Ulrich JN, Elizabeth Hartnett M, Shapiro MJ. Peripheral retinal nonperfusion in fellow eyes in coats disease. Retina. 2013;33:1694–9.
3. Jung EH, Kim JH, Kim SJ, Yu YS. Fluorescein angiographic abnormalities in the contralateral eye with Normal fundus in children with unilateral Coats' disease. Korean J Ophthalmol. 2018;32:65–9.
4. Kase S, Rao NA, Yoshikawa H, Fukuhara J, Noda K, Kanda A, Ishida S. Expression of vascular endothelial growth factor in eyes with Coats' disease. Invest Ophthalmol Vis Sci. 2013;54:57–62.
5. Black GC, Perveen R, Bonshek R, Cahill M, Clayton-Smith J, Lloyd IC, McLeod D. Coats' disease of the retina (unilateral retinal telangiectasis) caused by somatic mutation in the NDP gene: a role for norrin in retinal angiogenesis. Hum Mol Genet. 1999;8:2031–5.
6. Hasan SM, Azmeh A, Mostafa O, Megarbane A. Coat's like vasculopathy in leber congenital amaurosis secondary to homozygous mutations in CRB1: a case report and discussion of the management options. BMC Res Notes. 2016;9:91.
7. Gupta MP, Talcott KE, Kim DY, Agarwal S, Mukai S. Retinal findings and a novel TINF2 mutation in Revesz syndrome: clinical and molecular correlations with pediatric retinal vasculopathies. Ophthalmic Genet. 2017;38:51–60.
8. Sohn EH, Michaelides M, Bird AC, Roberts CJ, Moore AT, Smyth D, Brady AF, Hungerford JL. Novel mutation in PANK2 associated with retinal telangiectasis. Br J Ophthalmol. 2011;95:149–50.
9. Saatci AO, Ayhan Z, Yaman A, Bora E, Ulgenalp A, Kavukcu S. A 12-year-old girl with bilateral Coats disease and ABCA4 gene mutation. Case Rep Ophthalmol. 2018;9:375–80.
10. Shields JA, Shields CL, Honavar SG, Demirci H, Cater J. Classification and management of Coats disease: the 2000 Proctor Lecture. Am J Ophthalmol. 2001;131:572–83.
11. Sigler EJ, Randolph JC, Calzada JI, Wilson MW, Haik BG. Current management of Coats disease. Surv Ophthalmol. 2014;59:30–46.
12. Shields JA, Shields CL, Honavar SG, Demirci H. Clinical variations and complications of Coats disease in 150 cases: the 2000 Sanford Gifford Memorial Lecture. Am J Ophthalmol. 2001;131:561–71.
13. Levinson JD, Hubbard GB 3rd. 577-nm yellow laser photocoagulation for Coats disease. Retina. 2016;36:1388–94.
14. Ong SS, Buckley EG, McCuen BW 2nd, Jaffe GJ, Postel EA, Mahmoud TH, Stinnett SS, Toth CA, Vajzovic L, Mruthyunjaya P. Comparison of visual outcomes in Coats' disease: a 20-year experience. Ophthalmology. 2017;124:1368–76.

Chapter 2
Norrie Disease

2.1 Introduction

Norrie disease is a rare X-linked recessive disorder caused by mutations of *NDP* gene, which encodes a Wnt pathway protein, norrin. Patients with Norrie disease often present with blindness by incomplete vascularization, dysplastic retina and retinal detachment. Also, hearing loss and mental retardation are common in patients with Norrie disease.

2.2 Genetics

NDP is located on Xp11.3. Most patients have pathogenic mutations involving a cysteine residue in the cysteine-knot motif in the exon 3 [1, 2]. Many kinds of pathologic variants of *NDP* were associated with Norrie Disease including missense, null, splice-site, and deletions.

2.3 Ocular Features

Ophthalmic manifestations include leukocoria, retrolental fibroplasia, severe retinal dysplasia, and retinal detachment. Patients with Norrie disease present with blindness (no light perception) with bilateral retinal detachment at birth or shortly after birth (mostly by 3 months) [3].

In a retrospective case series by Drenser et al. [2], patients with Norrie disease presented with a similar retinal appearance of dense stalk tissue, globular dystrophic retina, and peripheral avascular retina with pigmentary changes.

U. Spandau, S. J. Kim, *Pediatric Retinal Vascular Diseases*,
https://doi.org/10.1007/978-3-030-13701-4_2

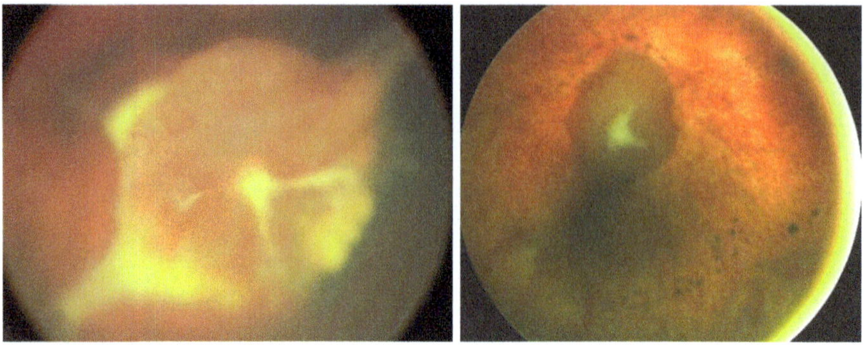

Fig. 2.1 Dysplastic retinas demonstrating the unique retinal structure associated with Norrie disease. Note the vascularized dysplastic retinal mass, called as "pumpkin" lesions. (Reprinted from Drenser et al. [2]. https://journals.lww.com/retinajournal/Abstract/2007/02000/A_CHARACTERISTIC_PHENOTYPIC_RETINAL_APPEARANCE_IN.16.aspx. Copyright (2007), with permission from Wolters Kluwer Health, Inc.)

Walsh et al. [3] described greyish-yellow masses (pseudogliomas) that consist of fibrovascular material behind the lens that disrupts the normal red reflex as "pumpkin" lesions (Fig. 2.1).

Non-retinal ocular manifestations include anterior chamber synechiae, cataract, hypoplasia of iris, hypotelorism, sclerocornea, nystagmus, ectopia lentis, shallow anterior chamber, and so on [4].

2.4 Extraocular Features

2.4.1 Auditory Findings

A knock-out mouse model with an Ndp gene disruption suggested that one of the principal functions of norrin in the ear is to regulate the interaction of the cochlea with its vasculature [5]. *NDP* mutations with subsequent defective norrin may cause progressive loss of vessels in the stria vascularis of the cochlea and lead to sensorineural hearing loss. Studies showed that almost all patients will eventually suffer some degree of hearing loss [6, 7].

2.4.2 Neurological Findings

Smith et al. study on 56 patients with IP showed that about one-third of patients had cognitive impairment. Also, behavioral disorders (such as autism) and chromic seizure disorder were also common [7].

2.4.3 Peripheral Vascular Disease

Smith et al. also showed 38% of Norrie disease patients reported issues with varicose veins, venous stasis ulcers, and/or erectile dysfunction [7].

2.5 Management

Patients with Norrie disease are recommended to have regular follow-up, even if no light perception, to monitor for a painful blind eye.

There is no standard established treatment for Norrie disease. However, laser photocoagulation and vitrectomy were reported to be useful in some cases.

A retrospective study of 14 boys with Norrie disease by Walsh et al. [3] in 2010 demonstrated that early vitrectomy (performed in the first 3–4 months of life) preserved at least light perception in at least one eye in 7 patients, 3 had no light perception bilaterally, and visual acuity data were not available for 4 patients. Also, only 2 of 24 eyes became phthisical [3]. The authors proposed elease of traction on the retina is likely to at least partly explain the benefit of vitrectomy for Norrie disease [3]. They also hypothesized that patients with complete retinal detachments should still be considered for vitrectomy to prevent development of phthisis bulbi [3].

In 2010, Chow et al. [8] reported the first case of laser photocoagulation to the avascular retina in a neonate born at 37 weeks. The mother had undergone prenatal amniocentesis fetal-genetic testing at 23 weeks of gestation [8]. A C520T (nonsense) mutation was found in the NDP gene [8]. After examination under anesthesia confirmed the diagnosis on the first day of life, laser photocoagulation was applied to the avascular retina bilaterally [8]. Complete regression of extraretinal fibrovascular proliferation was observed 1 month after laser treatment and no retinal detachment had occurred until 24 months [8].

In 2014, Sisk et al. [9] reported the first planned preterm delivery of a patient with a pathogenic *NDP* mutation identified by amniocentesis. Prompt laser photocoagulation at 34 weeks resulted in regression of neovascularization and resolution of hemorrhage [9].

These two cases suggest that there may be a chance to salvage eyes with Norrie disease several months before 40 weeks PMA.

References

1. Wu WC, Drenser K, Trese M, Capone A Jr, Dailey W. Retinal phenotype-genotype correlation of pediatric patients expressing mutations in the Norrie disease gene. Arch Ophthalmol. 2007;125:225–30.
2. Drenser KA, Fecko A, Dailey W, Trese MT. A characteristic phenotypic retinal appearance in Norrie disease. Retina. 2007;27:243–6.

3. Walsh MK, Drenser KA, Capone A Jr, Trese MT. Early vitrectomy effective for Norrie disease. Arch Ophthalmol. 2010;128:456–60.
4. From, https://rarediseases.info.nih.gov/diseases/7224/norrie-disease. Last accesses on 11 Nov 2018.
5. Rehm HL, Zhang DS, Brown MC, Burgess B, Halpin C, Berger W, Morton CC, Corey DP, Chen ZY. Vascular defects and sensorineural deafness in a mouse model of Norrie disease. J Neurosci. 2002;22:4286–92.
6. Halpin C, Owen G, Gutiérrez-Espeleta GA, Sims K, Rehm HL. Audiologic features of Norrie disease. Ann Otol Rhinol Laryngol. 2005;114:533–8.
7. Smith SE, Mullen TE, Graham D, Sims KB, Rehm HL. Norrie disease: extraocular clinical manifestations in 56 patients. Am J Med Genet A. 2012;158:1909–17.
8. Chow CC, Kiernan DF, Chau FY, Blair MP, Ticho BH, Galasso JM, Shapiro MJ. Laser photocoagulation at birth prevents blindness in Norrie's disease diagnosed using amniocentesis. Ophthalmology. 2010;117:2402–6.
9. Sisk RA, Hufnagel RB, Bandi S, Polzin WJ, Ahmed ZM. Planned preterm delivery and treatment of retinal neovascularization in Norrie disease. Ophthalmology. 2014;121:1312–3.

Chapter 3
Incontinentia Pigmenti

Incontinentia pigmenti (IP), also known as Bloch-Sulzberger syndrome, is a rare X-linked dominant disorder that involves skin, eye, central nervous system, hair, teeth and nails [1, 2]. Although characteristic skin lesions are crucial for diagnosis, blindness due to retinal vascular occlusion with neovascularization and psychomotor retardation are the two most serious complications of IP.

3.1 Pathophysiology and Genetics of IP

IP is caused by mutations, in *IKBKG* (inhibitor of nuclear factor kappa B kinase subunit gamma) (previously called *NEMO*) on Xq28. Because IP is an X-linked dominant disease, affected male fetuses usually do not survive, so majority of patients (>90%) with IP are female [2]. However, some male patients have also been reported: they are more severely affected than their female counterparts, with a significant occurrence of sex chromosome aneuploidy [3]. IP has high genetic penetrance and variable phenotypic expressivity. Most cases are sporadic; IP is familial in only 10–25% of cases [2]. Differences in expressivity may be explained by X-inactivation (also called lyonization) in females.

IKBKG encodes for the NEMO (nuclear factor kß essential modulator) protein or IKK-γ (inhibitor of nuclear factor kappa-ß kinase, subunit gamma). NEMO (or IKK-γ) is required for the activation of the nuclear factor kappa B (NF-κB) transcription factor. NF-κB upregulates the immune response and also prevents cellular apoptosis. Thus, mutations in IKBKG result in impaired NF- κB activation, which may leave cells susceptible to apoptosis from intrinsic factors [2].

The most common mutations in IP is a large deletion in the exons (4 through 10) of *IKBKG* gene, causing loss of function and reduced NF-κB activity [2]. This

U. Spandau, S. J. Kim, *Pediatric Retinal Vascular Diseases*,
https://doi.org/10.1007/978-3-030-13701-4_3

mutation accounts for about 60–80% of IP-causing mutations [4]. While most cases of IP are caused by frameshift or nonsense mutations, some may only involve a partial loss of NEMO (or IKK-γ) activity [2].

3.2 Clinical Features

3.2.1 Ocular Manifestations

Ocular manifestations occur from the neonatal period through the early infantile period [1]. Ocular involvements of IP patients have been reported in several studies with variable prevalence, from 16% to 77% [1]. In patients with suspicious IP, fundus examination should be performed early. More than half of ocular findings are considered vision-threatening [2].

Retinal abnormalities in incontinentia pigmenti range from avascular peripheral retina to tractional or exudative retinal detachment. Peripheral avascularity is a hallmark of retinal findings in IP. Progressive retinal vascular occlusion may result in neovascularization, hemorrhages foveal atrophy, macular vascular aneurysms, arteriovenous anastomoses, and exudative or tractional retinal detachments [2].

Fluorescein angiography is crucial in detecting avascular retina, retinal neovascularization and leakage (Figs. 3.1, 3.2, 3.3, and 3.4). Also, macular capillary nonperfusion may occur. Because retinal findings typically occur before age 2, most patients require EUA (examinations under anesthesia) including retinal photography, fluorescein angiography, and OCT, if possible. However, fluorescein angiography may be obtainable in an office setting with the use of non-contact ultra-widefield retinal imaging system with oral fluorescein (Figs. 3.5 and 3.6) [5].

Nonretinal ocular manifestations include strabismus, nystagmus, optic atrophy, cataract, uveitis, conjunctival pigmentation, corneal epithelial and stromal keratitis, and iris hypoplasia [2].

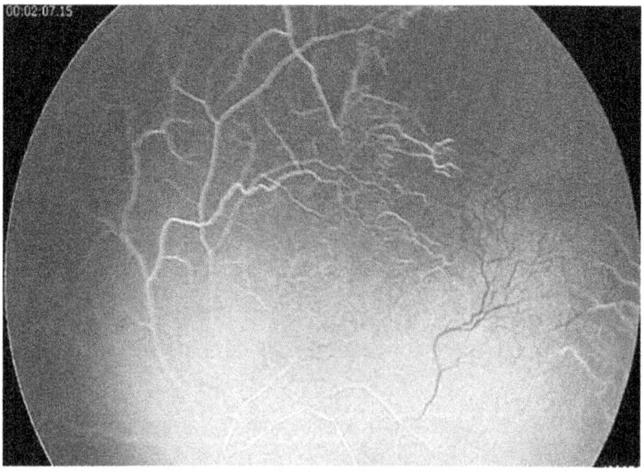

Fig. 3.1 Fluorescein angiography showing the abnormal retinal vessels and delayed venous filling. (Reprinted from O'Doherty et al. [9]. Copyright (2011) with permission from BMJ Publishing Group Ltd)

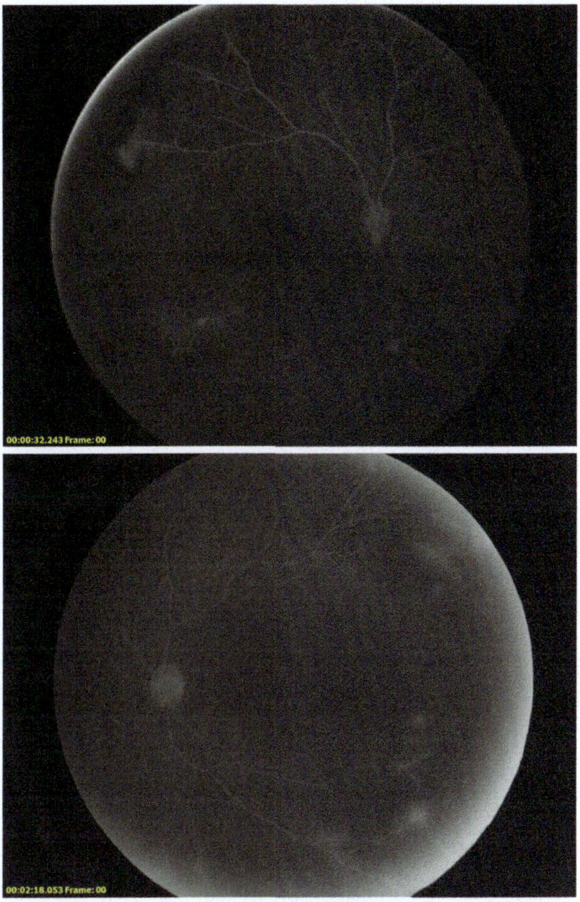

Fig. 3.2 Fluorescein angiography using RetCam in a 6-month baby with incontinentia pigmenti. (Courtesy of J. Peter Campbell, MD, MPH at Oregon Health and Science University Casey Eye Institute, Portland, Oregon, USA)

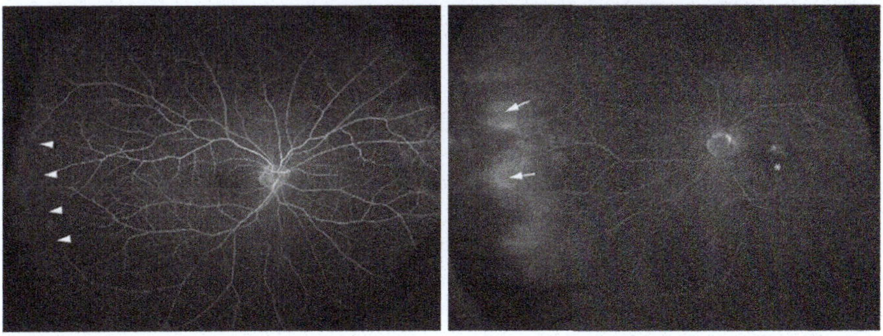

Fig. 3.3 Wide-field angiography showing mild nonperfusion temporally in the right eye (arrowheads) and nasal nonperfusion, arterio-venous loops, and mild late leakage (arrows) in a patient with IP. (Reprinted from Chen et al. [6]. https://journals.lww.com/retinajournal/Abstract/2015/12000/VARIABLE_EXPRESSION_OF_RETINOPATHY_IN_A_PEDIGREE.23.aspx. Copyright (2015), with permission from Wolters Kluwer Health, Inc)

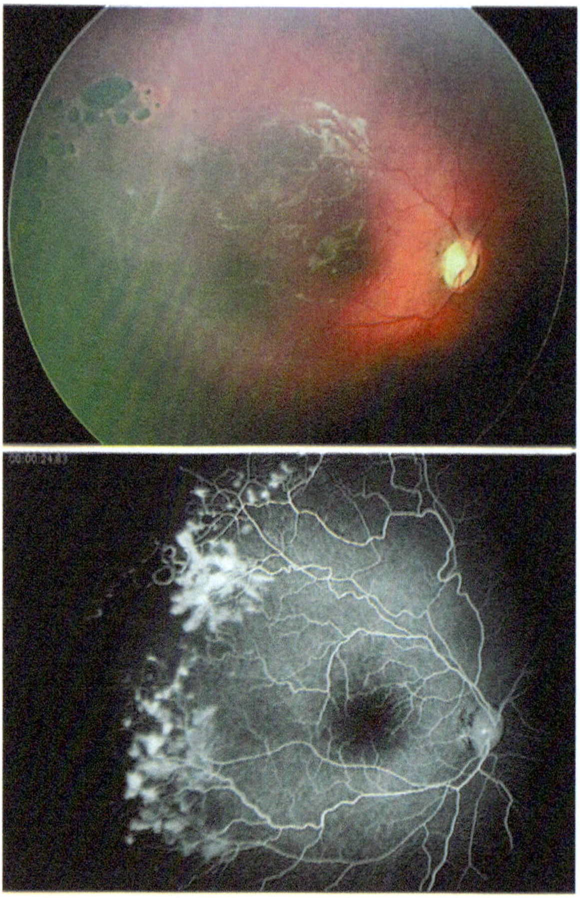

Fig. 3.4 Fundus photography and fluorescein angiography showing neovascularization and vascular leakage in a 4-year-old girl with IP. (Reprinted from Ranchod and Trese [7]. https://journals.lww.com/retinajournal/Citation/2010/04000/Regression_of_Retinal_Neovascularization_After.25.aspx. Copyright (2010), with permission from Wolters Kluwer Health, Inc)

3.2.2 Retinal Screening Protocol

In 2000, Holmström and Thorén [8] proposed the following schedule of monitoring: dilated eye examinations soon after birth, monthly for the first 4 months, every 3 months until 1 year of age, twice per year up to 3 years of age, and then annually throughout the childhood. However, in 2011, O'Doherty et al. [9] mentioned that if the retina is normal when examined under anesthesia, once the diagnosis has been fully established then it will remain normal. On the contrary, if the retina is abnormal at birth, then fluorescein angiography should be performed early to identify ischemic areas and retinal examinations should be frequent, every 2 weeks for the first 3 months, then monthly for 6 months then every 3 months for 1 year.

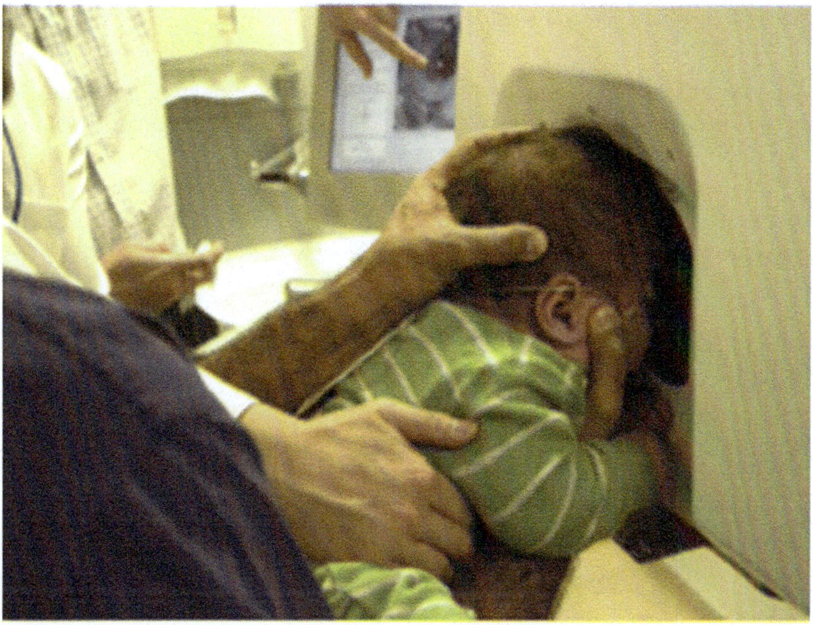

Fig. 3.5 Flying baby position to acquire fluorescein angiography in an office setting by using an ultra-widefield non-contact system with oral fluorescein. (Reprinted from Patel et al. [5]. Copyright (2013), with permission from Elsevier)

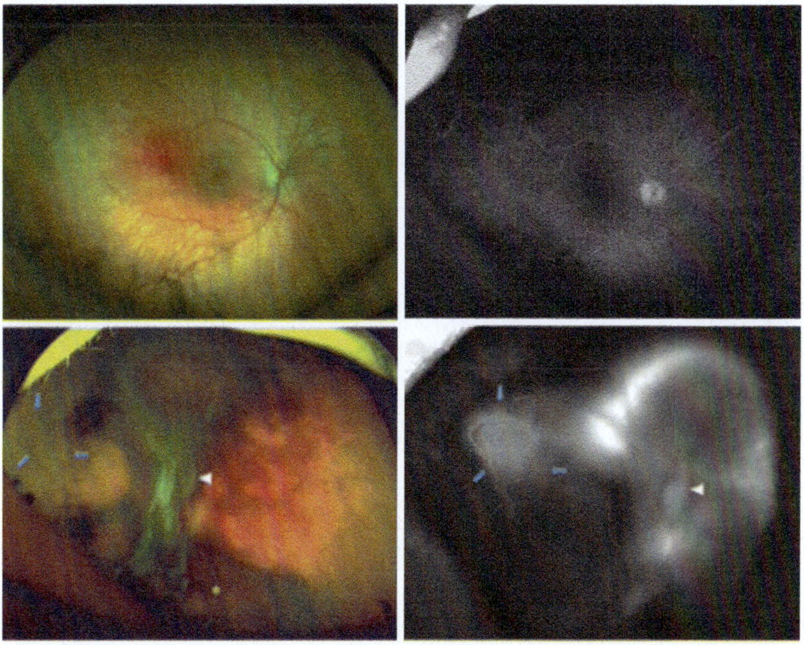

Fig. 3.6 Fluorescein angiography in an office setting by using an ultra-widefield non-contact system with oral fluorescein. (Reprinted from Patel et al. [5]. Copyright (2013), with permission from Elsevier)

3.3 Skin Manifestations

A rash starting within a few months of birth is the most common presenting sign. Skin lesions occur in nearly all IP patients and are considered to be nearly pathognomonic if they show the specific pattern and progression [2]. Stages of skin changes in IP are presented in Table 3.1. These skin lesions have a specific pattern of distribution along the Lines of Blaschko, which are patterns of dermal development during embryogenesis.

3.4 Neurologic Manifestations

Neurologic findings are present in about one third of IP cases. The neurological manifestations of IP include convulsive disorders, spastic paralysis, motor retardation, and mental retardation [2].

In a systematic review, the most frequent CNS types of anomalies were seizures, motor impairment, mental retardation and microcephaly [10].

3.5 Other Manifestations

Dental problems occur in more than half of affected individuals [2]. The most common dental abnormalities are absence of teeth or shape anomalies [2]. Alopecia, nail abnormalities and breast abnormalities may also be present [2].

3.6 Diagnostic Criteria of IP

In 1993 diagnostic criteria for IP were established by Landy and Donnai [11]. In 2014, Minić et al. proposed updated criteria of IP (Table 3.2) [1]. They proposed as major criteria one of the stages of IP skin lesions. As updated IP minor criteria, they included: dental, ocular; central nervous system, hair, nail, palate, breast and

Table 3.1 Stages of skin changes in IP

Stage	Skin changes
1. Vesiculo-bullous stage	Erythema and blistering
2. Verrucous stage	Hypertrophic rash
3. Hyperpigmented stage	Hyperpigmentation
4. Atrophic/ hypopigmented stage	Hypopigmentation and alopecia

Table 3.2 Updated diagnostic criteria of IP in 2014

<table>
<tr><th>Major criteria</th><th>Minor criteria (supportive evidence)</th><th>Conditions for establishing IP diagnosis</th></tr>
<tr><td rowspan="2">Typical IP skin stages distributed along Blaschko's lines:</td><td>Dental anomalies</td><td>No evidence of IP in a first-degree female relative:</td></tr>
<tr><td>Ocular anomalies</td><td rowspan="4">If lacking genetic IKBKG mutation data, at least two or more major criteria or one major and one or more minor criteria are necessary to make a diagnosis of sporadic IP</td></tr>
<tr><td>Vesiculo-bullous stage</td><td>CNS anomalies</td></tr>
<tr><td>Verrucous stage</td><td>Alopecia</td></tr>
<tr><td>Hyperpigmented stage</td><td>Abnormal hair (sparse hair, wooly hair, anomalies of eyebrows and eyelashes)</td></tr>
<tr><td rowspan="5">Atrophic/hypopigmented stage</td><td>Abnormal nails</td><td>In the case of confirmed IKBKG mutation typical for IP any single major or minor criterion is satisfactory for IP diagnosis</td></tr>
<tr><td>Palate anomalies</td><td rowspan="2">Evidence of IP in a first-degree female relative: Any single major or at least two minor criteria</td></tr>
<tr><td>Nipple and breast anomalies</td></tr>
<tr><td>Multiple male miscarriages</td><td rowspan="2">In all cases eosinophilia and skewed X-chromosome inactivation supports diagnosis</td></tr>
<tr><td>Typical skin pathohistological findings</td></tr>
</table>

nipple anomalies; multiple male miscarriages, and IP pathohistological findings. In the diagnosis of IP, the presence of *IKBKG* mutation typical for IP, and existence of family relatives with diagnosed IP can be considered.

References

1. Minić S, Trpinac D, Obradović M. Incontinentia pigmenti diagnostic criteria update. Clin Genet. 2014;85:536–42. Epub 2013 July 21.
2. Swinney CC, Han DP, Karth PA. Incontinentia pigmenti: a comprehensive review and update. Ophthalmic Surg Lasers Imaging Retina. 2015;46:650–7.
3. Scheuerle AE. Male cases of incontinentia pigmenti: case report and review. Am J Med Genet. 1998;77:201–18.
4. Fusco F, Pescatore A, Bal E, Ghoul A, Paciolla M, Lioi MB, D'Urso M, Rabia SH, Bodemer C, Bonnefont JP, Munnich A, Miano MG, Smahi A, Ursini MV. Alterations of the IKBKG locus and diseases: an update and a report of 13 novel mutations. Hum Mutat. 2008;29:595–604.
5. Patel CK, Fung TH, Muqit MM, Mordant DJ, Geh V. Non-contact ultra-widefield retinal imaging and fundus fluorescein angiography of an infant with incontinentia pigmenti without sedation in an ophthalmic office setting. J AAPOS. 2013;17:309–11.
6. Chen CJ, Han IC, Goldberg MF. Variable expression of retinopathy in a pedigree of patients with incontinentia pigmenti. Retina. 2015;35:2627–32.
7. Ranchod TM, Trese MT. Regression of retinal neovascularization after laser photocoagulation in incontinentia pigmenti. Retina. 2010;30:708–9.

8. Holmström G, Thorén K. Ocular manifestations of incontinentia pigmenti. Acta Ophthalmol Scand. 2000;78:348–53.
9. O'Doherty M, Mc Creery K, Green AJ, Tuwir I, Brosnahan D. Incontinentia pigmenti--ophthalmological observation of a series of cases and review of the literature. Br J Ophthalmol. 2011;95:11–6.
10. Minić S, Trpinac D, Obradović M. Systematic review of central nervous system anomalies in incontinentia pigmenti. Orphanet J Rare Dis. 2013;8:25.
11. Landy SJ, Donnai D. Incontinentia pigmenti (Bloch-Sulzberger syndrome). J Med Genet. 1993;30:53–9.

Chapter 4
Familial Exudative Vitreoretinopathy

4.1 Introduction

Familial exudative vitreoretinopathy (FEVR) is a rare hereditary vitreoretinal condition characterized by retinal avascular area, neovascularization, tractional retinal detachment, and exudation. These findings are similar to retinopathy of prematurity, but most patients with FEVR do not have a history of premature birth. So, FEVR has often been described as "similar to retinopathy of prematurity, but in full-term babies."

In 1969, Criswick and Schepens first described 6 patients (of 2 families) with FEVR.1 They described dragging of retinal vessels, macular ectopia, peripheral new vessels, exudation and so on [1]. In 1976, Canny and Oliver first reported fluorescein angiographic findings including peripheral nonperfusion in FEVR patients [2]. In 1998, Pendergast and Trese proposed a 5-stage classification system based on fundus findings [3]. In 2014, Trese and colleagues revised clinical staging system based on clinical and angiographic features [4].

4.2 Pathophysiology and Genetics

The primary pathology of FEVR is abnormal retinal vascular development of the peripheral retina, which is complicated by ischemia and retinal neovascularization. Abnormal retinal new vessels are prone to leakage and bleeding, with subsequent hemorrhage, exudates, retinal fold, retinal traction, followed by retinal detachment.

FEVR is genetically heterogenous. FEVR is inherited as an autosomal dominant, an autosomal recessive, or an X-linked recessive pattern [5]. Mutations in several genes have been implicated in the pathogenesis of FEVR: Wnt signaling pathway genes including *NDP, FZD4, LRP5,* and *TSPAN12*, have been reported to be associated with FEVR [5]. *FZD4* and *LRP5* encode the proteins that act as

U. Spandau, S. J. Kim, *Pediatric Retinal Vascular Diseases*,
https://doi.org/10.1007/978-3-030-13701-4_4

coreceptors for Wnt proteins and Norrin (encoded by *NDP* gene). FEVR patients with LRP5 mutations can have osteopenia and osteoporosis, and those with severe NDP mutations are likely to have progressive deafness and mental retardation [5]. In addition, *ZNF408* was reported to be a new causative gene of FEVR [6]. The knock-down of *znf408* in zebrafish revealed that it is important in retinal vasculogenesis [6]. Mutations in *KIF11* gene have also been associated with FEVR with or without microcephaly, and mental retardation [7–9].

4.3 Diagnosis of Familial Exudative Vitreoretinopathy

4.3.1 Clinical Features

FEVR can be diagnosed based on fundus findings. In addition, the role of fluorescein angiographic evaluation has been increasing. The most characteristic feature of FEVR is peripheral retinal avascularity, most commonly in the temporal periphery. In mild cases, these peripheral retinal changes do not cause any symptoms. As the disease progresses, exudation and neovascularization may develop at the vascular-avascular junction. These changes may result in retinal fold, ectopic macula, and retinal detachment (Figs. 4.1 and 4.2). In a large-scale study by Ranchod et al. [10], 77 of 273 eyes (28%) showed radial retinal folds. The majority of retinal folds extended radially in the temporal quadrants, but radial folds were seen in almost all quadrants [10]. The radial folds in the retina are sometimes described as 'falciform'. These folds represent one of the classic features of FEVR. Less common findings are secondary epiretinal membrane formation (Fig. 4.3), peripheral retinoschisis, vitreous hemorrhage, secondary glaucoma, retinal capillary angioma, retained hyaloid vascular remnants, and persistent fetal vasculature [5].

Fig. 4.1 Retinal fold with disc dragging in FEVR

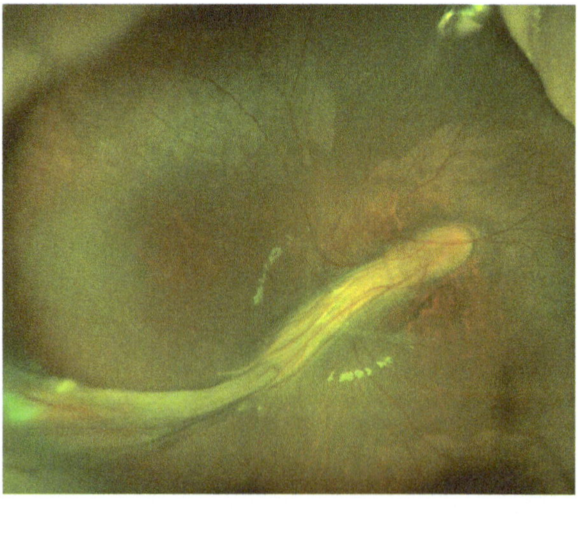

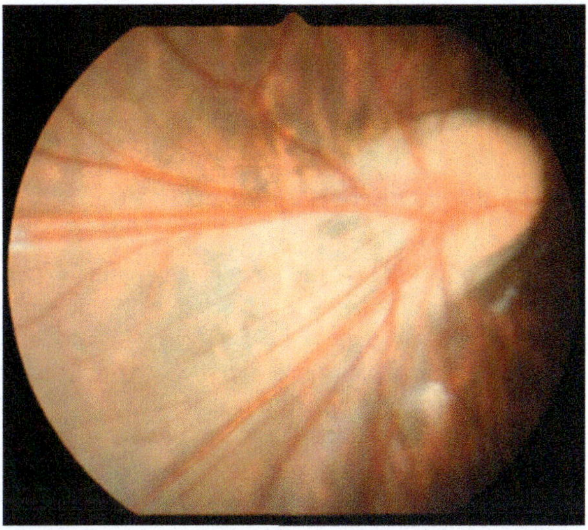

Fig. 4.2 Disc dragging in FEVR

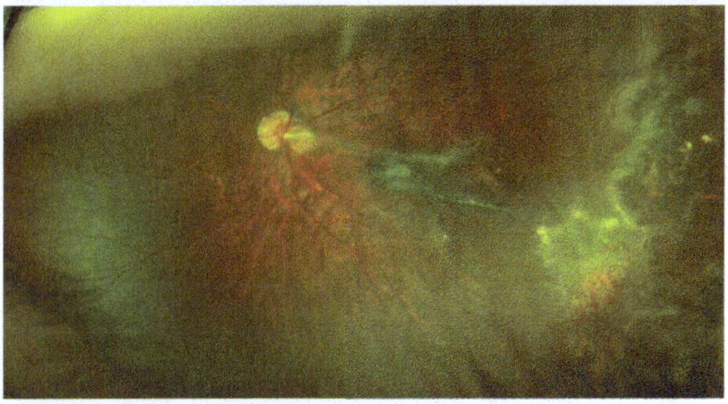

Fig. 4.3 Epiretinal membrane in an eye with FEVR after cryotherapy

In several clinical studies on FEVR by Trese and colleagues, the following diagnostic criteria for FEVR were used: (1) incomplete peripheral retinal vascular development, (2) full-term or preterm birth with a disease tempo not consistent with ROP, and (3) variable degrees of nonperfusion, vitreoretinal traction, subretinal exudation, or retinal neovascularization occurring at any age [4, 10, 11].

It's sometimes not easy to differentiate FEVR from ROP. Classically, positive family history, full-term birth, and no oxygen therapy favours FEVR. In contrast, preterm birth and oxygen supplementation favours ROP. However, there are some infants with FEVR but born prematurely. Berrocal and colleagues reported clinical and angiographic findings of 9 premature infants with FEVR-like retinal findings and proposed a new classification system called "ROPER" (ROP vs. FEVR) [12]. The authors reported several distinguishing angiographic features of ROPER compared to typical ROP. In eyes with typical ROP, abnormal branching patterns at the vascular/avascular junction included tangles or circumferential vessels, hyperfluorescent lesions, focal capillary dilatation, new vessels and fluorescein leakage [12]. In contrast, eyes with FEVR showed bulbous vascular terminals, capillary dropout, venous/venous shunting (not AV shunting), and irregular sprouts of vascularization at the vascular/avascular junction (rather than homogenous vascular advancing front in ROP) [12]. Differentiating FEVR from ROP is important in that FEVR is progressive disease and early diagnosis with treatment is crucial to prevent worse visual outcome.

4.3.2 Fluorescein Angiography Findings

The role of wide-field fluorescein angiography (e.g. RetCam, Natus or ultra-widefield retinal imaging devices, Optos) is important for proper diagnosis and monitoring disease activity in FEVR (Figs. 4.4 and 4.5).

Kashani et al. [4] described wide-field angiographic findings in 87 FEVR patients. This study reported a broad spectrum of angiographic findings including anatomic

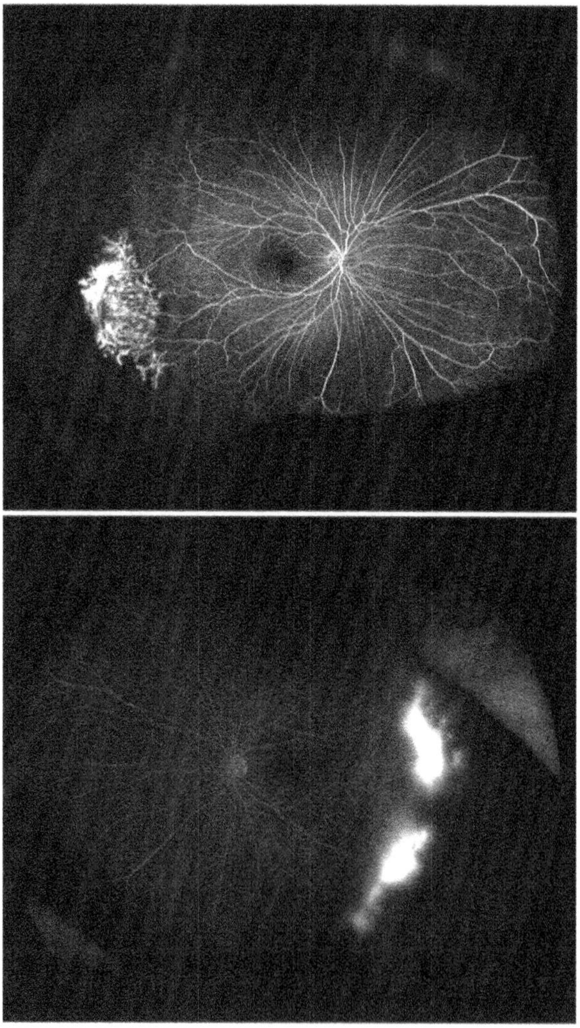

Fig. 4.4 Ultra-wide field fluorescein angiography in a 12-year old patient with stage 2 FEVR. (Courtesy of Dr. J. Peter Campbell, MD, MPH at Oregon Health and Science University Casey Eye Institute, Portland, Oregon, USA)

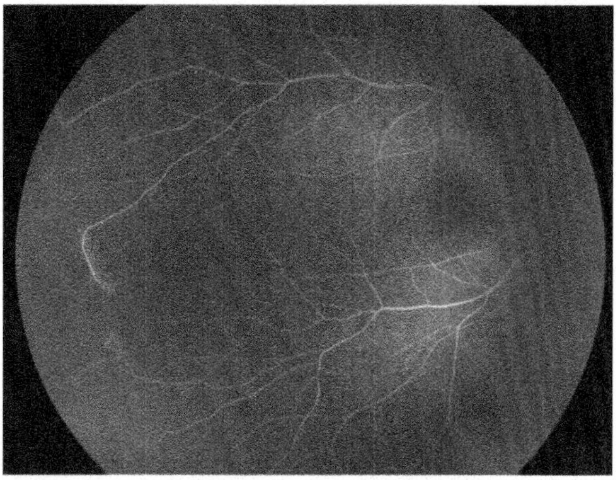

Fig. 4.5 Wide field fluorescein angiography in a 10-month old patient with stage 1 FEVR

changes (central and peripheral bulbous vascular endings with or without fluorescein leakage, arterial tortuosity, optic nerve head leakage, aberrant circumferential vessels in the far periphery, and capillary anomalies and agenesis) and functional changes (delayed arteriovenous transit, delayed or absent choroidal perfusion, and venous-venous shunting.) The authors mentioned that angiographic leakage, especially at the vascular-avascular junction, warrants immediate laser ablation and close observation [4].

Considerable proportion of asymptomatic family members of patients with FEVR have some degree of disease. Kashani et al. [11] investigated clinical and angiographic findings in 57 family members of symptomatic FEVR patients at a single tertiary referral vitreoretinal practice in United States. Among 114 eyes of 57 subjects, only 21% showed normal findings on both clinical and angiographic examinations. Among them, 58% demonstrated clinical or angiographic stage 1 or 2 FEVR and 21% demonstrated stage 3, 4, or 5 FEVR. Therefore, the authors suggested that clinical and wide-field angiographic screening be performed on family members [11]. This may be helpful for early detection of treatment-requiring disease and genetic counselling.

4.3.3 OCT Features

Evaluation of FEVR patients with OCT may be helpful for treatment and understanding vitreoretinal relationships.

Shimouchi et al. [13] reported two cases with FEVR patients and showed that SD-OCT revealed perifoveal posterior vitreous detachment with vitreofoveal adhesion and small deposits that appeared as rod-shaped attachments perpendicular to the parafoveal face without intraretinal and subretinal materials beneath the posterior hyaloid face that corresponded to white material on the fundus examination (Fig. 4.6).

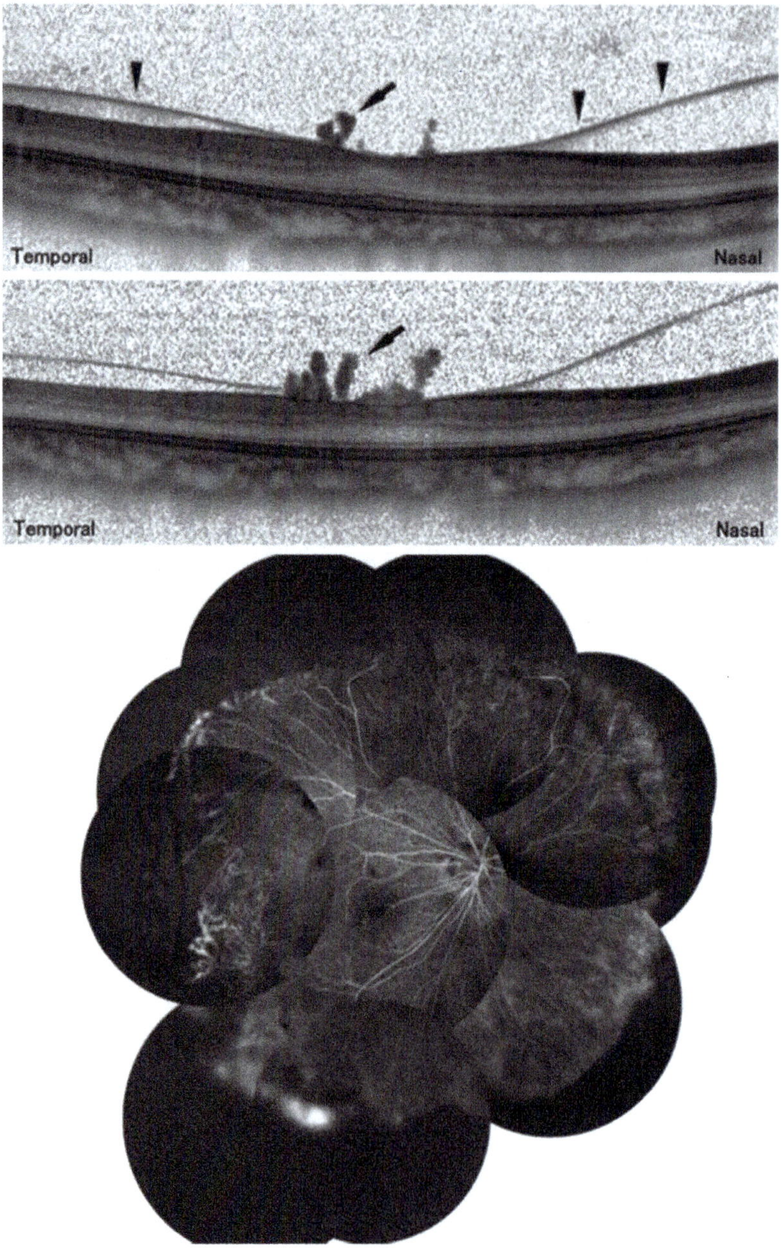

Fig. 4.6 SD-OCT and fluorescein angiography in a 14-year old patient with FEVR. Note the perifoveal PVD (arrowheads) and numerous small deposits (arrows) that appear as rod-shaped attachments perpendicular to the parafoveal face without intraretinal and subretinal material beneath the posterior hyaloid face. Fluorescein angiography shows a circumferential peripheral avascular area and peripheral neovascularization temporally. (Reprinted by permission from Springer Nature, Shimouchi et al. [13]. Copyright (2013))

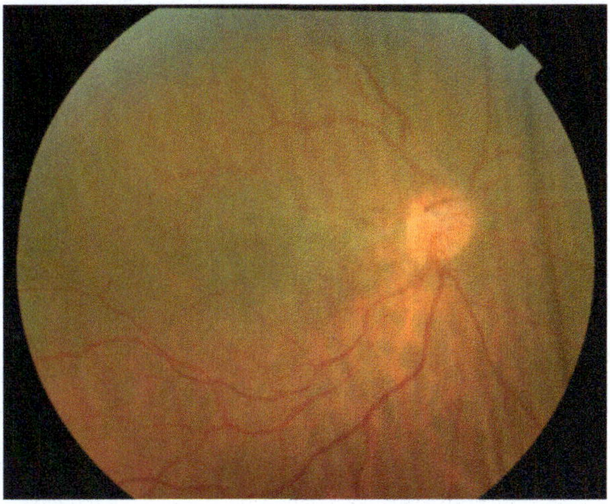

Fig. 4.7 SD-OCT reveals macular epiretinal membrane formation. (Reprinted by permission from Springer Nature, Gilmour [5]. Copyright (2015))

Yonekawa et al. [14] investigated SD-OCT findings in 74 eyes from 41 FEVR patients. This study revealed a broad spectrum of features: various forms of posterior hyaloidal organization (ranging from thinner epiretinal membrane-like hyperreflective layers to thicker opacities), vitreomacular traction, vitreopapillary traction, vitreo-fold traction, vitreo-laser scar adhesion, diminished foveal contour, persistent fetal foveal architecture, cystoid macular edema, intraretinal exudates and subretinal lipid aggregation, dry or edematous radial folds, and disruption of the ellipsoid zone [14].

These OCT findings may be helpful in identifying potential treatment targets including epiretinal membrane, vitreomacular traction, and macular edema (Fig. 4.7). In addition, because abnormal foveal development (persistence of inner retinal layers in fovea) might be related to visual prognosis, further investigations are warranted.

4.4 Classification of Familial Exudative Vitreoretinopathy

Several classification systems of FEVR have been proposed. In 1980, Laqua [15] proposed a 3-level staging system. In stage 1, the patient is asymptomatic, and all the pathology is confined to the peripheral retina [15]. Stage 2 describes a peripheral fibrovascular mass with dragging of the posterior pole structures [15]. In stage 3, complications that result in severe visual loss are present (e.g. total RD) [15].

In 1984, Miyakubo et al. [16] suggested a 5-stage system: type 1, simple type (avascular zone less than 2 disc diameters in the periphery); type 2, arcuate type (avascular zone more than 2 disc diameters in the periphery); type 3, V-shaped type (wedge-shaped avascular zone in the temporal periphery); type 4, proliferative type (retinal neovascularization, fluorescein leakage); and type 5, cicatricial type (solid cicatricial mass in pars plana and tractional, falciform retinal detachment).

Table 4.1 Clinical and angiographic classification of FEVR

Stage	Clinical Staging (proposed in 1998)	Revised Clinical and Angiographic staging (proposed in 2014)
1	Avascular retinal periphery without extraretinal vascularization	Avascular retinal periphery or anomalous intraretinal vascularization
1A		Without exudation or fluorescein leakage
1B		With exudation or fluorescein leakage
2	Avascular retinal periphery with extraretinal vascularization	Avascular retinal periphery with extraretinal vascularization
2A	Without exudate	Without exudation or fluorescein leakage
2B	With exudate	With exudation or fluorescein leakage
3	Extramacular retinal detachment	Extramacular retinal detachment
3A	Primarily exudative	Without exudation or fluorescein leakage
3B	Primarily tractional	With exudation or fluorescein leakage
4	Macula-involving retinal detachment	Macula-involving retinal detachment
4A	Primarily exudative	Without exudation or fluorescein leakage
4B	Primarily tractional	With exudation or fluorescein leakage
5	Total retinal detachment	Total retinal detachment
5A	Open funnel	Open funnel
5B	Closed funnel	Closed funnel

In 1998, Pendergast and Trese proposed a 5-stage classification system based on fundus findings (Table 4.1) [3]. This system is based on critical findings (macular involvement, presence of exudation, exudative vs. tractional) that may be important in selecting treatment methods [3].

In 2014, Trese and colleagues revised the clinical staging system based on clinical and angiographic features (Table 4.1) [4]. Based on their findings that angiographic leakage is a precursor to clinical exudation, they modified the staging system to include angiographic leakage [4]. Also, they suggested eyes with stage 1B or 2B receive immediate laser ablation of the leaking lesion and peripheral avascular retina [4].

References

1. Criswick VG, Schepens CL. Familial exudative vitreoretinopathy. Am J Ophthalmol. 1969;68:578–94.
2. Canny CL, Oliver GL. Fluorescein angiographic findings in familial exudative vitreoretinopathy. Arch Ophthalmol. 1976;94:1114–20.
3. Pendergast SD, Trese MT. Familial exudative vitreoretinopathy. Results of surgical management. Ophthalmology. 1998;105:1015–23.
4. Kashani AH, Brown KT, Chang E, Drenser KA, Capone A, Trese MT. Diversity of retinal vascular anomalies in patients with familial exudative vitreoretinopathy. Ophthalmology. 2014;121:2220–7.

5. Gilmour DF. Familial exudative vitreoretinopathy and related retinopathies. Eye (Lond). 2015;29:1–14. Epub 2014 Oct 17.
6. Collin RW, Nikopoulos K, Dona M, Gilissen C, Hoischen A, Boonstra FN, Poulter JA, Kondo H, Berger W, Toomes C, Tahira T, Mohn LR, Blokland EA, Hetterschijt L, Ali M, Groothuismink JM, Duijkers L, Inglehearn CF, Sollfrank L, Strom TM, Uchio E, van Nouhuys CE, Kremer H, Veltman JA, van Wijk E, Cremers FP. ZNF408 is mutated in familial exudative vitreoretinopathy and is crucial for the development of zebrafish retinal vasculature. Proc Natl Acad Sci U S A. 2013;110:9856–61.
7. Robitaille JM, Gillett RM, LeBlanc MA, Gaston D, Nightingale M, Mackley MP, Parkash S, Hathaway J, Thomas A, Ells A, Traboulsi EI, Héon E, Roy M, Shalev S, Fernandez CV, MacGillivray C, Wallace K, Fahiminiya S, Majewski J, McMaster CR, Bedard K. Phenotypic overlap between familial exudative vitreoretinopathy and microcephaly, lymphedema, and chorioretinal dysplasia caused by KIF11 mutations. JAMA Ophthalmol. 2014;132:1393–9.
8. Hu H, Xiao X, Li S, Jia X, Guo X, Zhang Q. KIF11 mutations are a common cause of autosomal dominant familial exudative vitreoretinopathy. Br J Ophthalmol. 2016;100:278–83.
9. Karjosukarso DW, Cremers FPM, van Nouhuys CE, Collin RWJ. Detection and quantification of a KIF11 mosaicism in a subject presenting familial exudative vitreoretinopathy with microcephaly. Eur J Hum Genet. 2018;26:1819–23. https://doi.org/10.1038/s41431-018-0243-y. (E-pub).
10. Ranchod TM, Ho LY, Drenser KA, Capone A Jr, Trese MT. Clinical presentation of familial exudative vitreoretinopathy. Ophthalmology. 2011;118:2070–5.
11. Kashani AH, Learned D, Nudleman E, Drenser KA, Capone A, Trese MT. High prevalence of peripheral retinal vascular anomalies in family members of patients with familial exudative vitreoretinopathy. Ophthalmology. 2014;121:262–8.
12. John VJ, McClintic JI, Hess DJ, Berrocal AM. Retinopathy of prematurity versus familial exudative vitreoretinopathy: report on clinical and angiographic findings. Ophthalmic Surg Lasers Imaging Retina. 2016;47:14–9.
13. Shimouchi A, Takahashi A, Nagaoka T, Ishibazawa A, Yoshida A. Vitreomacular interface in patients with familial exudative vitreoretinopathy. Int Ophthalmol. 2013;33:711–5.
14. Yonekawa Y, Thomas BJ, Drenser KA, Trese MT, Capone A Jr. Familial exudative vitreoretinopathy: spectral-domain optical coherence tomography of the vitreoretinal interface, retina, and choroid. Ophthalmology. 2015;122:2270–7.
15. Laqua H. Familial exudative vitreoretinopathy. Albrecht Von Graefes Arch Klin Exp Ophthalmol. 1980;213:121–33.
16. Miyakubo H, Hashimoto K, Miyakubo S. Retinal vascular pattern in familial exudative vitreoretinopathy. Ophthalmology. 1984;91:1524–30.

Chapter 5
Retinopathy of Prematurity (ROP)

Severe retinopathy of prematurity is a serious complication of neonatal intensive care for preterm infants. The disease was first described in a premature baby in 1942. Between 1941–1953, over 12,000 babies worldwide were affected by it such as soul musician Stevie Wonder. The cause for the fast growth of this blinding disease was the increased usage of incubators for premature babies. Oxygen was given freely until the end of the 1950s to prevent brain damage. The deleterious effects of high oxygen were yet unknown.

Two women, Kate Campbell from Australia and Mary Crosse from England, suggested that it was oxygen toxicity that caused the disease. The hypothesis was eventually confirmed by a controversial study undertaken in the USA [1]. The study involved two groups of babies. In a randomised fashion, one group was given the usual oxygen concentrations, while the other group received reduced oxygen levels. The latter group had a significant lower incidence of the ROP disease. As a result, oxygen levels in incubators were lowered and consequently the epidemic was halted within 1 year.

5.1 Pathophysiology of Retinopathy of Prematurity (ROP)

An animal model was developed which mimics very closely retinopathy of prematurity [2]. In this animal model mice are placed in an incubator from day 7 to day 12 and exposed to 75% oxygen (hyperoxia) (Fig. 5.1). Then the mice are removed from the incubator and exposed to room air. The re-exposure to room air is equivalent to hypoxia. After 6–12 hours in room air the eyes express excessive amounts of VEGF. Immunhistology demonstrates that VEGF is expressed in the inner nuclear layer by Mueller cells. Shortly thereafter, retinal neovascularizations develop (Figs. 5.2 and 5.3). After 26 days the VEGF levels subside and retinal neovascularizations decrease.

These results prove that hypoxia triggers VEGF production. And VEGF itself upregulates retinal proliferations. This pathophysiologic cascade can be blocked if

U. Spandau, S. J. Kim, *Pediatric Retinal Vascular Diseases*,
https://doi.org/10.1007/978-3-030-13701-4_5

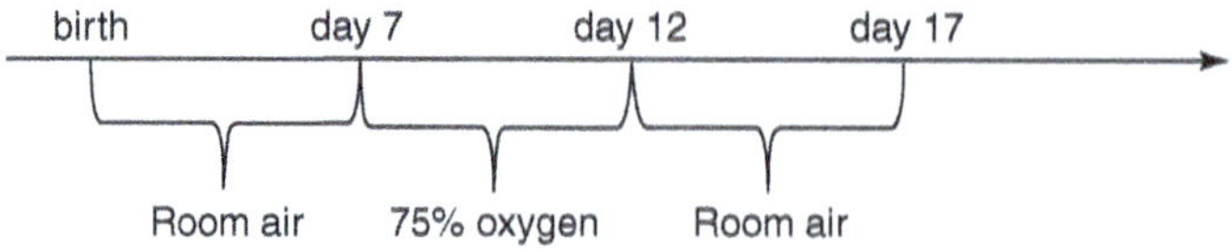

Fig. 5.1 Animal model of ROP. Mice are in room air from birth to day 7 after birth. From day 7 to day 12 after birth the mice are placed in an incubator with 75% oxygen. From day 12 the mice are removed from the incubator and remain in room air until they are sacrificed and examined at day 17

Fig. 5.2 A mouse eye after exposure to 75 oxygen. Note the big lens

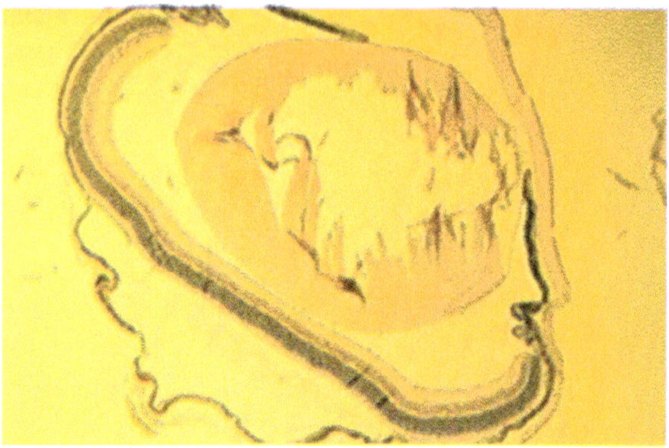

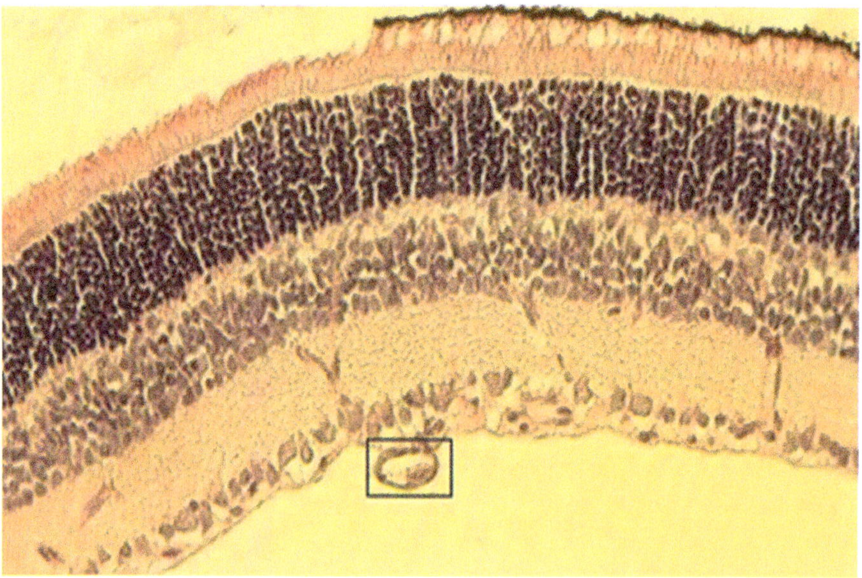

Fig. 5.3 A mouse retina after exposure to 75% oxygen. The black box encloses a retinal proliferation

an intraocular injection of VEGF is made at the same day when the mice are placed in the incubators [3].

5.2 Classification of ROP

5.2.1 Classification System of Retinopathy of Prematurity (ROP)

In 1984, an international group of ROP experts published a classification system of ROP (International Classification of Retinopathy of Prematurity; ICROP), which included the location of retinal involvement by zone, the extent of retinal involvement by clock hour, the stage or severity of retinopathy at the junction of the vascularized and avascular retina, and the presence or absence of plus disease [4]. The original ICROP mentioned that "the unifying principle underlying this classification is the following: the more posterior the disease and the greater the amount of involved retinal vascular tissue, the more serious the disease." The original ICROP was expanded in 1987 and updated in 2005 [5, 6]. In the updated version of ICROP in 2005, several changes were made including the concept of aggressive posterior ROP (AP-ROP) and pre-plus disease [6]. In this chapter, this classification system will be introduced.

5.2.2 Location and Extent of Disease

To define the location of disease, 3 concentric zones have been described (zone I, II and III). In Fig. 5.4, zone I consists of a circle, the radius of which extends from the center of the optic disc to twice the distance from the center of the optic disc to the macular center [6]. The zone II retinal area extends from the edge of zone I to the nasal ora serrata. Zone III is the residual retinal area anterior to zone II [6].

When using a 25- or 28-diopter lens during indirect ophthalmoscopic examinations, by placing the nasal edge of the optic disc at one edge of the field of view, the limit of zone I is at the temporal field of view [6].

The extent of disease is recorded as hours of the clock (e.g. 5 clock hours of extraretinal fibrovascular proliferation) or as 30° sectors (Fig. 5.4) [6].

5.2.3 Stage of ROP (Table 5.1)

There are 5 stages that are used to describe the vascular pathology at the junction of the vascularized and avascular retina (Figs. 5.5, 5.6, 5.7, 5.8, 5.9, 5.10, and 5.11) [6]. Because more than one ROP stage may be present in the same eye, staging for the eye as a whole is based on the most severe stage.

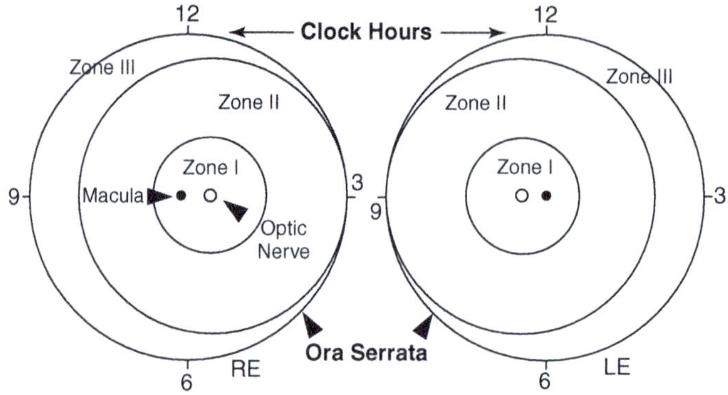

Fig. 5.4 Scheme of retina showing zone borders and clock hours used to describe the location and extent of ROP. (Reproduced with permission from International Committee for the Classification of Retinopathy of Prematurity [6]. Copyright© (2005) American Medical Association. All rights reserved)

Table 5.1 Staging system of ROP [6]

Stage	Description
1. Demarcation Line	Thin structure that separates the avascular retina anteriorly from the vascularized retina posteriorly.
2. Ridge	It arises in the region of the demarcation line, has height and width, and extends above the plane of the retina. Small isolated tufts of neovascular tissue lying on the surface of the retina may be seen posterior to this ridge structure.
3. Extraretinal Fibrovascular Proliferation (EFP)	Neovascularization extends from the ridge into the vitreous.
4. Partial retinal detachment	Extrafoveal (stage 4A) and foveal (stage 4B) partial retinal detachment.
5. Total retinal detachment	Generally tractional and may occasionally be exudative. They are usually funnel shaped. The configuration of the funnel: open or narrow/anteriorly or posteriorly

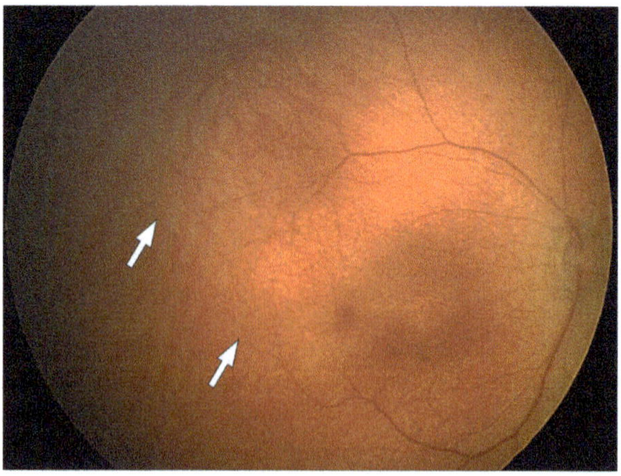

Fig. 5.5 Fundus photograph to demonstrate immature retinal vascularization (Stage 0). (Reproduced with permission from International Committee for the Classification of Retinopathy of Prematurity [6]. Copyright© (2005) American Medical Association. All rights reserved)

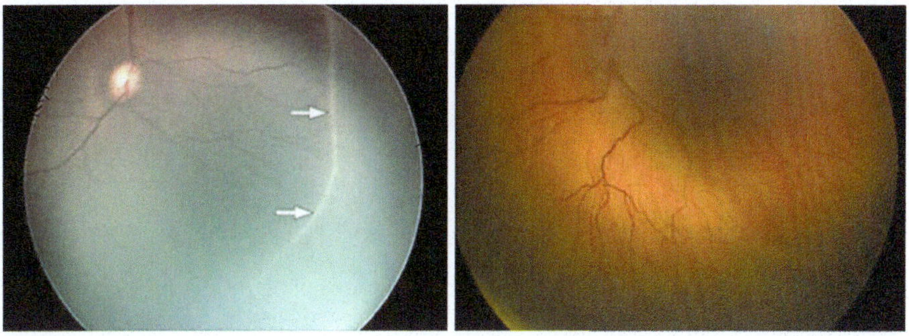

Fig. 5.6 Fundus photograph to illustrate the demarcation line of stage 1. (Reproduced with permission from International Committee for the Classification of Retinopathy of Prematurity [6]. Copyright© (2005) American Medical Association. All rights reserved)

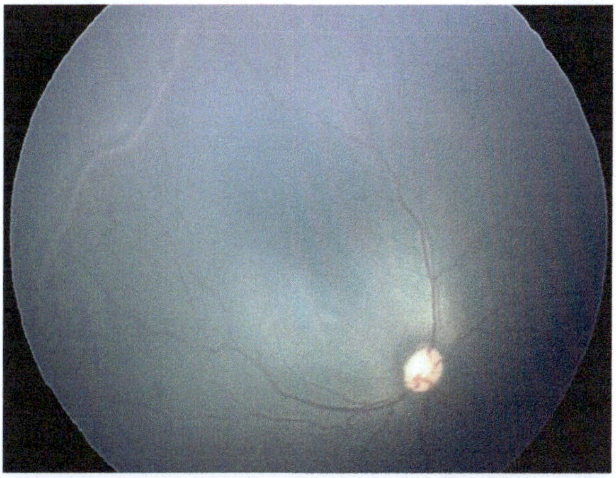

Fig. 5.7 Pigmented fundus photograph showing stage 2 retinopathy of prematurity at the junction between vascularized and avascular retina. (Reproduced with permission from International Committee for the Classification of Retinopathy of Prematurity [6]. Copyright© (2005) American Medical Association. All rights reserved)

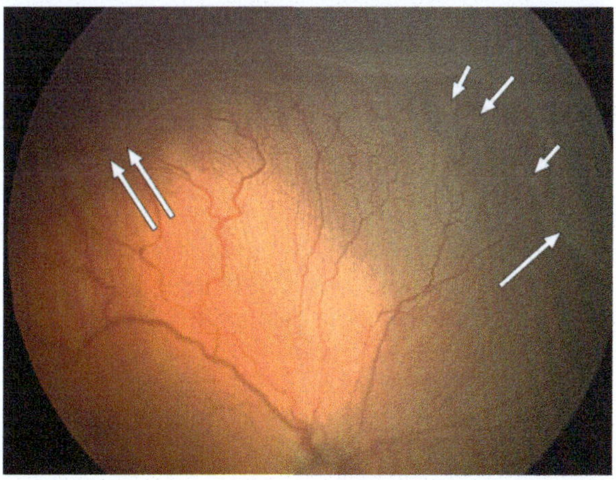

Fig. 5.8 Fundus photograph showing the ridge between vascularized and avascular retina characteristic of stage 2 retinopathy of prematurity (single long arrow). (Reproduced with permission from International Committee for the Classification of Retinopathy of Prematurity [6]. Copyright© (2005) American Medical Association. All rights reserved)

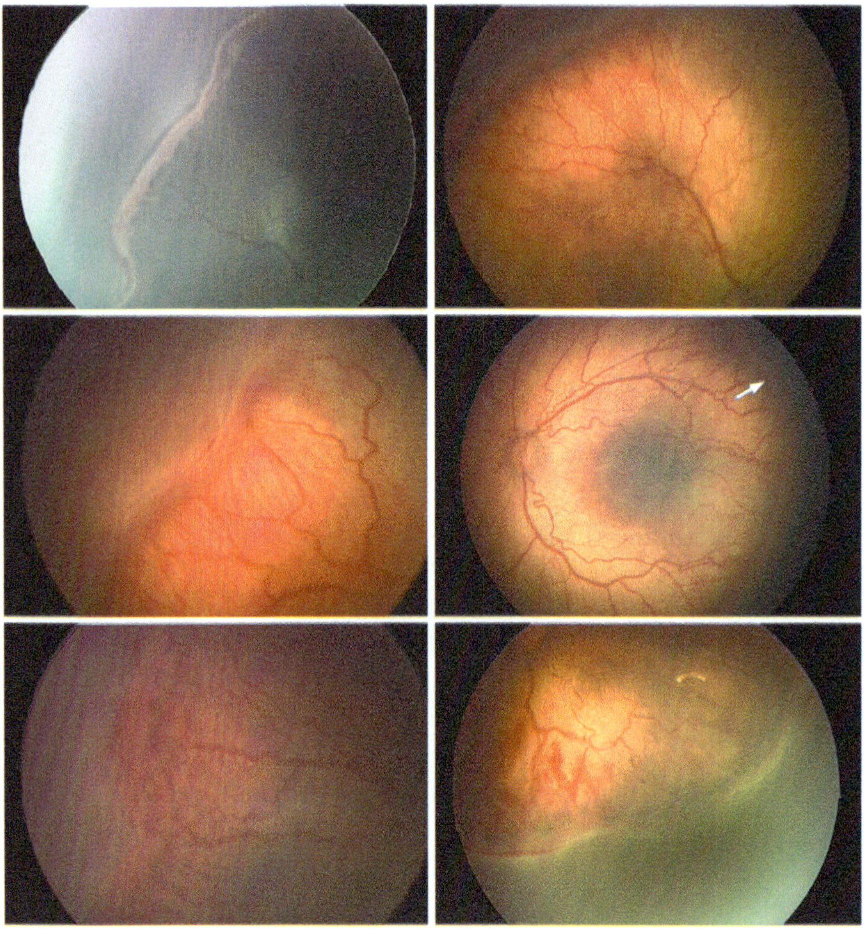

Fig. 5.9 Fundus photographs of mild to severe stage 3 retinopathy of prematurity (ROP). (Reproduced with permission from International Committee for the Classification of Retinopathy of Prematurity [6].)

5.2.4 *Plus Disease*

Defined as "increased venous dilatation and arterial tortuosity of the posterior retinal vessels in at least 2 quadrants of the eye (Figs. 5.12 and 5.13) [6]. A "+" symbol is added to the ROP stage number to designate the presence of plus disease (e.g. "stage 3+").

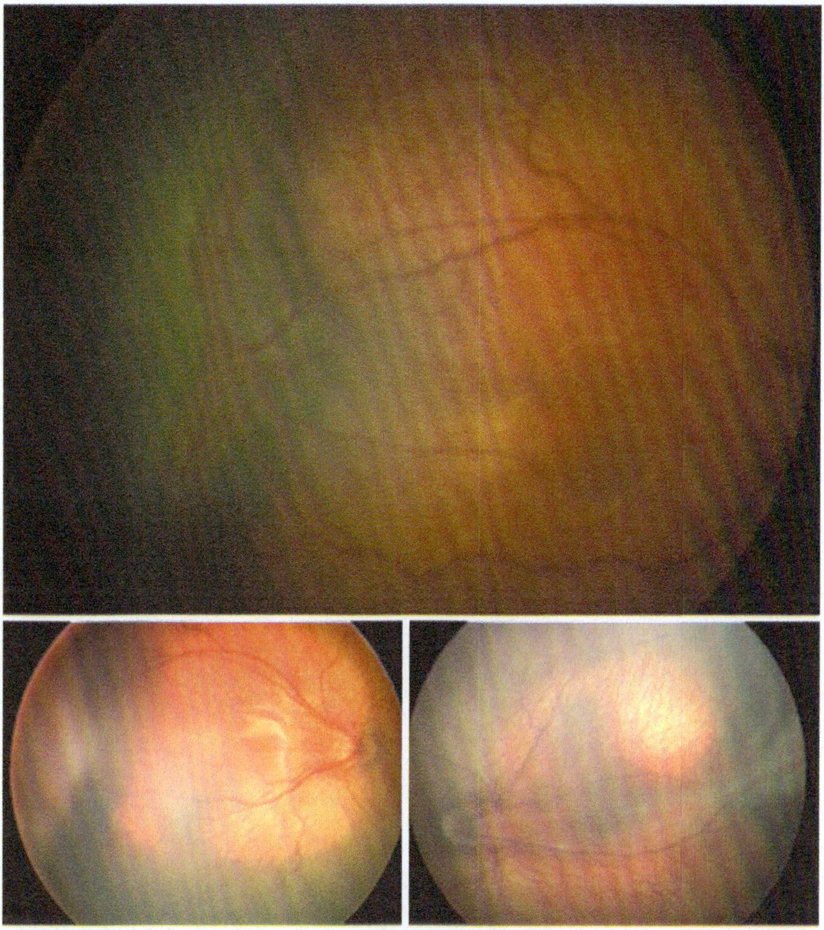

Fig. 5.10 Examples of stages 4A and B retinopathy of prematurity. (Reproduced with permission from International Committee for the Classification of Retinopathy of Prematurity [6]. Copyright© (2005) American Medical Association. All rights reserved)

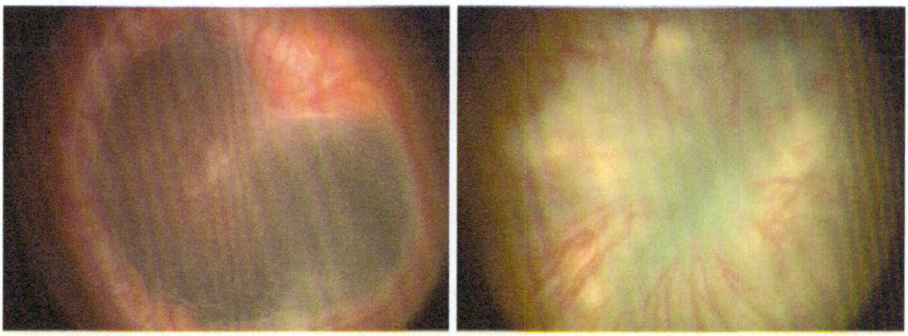

Fig. 5.11 Stage 5 retinopathy of prematurity. (Reproduced with permission from International Committee for the Classification of Retinopathy of Prematurity [6]. Copyright© (2005) American Medical Association. All rights reserved)

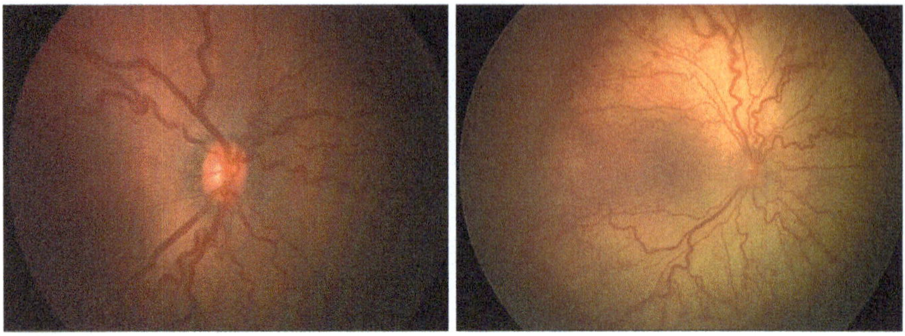

Fig. 5.12 Examples of plus disease. (Reproduced with permission from International Committee for the Classification of Retinopathy of Prematurity [6]. Copyright© (2005) American Medical Association. All rights reserved)

Fig. 5.13 Standard fundus photograph of posterior venous dilatation and arteriolar tortuosity characteristic of plus disease from original International Committee for the Retinopathy of Prematurity. (Reproduced with permission from International Committee for the Classification of Retinopathy of Prematurity [6]. Copyright© (2005) American Medical Association. All rights reserved)

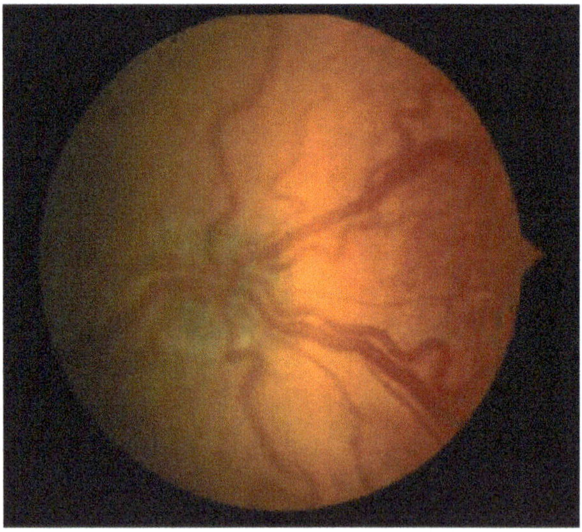

5.2.5 *Pre-plus Disease*

Defined as vascular abnormalities of the posterior pole that are insufficient for the diagnosis of plus disease but that demonstrate more arterial tortuosity and more venous dilatation than normal (Fig. 5.14) [6].

5.2.6 *Aggressive Posterior ROP (AP-ROP)*

AP-ROP is a rapidly progressing, severe form of ROP (Fig. 5.15), characterized by posterior location, prominence of plus disease, and the ill-defined nature of the retinopathy [6].

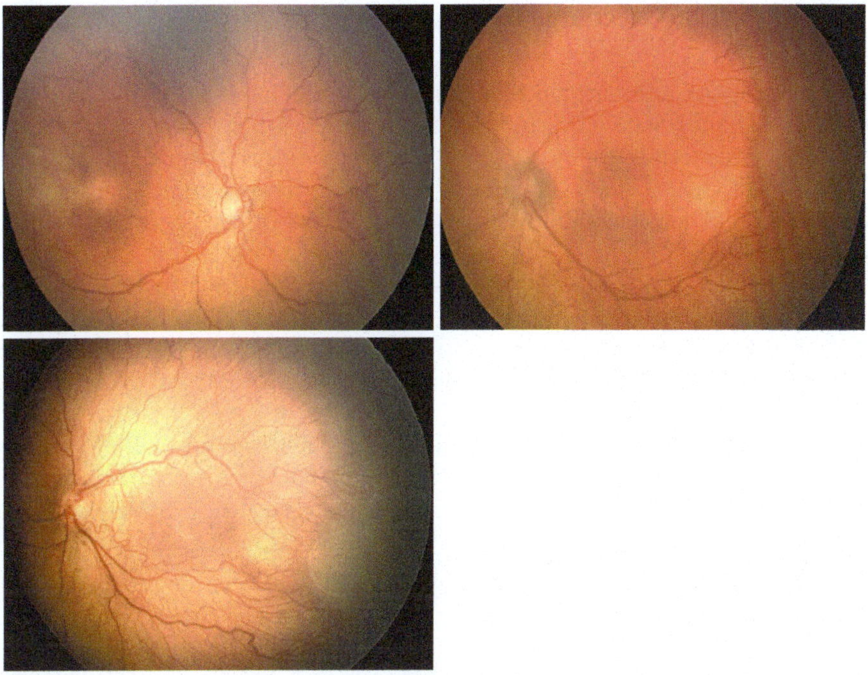

Fig. 5.14 Examples of pre-plus disease. (Reproduced with permission from International Committee for the Classification of Retinopathy of Prematurity [6]. Copyright© (2005) American Medical Association. All rights reserved)

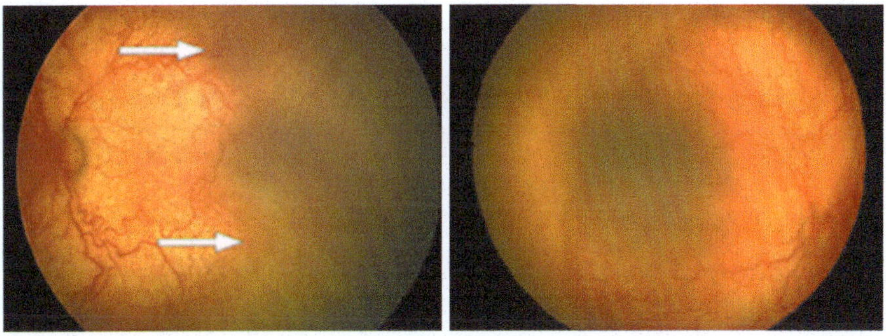

Fig. 5.15 Examples of aggressive posterior retinopathy of prematurity (AP-ROP). (Reproduced with permission from International Committee for the Classification of Retinopathy of Prematurity [6]. Copyright© (2005) American Medical Association. All rights reserved)

AP-ROP is observed most commonly in zone I, but may also occur in posterior zone II. Early in the development of AP-ROP, the posterior retinal vessels show increased dilation and tortuosity that is out of proportion to the peripheral retinopathy [6]. There may also be retinal hemorrhages at the junction between the vascularized and avascular retina. Also, AP-ROP usually does not progress through the classic stages 1–3.

5.3 Screening Recommendations

There are several screening guidelines or recommendations. The most widely used one is the United States (US) recommendations. The US recommendations were made by American academy of pediatrics section on ophthalmology, American Academy of Ophthalmology, American Association for Pediatric Ophthalmology and Strabismus, and American Association of Certified Orthoptists, which was last updated in 2013 [7].

The United Kingdom (UK) guideline was developed by a multidisciplinary guideline development group (GDG) of the Royal College of Paediatrics & Child Health (RCPCH) in collaboration with the Royal College of Ophthalmologists (RCOphth), British Association of Perinatal Medicine (BAPM) and the premature baby charity BLISS in 2008 [8].

In 2015, New Zealand recommendations were published on behalf of the New Zealand Paediatric Ophthalmology Interest Group, the Newborn Network and the Fetus and Newborn Special Interest Group of the Paediatric Society of New Zealand [9].

1. **Which babies are recommended to be examined?**

The screening criteria of the 3 guidelines are shown in Table 5.2. The GA and BW criteria slightly differ among the three. The New Zealand recommendations describe the unstable clinical course in detail (Table 5.2) [9].

Table 5.2 ROP screening criteria

Guidelines or recommendations	Criteria
United States (2013) [7]	All infants with a birth weight of ≤1500 g or GA of 30 weeks or less (as defined by the attending neonatologist) Selected infants with a birth weight between 1500 and 2000 g or GA age of >30 weeks with an unstable clinical course, including those requiring cardiorespiratory support and who are believed by their attending pediatrician or neonatologist to be at high risk for ROP
United Kingdom (2008) [8]	All babies less than 32 weeks GA (up to 31 weeks and 6 days) or less than 1501 g BW
New Zealand (2015) [9]	All infants less than 30 weeks gestation or less than 1250 g birthweight Selected infants ≥1250 g and ≥30 weeks with an unstable clinical course who are believed to be at high risk by their attending neonatologist. The conditions/treatment to consider screening include, but not limited to: *In utero* hydrops, when gestation uncertain; Grade 3/4 intraventricular hemorrhage or post-hemorrhagic hydrocephalus; Severe sepsis; Treatment with nitric oxide for pulmonary hypertension; Affected twin-to-twin transfusion infants Prolonged period in high inspired oxygen.

GA gestational age, *BW* birth weight

2. **How to exam**

ROP screening is performed by dilated indirect ophthalmoscopic examinations with an eyelid speculum and scleral depression (Fig. 5.16). Sterile instruments are used to examine each infant to avoid possible cross-contamination. To minimize the discomfort, a topical anesthetic agent such as proparacaine is often used and consideration also may be given to the use of pacifiers, oral sucrose, and so on.

3. **The timing of initial screening**

The timing of initial screening is similar in all the 3 guidelines (Table 5.3). In extremely preterm infants (i.e. born before 25 weeks' gestation), initial screening exam can be done before 31 weeks' PMA, if possible. Although US guideline recommends initial screening at 31 weeks' PMA (Table 5.3), they mentioned that it should be appreciated that infants born before 25 weeks' gestational age should be considered for earlier screening on the basis of severity of comorbidities (even if before 31 weeks' postmenstrual age to enable earlier identification and treatment of aggressive posterior ROP that is more likely to occur in this extremely high-risk population) [7].

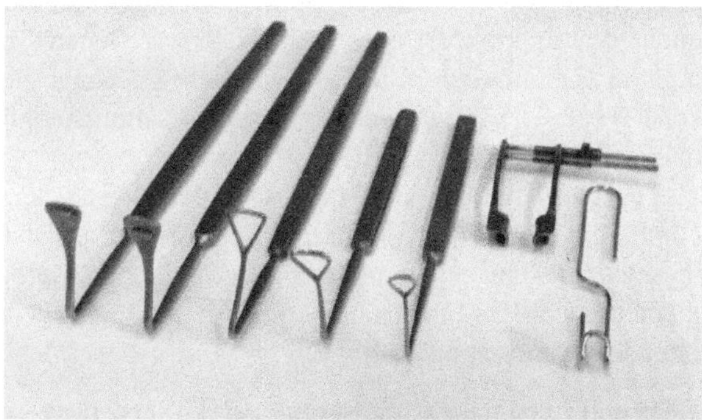

Fig. 5.16 Examples of ROP screening instruments including an eyelid speculum and various sizes of retractor (Morizane and Igarashi, INAMI, Tokyo, Japan) for eyeball rotation and scleral depression

Table 5.3 Timing of initial ROP screening in US, UK, and New Zealand guidelines

	United States (2013) [7]		United Kingdom (2008) [8]	New Zealand (2015) [9]
GA	PMA	CA	PMA (week)	
22	31	9	30–31	30–31 weeks PMA
23		8		
24		7		
25		6		
26		5		4 weeks CA
27		4	31–32	
28	32	4	32–33	
29	33	4	33–34	
30	34	4	34–35	
31			35–36	

GA gestational age, *PMA* postmenstrual age, *CA* chronological age

4. **Follow-up schedule After initial exams**

Suggested follow-up schedule by US recommendations is shown in Table 5.4. In their revised screening recommendations in 2013, more frequent examinations were recommended in eyes with posteriorly located disease (zone I or posterior zone II) [7].

In UK screening protocol, minimum frequencies of screening should be weekly when 1) the vessels end in zone I or posterior zone II, or 2) there is any plus or pre-plus disease, or 3) there is ant stage 3 disease in any zone [8]. Minimum frequencies of screening should be every 2 weeks in all other circumstances until the criteria for termination have been reached. UK screening protocol also recommends that all babies <32 weeks' gestation or BW <1501 g should have their first ROP screening examination prior to discharge.

In New Zealand follow-up recommendations, timing of follow-up is <1 week when there are early features of possible AP-ROP, 1 week when there is any ROP in zone I, regressing ROP zone I, immature vascularization in zone I, stage 3 in zone 2, pre-plus disease in any zone, or hazy view of retina, and 2 weeks when there is any stage ROP except stage 3 in zone II, regressing ROP zone II, stage 1 or 2 ROP in zone III, or regressing ROP zone III [9].

Compared to the other two guidelines, the US recommendations emphasizes frequent examinations in eyes with posteriorly located disease (e.g. 1 week of less interval for immature retina extends into posterior zone II, near the boundary of zone I) [7]. The New Zealand recommendations emphasizes short-term follow-up in eyes with possible AP-ROP [9].

The UK guideline also mentioned that "it is acknowledged that there may be clinical or organizational circumstances which prevent following the protocol. In these circumstances, the reasons for doing so should be clearly stated in the baby's medical record and the examination should be rescheduled within one week of the intended examination." [8]

5. **When to conclude acute-phase ROP screening examinations**

The termination of acute phase ROP retinal screening examinations should be based on PMA and findings (Table 5.5). It should be noted that "full retinal

Table 5.4 Suggested follow-up schedule by US recommendations in 2013 [7]

	Zone I	Posterior Zone II	Zone II	Zone III
No ROP	1 week or less	1–2 week[a]	2 week	
Stage 1	1 week or less		2 week	2–3 week
Stage 2	1 week or less		1–2 week	2–3 week
Stage 3		1 week or less		
Unequivocally regressing ROP	1–2 week		2 week	2–3 week
AP-ROP	1. Week or less			

[a]"1 week of less" for immature retina extends into posterior zone II, near the boundary of zone I

Table 5.5 Termination of ROP screening criteria

Guidelines or recommendations	Criteria
United States (2013) [7]	Zone III retinal vascularization attained without previous zone I or II ROP Full retinal vascularization in close proximity to the ora serrata for 360°—That is, the normal distance found in mature retina between the end of vascularization and the ora serrata. Postmenstrual age of 50 weeks and no prethreshold disease or worse ROP is present Regression of ROP
United Kingdom (2008) [8]	In babies without ROP, there is minimal risk of developing sight-threatening ROP when vascularization has extended into zone III and eye examinations may be stopped when this happens, usually after 36 completed weeks postmenstrual age. In the presence of ROP, screening for progressive active disease may be discontinued when any of the following characteristics of regression are seen on at least 2 successive examinations: lack of increase in severity partial resolution progressing towards complete resolution change in color in the ridge from salmon pink to white transgression of vessels through the demarcation line commencement of the process of replacement of active ROP lesions by scar tissue
New Zealand (2015) [9]	Retinal vascularization reached zone 3 without previous ROP. Regressed ROP, either spontaneously or after treatment, indicated by development of dry white ridges/line from active pink ridges, development of laser-induced scar tissue and transgression of vessels across the demarcation line. PMA 45 weeks with no type 1 ROP

vascularization in close proximity to the ora serrata for 360°" should be used for all cases treated with bevacizumab monotherapy according to the US recommendations [7].

Key Points

- A good screening is essential for a successfull treatment
- A poor screening results in a poor treatment
- Examine the neonates in weekly intervals until stage 3
- Examine the neonates twice a week if stage 3 is present
- After the diagnosis has been made, the treatment must be carried out after 72 hours at the latest.

References

1. Silverman WA. Chapter 8: The consequences of oxygen restriction. In: Retrolental fibroplasia: a modern parable. New York: Grune & Stratton; 1980. Retrieved 21 September 2013.
2. Pierce EA, Avery RL, Foley ED, Aiello LP, Smith LE. Vascular endothelial growth factor/vascular permeability factor expression in a mouse model of retinal neovascularization. Proc Natl Acad Sci U S A. 1995;92(3):905–9.
3. Alon T, Hemo I, Itin A, Pe'er J, Stone J, Keshet E. Vascular endothelial growth factor acts as a survival factor for newly formed retinal vessels and has implications for retinopathy of prematurity. Nat Med. 1995;1(10):1024–8.
4. An International Classification of retinopathy of Prematurity. The committee for the classification of retinopathy of prematurity. Arch Ophthalmol. 1984;102:1130–4.
5. An International Classification of Retinopathy of Prematurity. II. The classification of retinal detachment. The International Committee for the Classification of the late stages of retinopathy of prematurity. Arch Ophthalmol. 1987;105:906–12.
6. International Committee for the Classification of Retinopathy of Prematurity. The international classification of retinopathy of prematurity revisited. Arch Ophthalmol. 2005;123:991–9.
7. Fierson WM, American Academy of Pediatrics section on ophthalmology; American Academy of ophthalmology; American Association for Pediatric Ophthalmology and Strabismus; American Association of Certified Orthoptists. Screening examination of premature infants for retinopathy of prematurity. Pediatrics. 2013;131:189–95.
8. Wilkinson AR, Haines L, Head K, Fielder AR. UK retinopathy of prematurity guideline. Early Hum Dev. 2008;84:71–4.
9. Dai S, Austin N, Darlow B, New Zealand Paediatric Ophthalmology Interest Group; Newborn Network; Fetus and Newborn Special Interest Group; Paediatric Society of New Zealand. Retinopathy of prematurity: New Zealand recommendations for case detection and treatment. J Paediatr Child Health. 2015;51:955–9.

Part II
Examination

Chapter 6
Fundus Examination

6.1 Small Pupil

It is a common problem that the pupil of the newborn is small at the beginning of an examination or surgical treatment. This problem can be solved with intensive treatment of pupils with dilating drops. We NEVER experienced an eye which was not sufficiently dilated for laser coagulation. Our drop algorithm is as follows:

One hour before surgery we drop the newborn every 15 min with cyclopentolate + phenylephrine, 0.5% + 0.5%. When arriving at the operation room the newborn has been dropped 4 times.

If the pupil is still too small then drop the eye EVERY minute with ALL pupil-dilating drops you have available: tropicamide 0.5%, phenylephrine 10%, atropine 0.5% and cyclopentolate 1%.

- Drop the first minute tropicamide 0.5%.
- Drop the second minute phenylephrine 10%.
- Drop the third minute atropine 0.5%.
- Drop the fourth minute cyclopentolate 1%.
- and so on.

After maximal 20 min the pupil will be maximally dilated.

6.2 Indirect Binocular Ophthalmoscopy

The examination of ROP newborn is performed with a binocular indirect ophthalmoscope (Fig. 6.1). It is essential to master this technique for examination of the retina before you start with laser photocoagulation. The laser coagulation with binocular indirect ophthalmoscope is called Laser Indirect Ophthalmoscope (LIO).

U. Spandau, S. J. Kim, *Pediatric Retinal Vascular Diseases*,
https://doi.org/10.1007/978-3-030-13701-4_6

First you must learn to examine adults with the binocular indirect ophthalmoscope. If you are able to examine adults with ease, then start to examine newborns on the weekly ROP examinations. The examination of a newborn is much more difficult (Fig. 6.2). This training requires approximately 12 months.

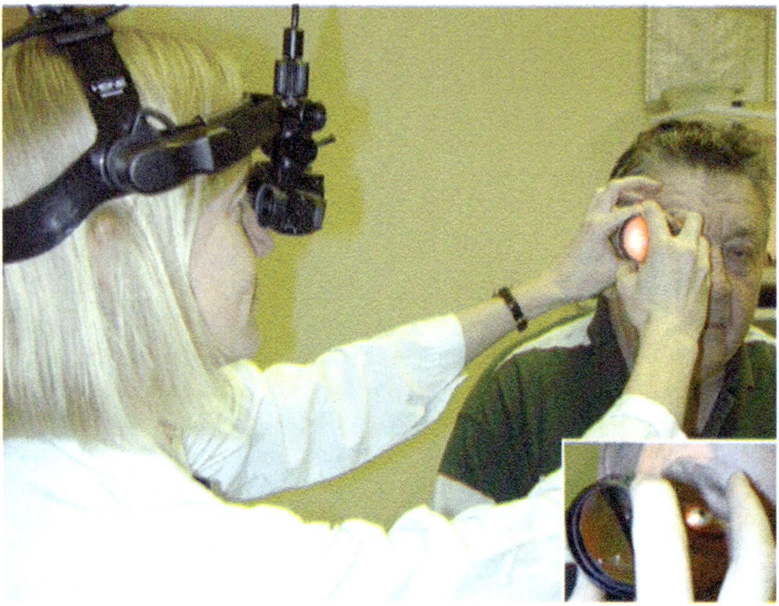

Fig. 6.1 Examination of an adult with a binocular indirect ophthalmoscope

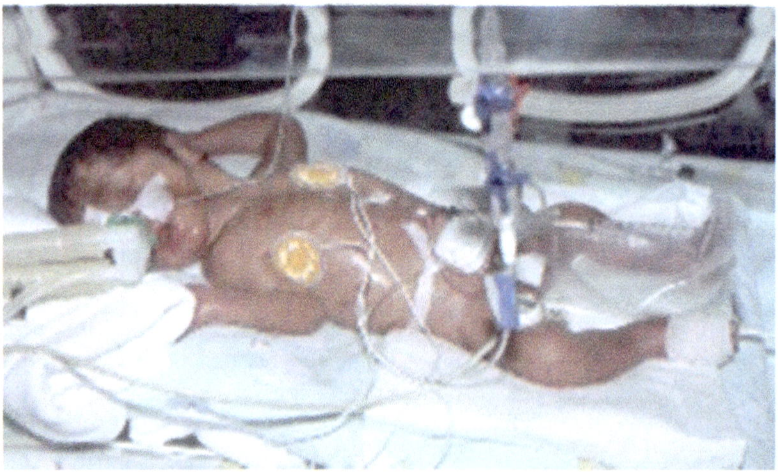

Fig. 6.2 The examination of a ROP newborn is much more difficult

6.2.1 Examination Technique

In indirect ophthalmoscopy the lens is held close to the eye of the patient (Fig. 6.1). If you increase the lens power (25D or 30D) you decrease the image size but increase the field of view (Fig. 6.3). If you choose a lens with less power (15D or 20D) you increase the image size but decrease the field of view. The most suitable lenses for examination of ROP neonates are the 20D and especially the 25D lenses (Fig. 6.4). When examining the retina of a newborn, you see the central retina called zone I (Fig. 6.5). The main pathologies of ROP, however, are located on the height of the equator (zone II).

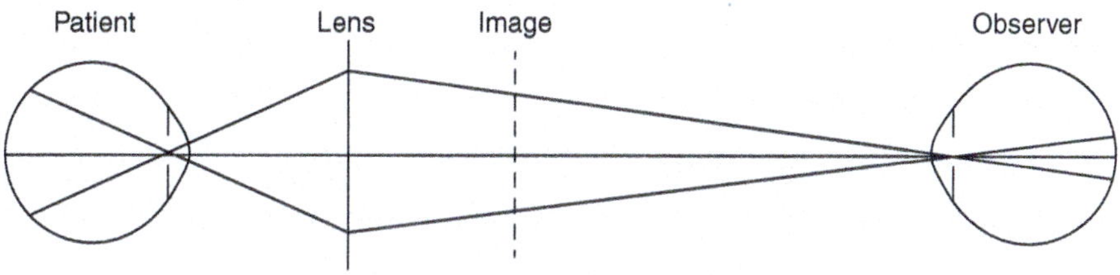

Fig. 6.3 A diagram of rays in indirect ophthalmoscopy

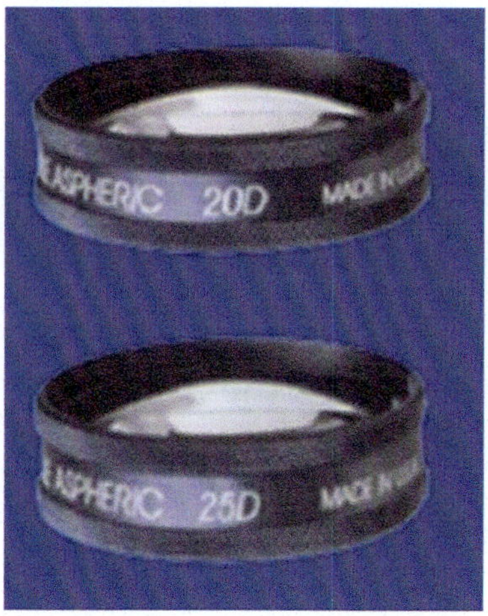

Fig 6.4 A 20D and 25D lenses are the most common lenses used for ROP examination

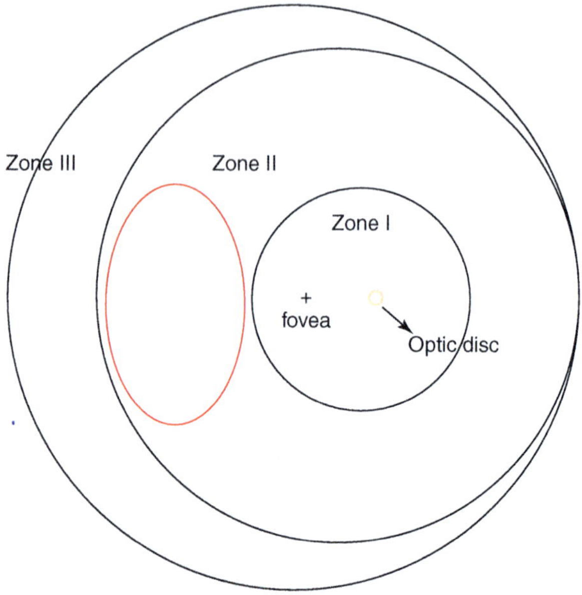

Fig. 6.5 If you look central into a newborn eye you see zone I. But the pathological changes in ROP occur in the periphery; mostly in the temporal part of zone II (red circle). (Reprinted from, *Arch Ophthalmol.* 2005;123:991–9. with permission)

Chapter 7
Wide-Field Fundus Photography

Fundus imaging is helpful for detection of various retinal conditions and monitoring of disease progression in infantile retinal diseases including retinopathy of prematurity (ROP). Retinal imaging is not easy in young children such as neonates because of small eyeball size, uncooperativeness, supine position, and so on. However, several fundus camera systems are currently available in many countries. Several types of wide-filed cameras that are commercially available are listed in Table 7.1. New camera systems are emerging, so readers of this book may be able to obtain the most up-to-date information on the camera systems by contacting the vendors. All products are not available in every country.

Table 7.1 Commercially available fundus cameras for fundus imaging in very young children including premature infants

Product	RetCam	Panocam™	3nethra neo	Pictor plus	Icon
Vendor	Natus Medical Inc.	Visunex Medical Systems, Inc.	Forus Health	Volk Optical, Inc.	Phoenix
Field of view (degree)	130	130	120	40	100
Hand-held	+	+	+	+	+
Contact or non-contact	Contact	Contact	Contact	Non-contact	Contact
Fluorescein angiography	+ (RetCam 3)	+ (Panocam Pro)	–	+	+
Portability	Moderate (RetCam shuttle)	Good (Panocam LT)	Good	Good	–
Lens	Interchangeable lenses (30–130°)	130° and 80°			100° and 30°

U. Spandau, S. J. Kim, *Pediatric Retinal Vascular Diseases*,
https://doi.org/10.1007/978-3-030-13701-4_7

7.1 RetCam 3 (Natus, https://newborncare.natus.com/products-services/newborn-care-products/eye-imaging)

RetCam is the first commercially available digital wide-field fundus imaging system that are the most widely used for infants worldwide (Fig. 7.1). RetCam systems have long been used in real clinical practices (in NICUs) and many ROP studies including telemedicine studies and image analysis studies. Retcam is a handheld contact fundus camera system with an interchangeable lens (30–130°) (Fig. 7.2). Retinal imaging can be done in video or still image mode. Taking

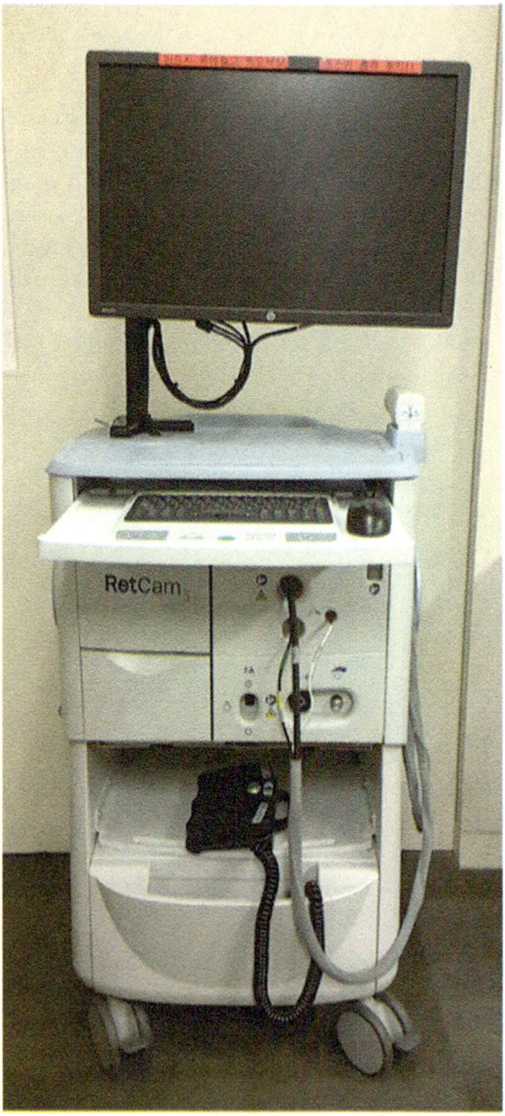

Fig. 7.1 RetCam3 unit

a video and capturing still images while reviewing the video is preferred by some ROP experts. It also has a review software for easy review and comparison between exam sessions. RetCam Shuttle is a compact model without fluorescein angiography capability. RetCam Shuttle is cheaper than RetCam 3, but has better portability.

To obtain fundus images, a coupling gel is applied on corneal surface after topical anesthesia, and the lens piece is placed on cornea. The photographer can move the lens piece while looking at the computer screen to take photos of retinal areas of interest. The photographer can adjust brightness and focusing with a foot pedal.

Examples of color fundus photographs using RetCam3 in preterm babies are shown in Figs. 7.3 and 7.4.

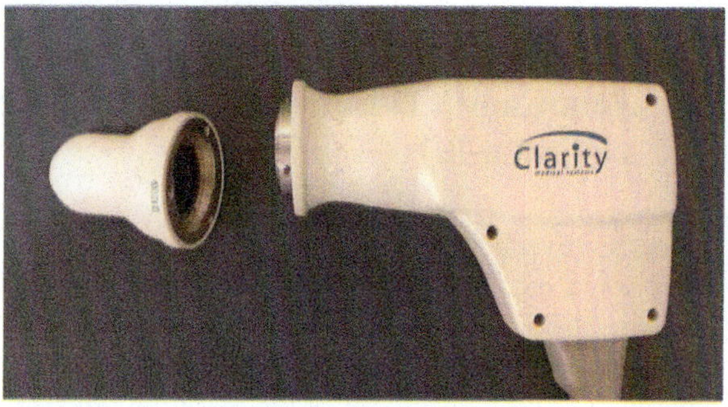

Fig. 7.2 A RetCam3 handpiece. The lens is interchangeable

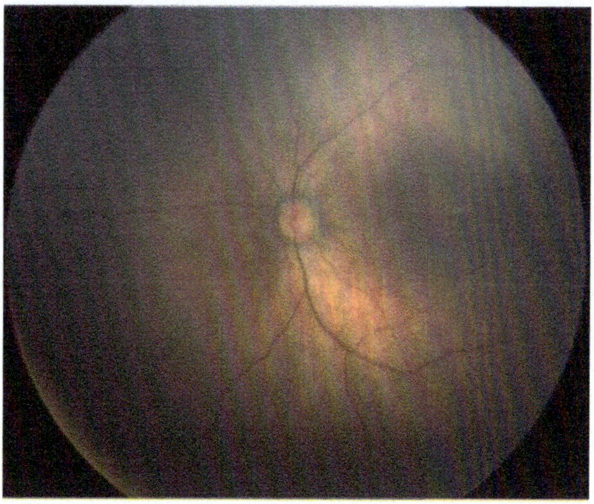

Fig. 7.3 A fundus photograph obtained by using RetCam3. This is an optic disc-centered image to evaluate plus disease in ROP

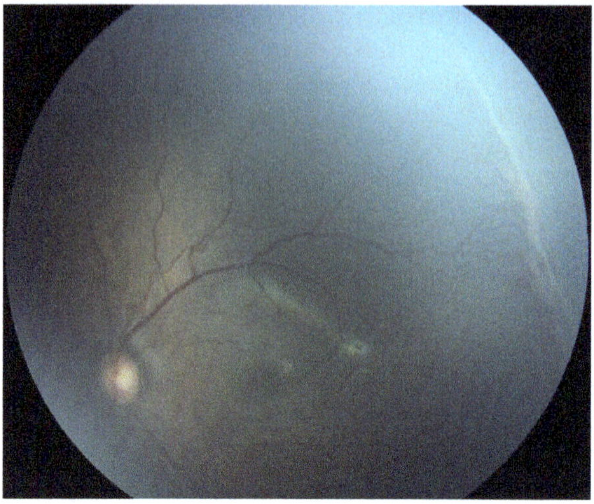

Fig. 7.4 A fundus photograph obtained by using RetCam3. This shows extraretinal fibrovascular proliferation in temporal mid-periphery

7.2 PanoCam™ (Visunex, http://visunex.com/products/panocam-lt/)

Recently, several wide-field fundus cameras became commercially available in many countries. PanoCam™ is one of the new cameras. PanoCam™ is similar to RetCam (the same field of view, etc.), but has several distinct features. The most distinct feature is the handpiece. There is a screen on the handpiece which enables a photographer to easily look at the real-time fundus image. Also, the handpiece is wireless. The HiMag™ 80° lens can be used for higher magnification.

7.3 3nethra neo (Forus, http://www.forushealth.com/3nethra-neo.html)

3nethra neo is a portable and compact wide-field digital imaging system with a 120° field-of-view lens (Fig. 7.5). Still images and burst mode images can be obtained.

Examples of color fundus photographs using 3nethra neo are shown in Figs. 7.6 and 7.7.

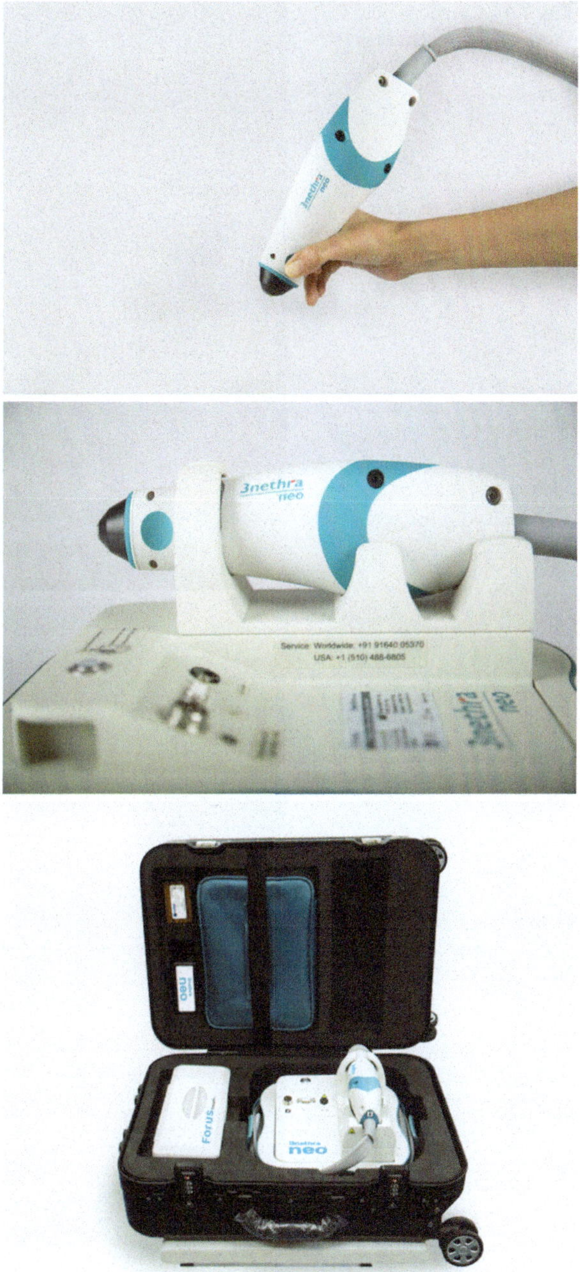

Fig. 7.5 3nethra neo. (Photos courtesy of Forus Health)

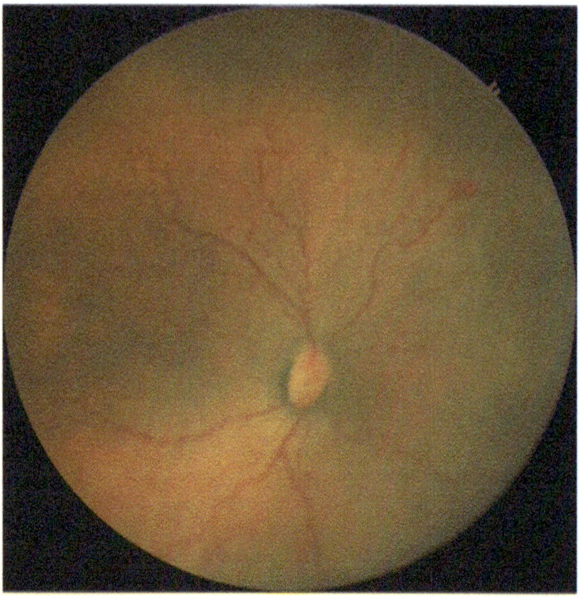

Fig. 7.6 A fundus photo showing plus disease in ROP. (Courtesy of Forus Health)

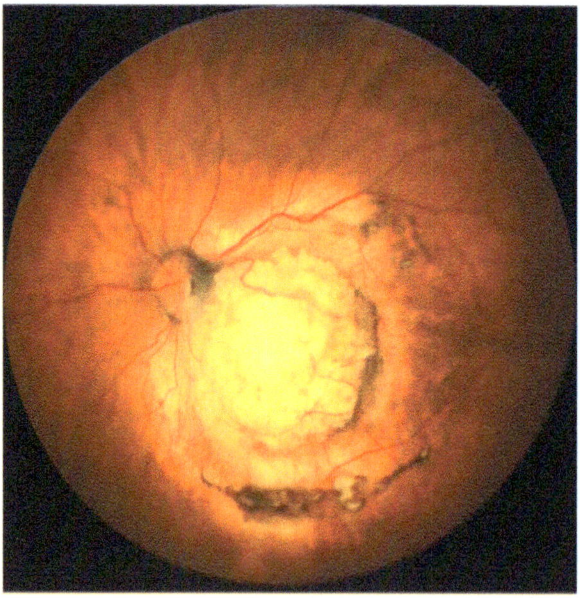

Fig. 7.7 A fundus photo showing retinoblastoma. (Courtesy of Forus Health)

7.4 Pictor (Volk, https://volk.com/index.php/volk-products/ophthalmic-cameras/volk-pictor-plus-digital-ophthalmic-imager.html)

Pictor is a portable, non-contact digital fundus camera system (Fig. 7.8). Although field of view is not large (40°), Pictor is easy to use in outpatient clinics and as well as in NICUs (Fig. 7.9).

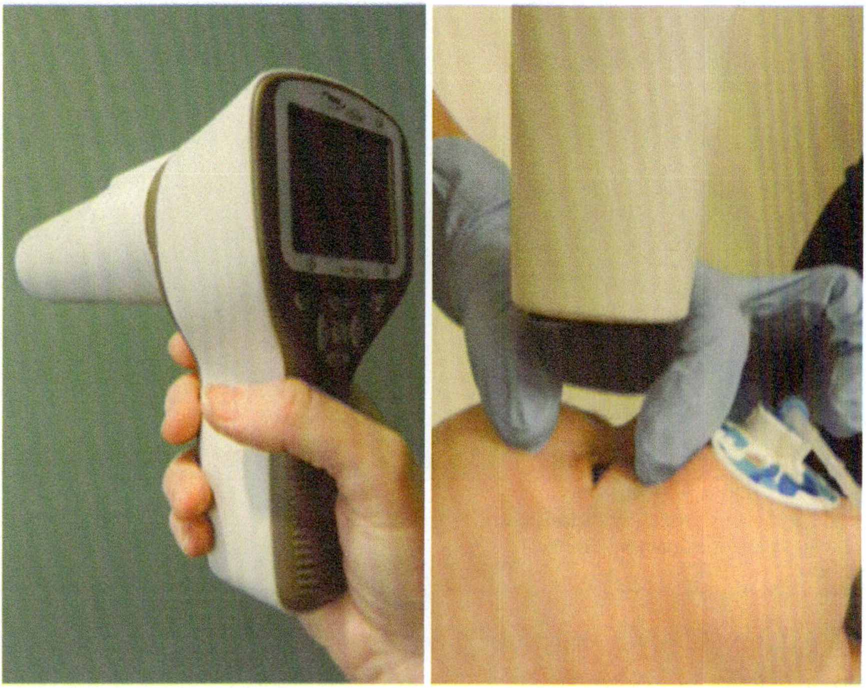

Fig. 7.8 Pictor camera. (Reprinted from Prakalapakorn et al. [1]. Copyright (2014) with permission from Elsevier)

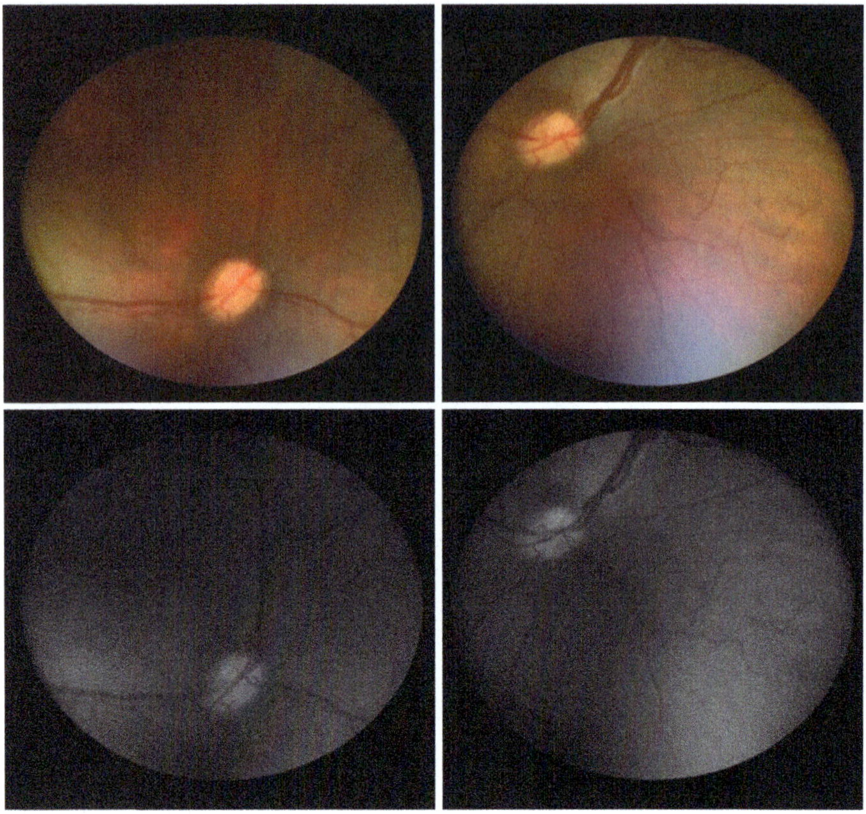

Fig. 7.9 Fundus images by Pictor camera. (Reprinted from Prakalapakorn et al. [1]. Copyright (2014) with permission from Elsevier)

7.5 Icon (Phoenix, http://phoenix-clinical.com/)

Icon is a new wide-field (Field-of-view, 100°) digital fundus camera with fluorescein angiography capability (Figs. 7.10 and 7.11). According to the vendor, darkly pigmented retinas benefit from the Phoenix Direct Illumination™, designed for high resolution and high contrast imaging while reducing scatter at the edge of the field of view.

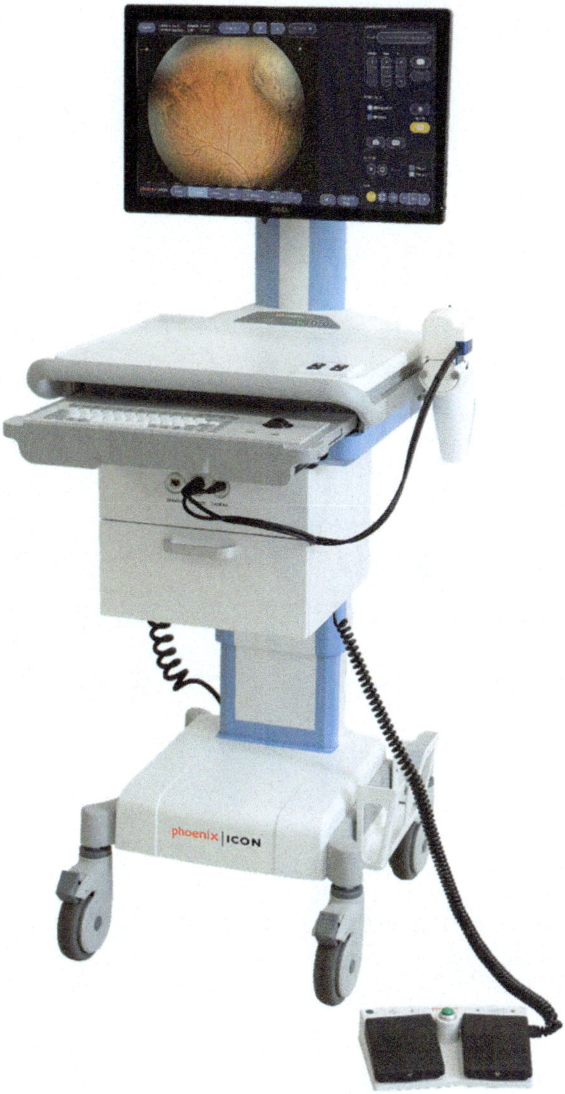

Fig. 7.10 Phoenix Icon. (Courtesy of Phoenix)

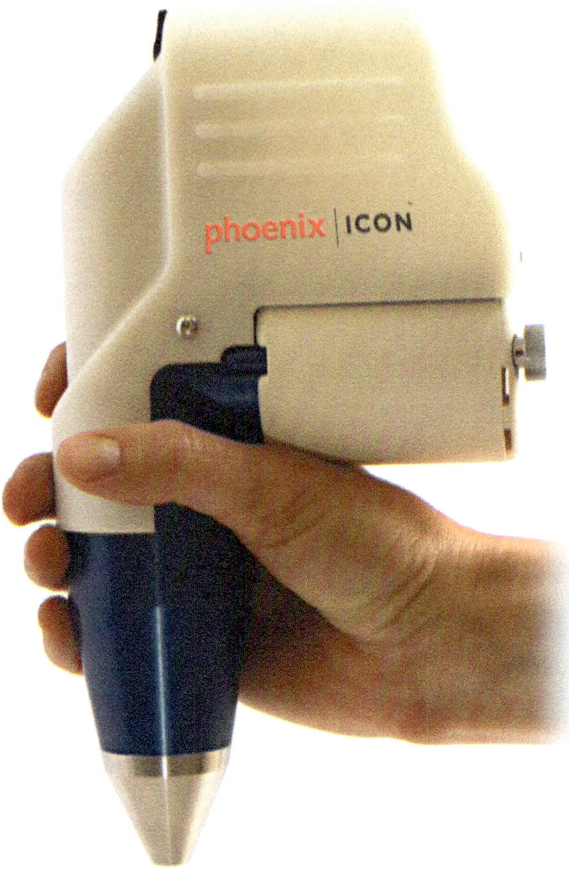

Fig. 7.11 A handpiece of Phoenix Icon. (Courtesy of Phoenix)

Reference

1. Prakalapakorn SG, Wallace DK, Freedman SF. Retinal imaging in premature infants using the Pictor noncontact digital camera. J AAPOS. 2014;18:321–6.

Chapter 8
Angiography of Newborn

An angiography examination of newborn is possible with the Retcam III (Clarity Medical System Inc., USA), the Panocam (Visunex Medical Systems, USA) and the Optos California (Optos, Scotland). The Retcam camera has a central viewing field of 30°. The viewing field is 130° with all peripheral pictures. The Optos camera has a central viewing field of 200°.

The most commonly used angiography machine for newborn is the Retcam device. But an examination of newborn with the Optos machine is also possible [1]. For the Optos examination, the newborn is sedated and positioned behind the device.

8.1 Technique of Retcam Angiography

The dose of **fluorescein** is 0.08–0.1 ml per kg body weight. We perform the examination in general anaesthesia. An IV line is required for injection of the fluorescein. We take first colour pictures and then continue with angiography. A few adjustments have to made prior to start: (1) Place a yellow filter in the handpiece of the camera (Fig. 8.1). (2) Then insert the fiber optic cable into the FA fiber connection and (3) activate the FA switch (Fig. 8.2).

Decide which eye to examine first with angiography. Activate the "FA ON" icon on the screen. Then the anaesthetist injects the fluorescein intravenously. Now start the timer. After approximately 10 seconds the fluorescein has reached the eye and you can take pictures.

U. Spandau, S. J. Kim, *Pediatric Retinal Vascular Diseases*,
https://doi.org/10.1007/978-3-030-13701-4_8

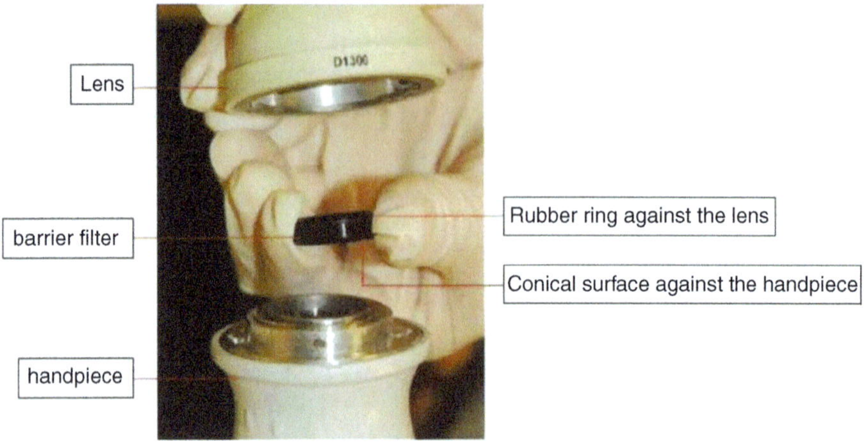

Fig. 8.1 Insert a yellow filter in the handpiece of the Retcam machine. (Photocourtesy Clarity Medical System Inc)

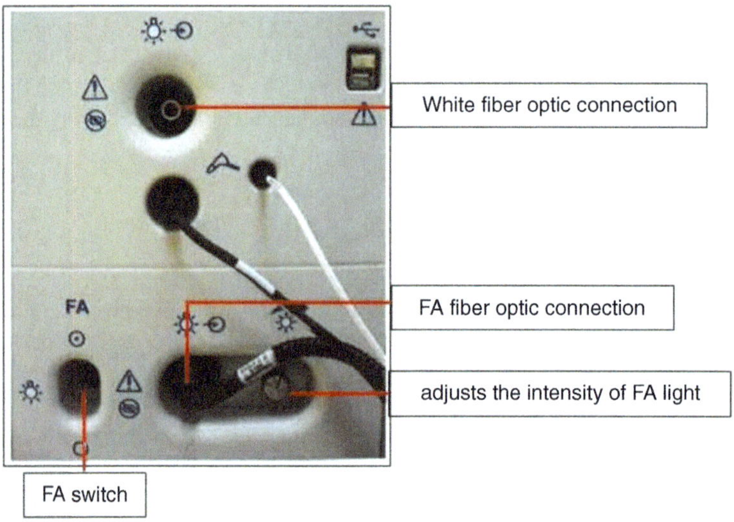

Fig. 8.2 Remove the fiber optic from the white fiber optic connection and insert it into the FA fiber connection. Then activate the FA switch. You can adjust the intensity of FA light; we recommend leaving it at maximal intensity. (Photocourtesy Clarity Medical System Inc)

8.2 Retcam Angiography Atlas

In the following, Retcam angiographies of different pathologies are demonstrated:

8.2.1 *ROP 3 in zone I* (Fig. 8.3)

A neonate born in week 23 and now in week 32 GA. A fast progressing ROP occurred and a ROP stage 3 in zone I was detected. An angiography with Retcam was performed (Fig. 8.3).

8.2.2 *Incomplete Laser Photocoagulation for ROP Newborn* (Figs. 8.4 and 8.5)

A ROP 3+ in zone II is an indication for laser photocoagulation. The laser treatment is done in both eyes and covers the complete ischemic retina from the ridge to the ora serrata. In case of an incomplete laser photocoagulation a progression of the retinopathy may occur. In this specific case an undertreatment and overtreatment has been performed (Figs. 8.4 and 8.5); undertreatment because ischemic retina is clearly visible under angiography and overtreatment because laser spots extend over the ridge.

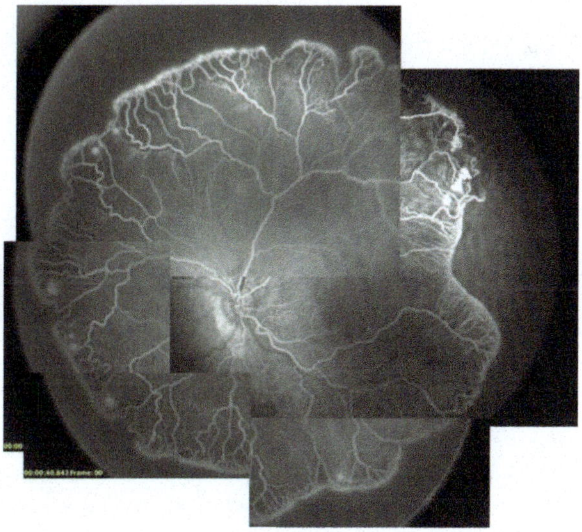

Fig. 8.3 A 360° fundus picture of a neonate born in week 32 gestational age (GA). A ROP stage 3 in zone I is present, the vessels are thick and little tortuous. Observe the proliferations and vessel malformations at the ridge

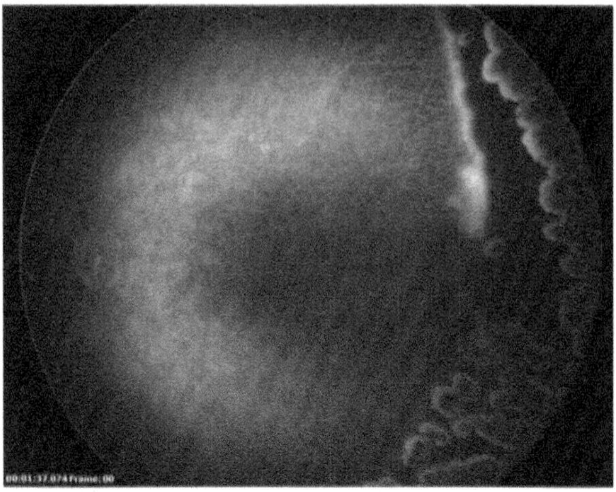

Fig. 8.4 A skip lesion at the ridge after laser photocoagulation from 2–4 o'clock. An increased leakage from retinal proliferations is present. Note also the overtreatment from 4–5 o'clock

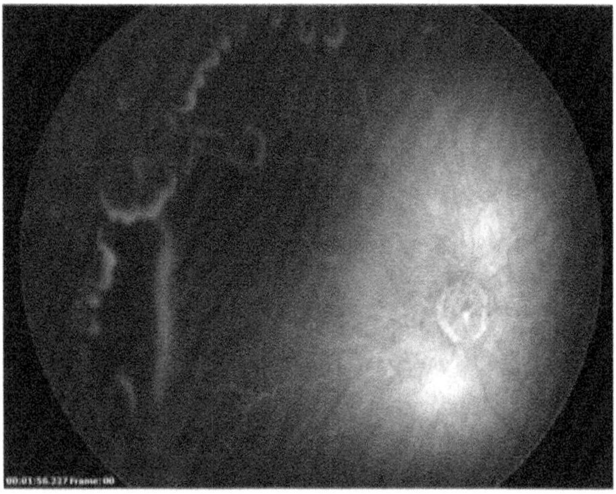

Fig. 8.5 A skip lesion at the ridge after incomplete laser photocoagulation. Note also the overtreatment from 10–12 o'clock

8.2.3 ROP Stage 4 (Figs. 8.6 and 8.7)

ROP stage 4 is defined as a retinal detachment. In stage 4A the macula is attached and in stage 4B the macula is detached. In this specific case the temporal retina is shallow detached and extensive proliferations along the ridge are visible (Figs. 8.6, 8.7, 8.8, and 8.9). This is a stage 4A detachment.

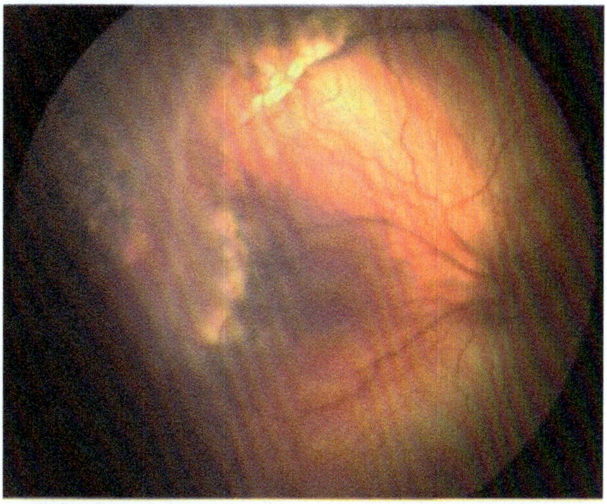

Fig. 8.6 Progression to stage 4A after laserphotocoagulation for ROP zone I

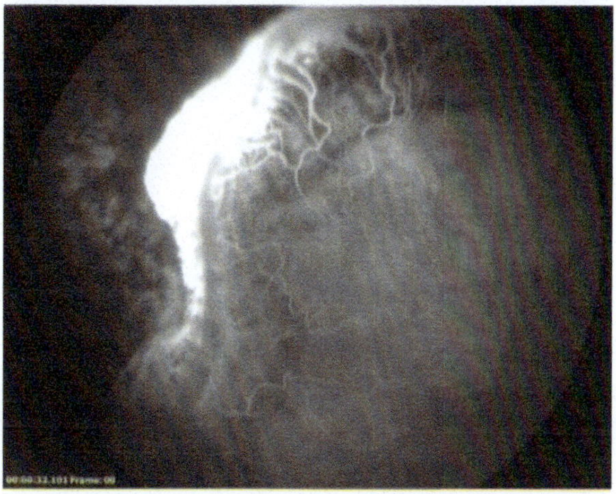

Fig. 8.7 Fluoresceine angiography demonstrates extensive leakage from proliferations

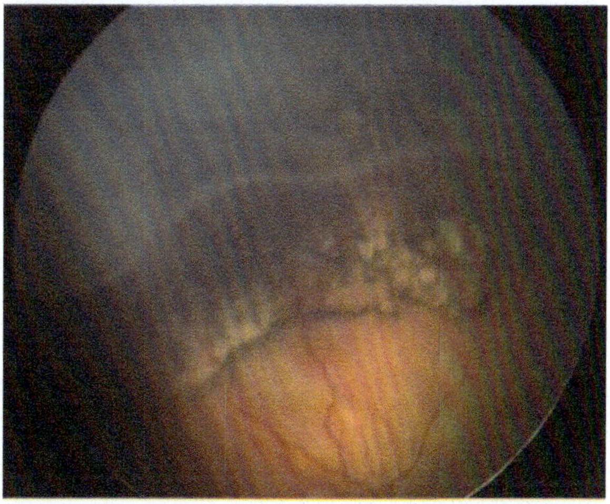

Fig. 8.8 The same eye. Note the proliferations anterior to the ridge

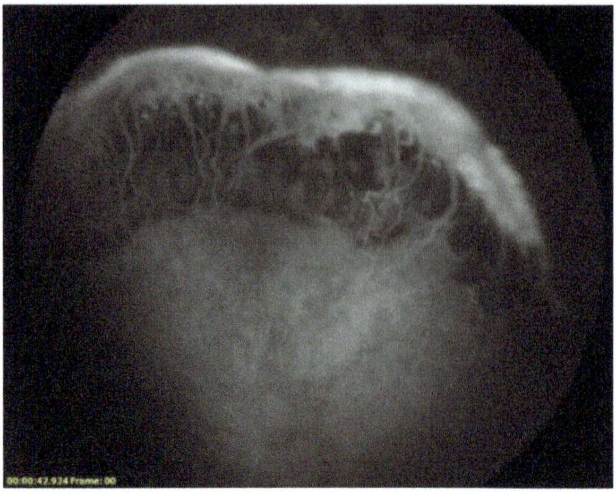

Fig. 8.9 The retina is well laser treated. No skip lesion is visible

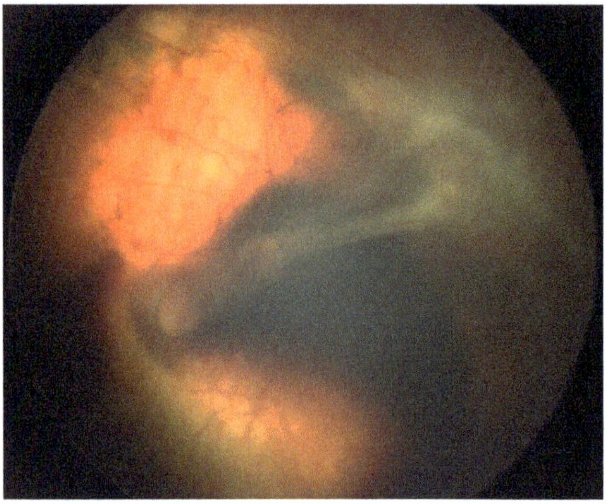

Fig. 8.10 A colour picture of a stage 4B detachment. An extensive subretinal bleeding at the posterior pole is present and a retinal fold extends from the optic disc to the periphery

8.2.4 ROP Stage 4B (Figs. 8.10 and 8.11)

ROP stage 4B is defined as a retinal detachment with detached macula. In this case the temporal retina is detached and a retinal fold extending up to the lens has developed (Figs. 8.10 and 8.11).

8.2.5 Incontinentia Pigmenti (Figs. 8.12, 8.13, 8.14, 8.15, and 8.16)

Incontinentia pigmenti is a rare congenital skin disease with eye affection. A retinal ischemia may be present resulting in a retinal detachment [2, 6]. In this case, colour photography shows no sign of vessel pathology. But fluorescein angiography shows peripheral ischemia and leakage.

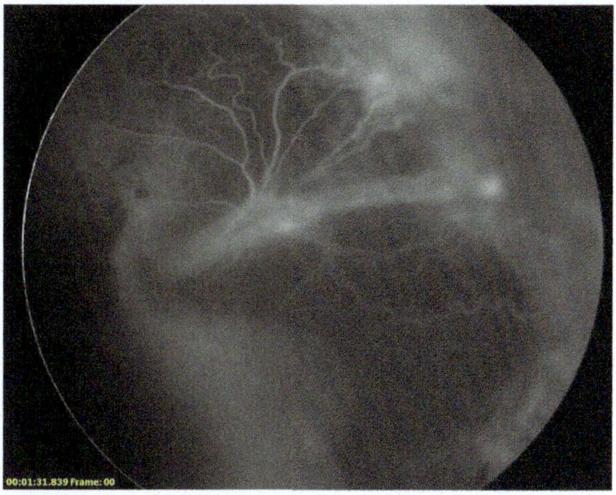

Fig. 8.11 A hyperfluorescence within the retinal fold and within the peripheral detached retina is visible. A fibrovascular membrane from the ridge to the posterior lens detaches the retina (visible in the far upper right of this picture)

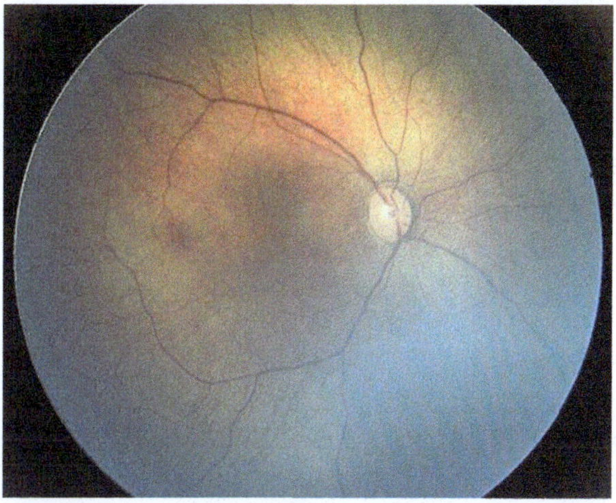

Fig. 8.12 RE: The colour picture shows no pathology

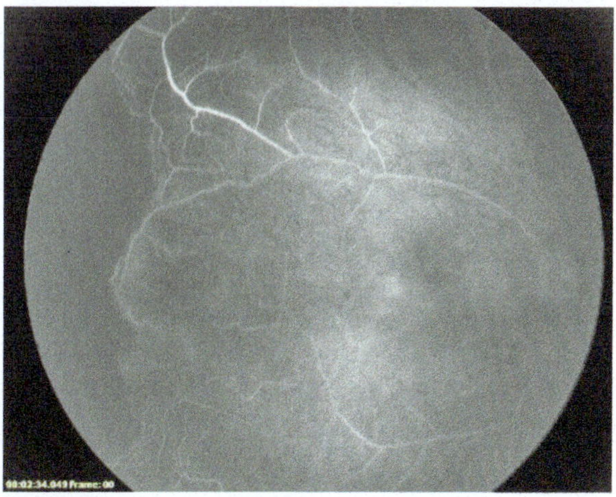

Fig. 8.13 RE: The retinal pathology can only be visualized with fluorescein angiography

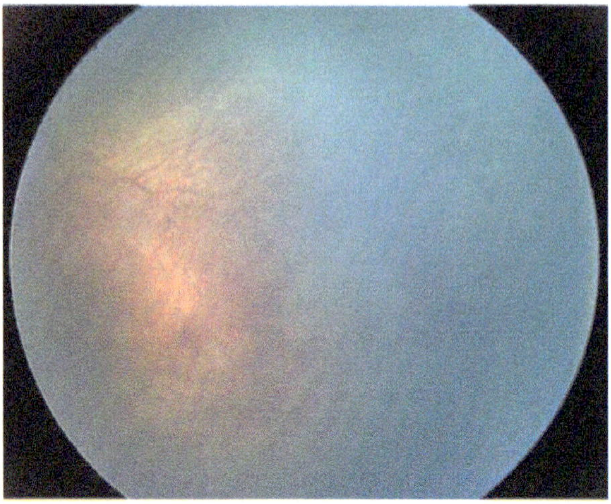

Fig. 8.14 LE: Colour photography shows the left eye with "normal" retina

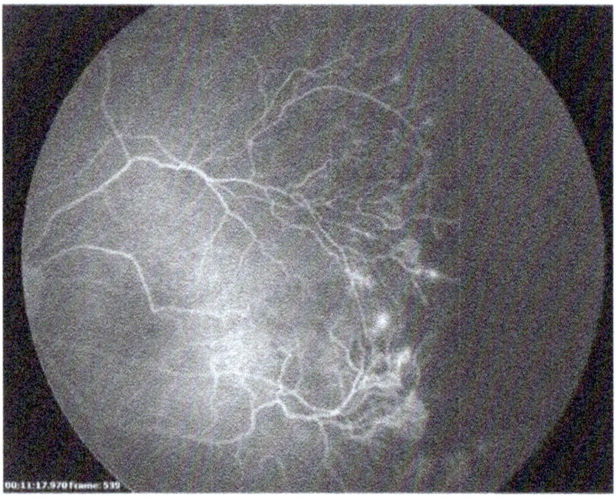

Fig. 8.15 LE: Fluorescein angiography demonstrates vessel malformation and leakage

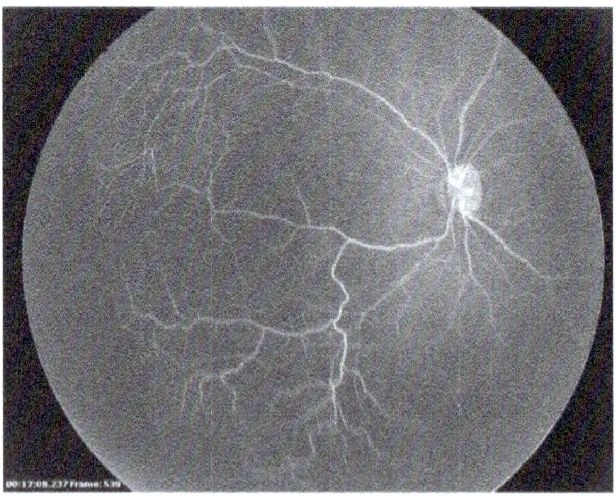

Fig. 8.16 LE: Fluorescein angiography shows an ischemic retina and leakage from the vessels on the nasal pole

8.2.6 *Microcephalus* (Fig. 8.17)

Microcephalus is a rare disease which may be caused by an infection (Zika), Crystal Meth or alcohol abuse during pregnancy [4]. Angiography shows a very immature retina with ischemia in the periphery.

8.2.7 *FEVR or ROP* (Figs. 8.18 and 8.19)

If a macular dragging or retinal fold is observed in a neonate which is born premature then the diagnosis may be FEVR or ROP. In this specific case a temporal macular dragging at the temporal pole and a normal retina on the nasal pole speaks for FEVR. In unclear cases John and collagues suggest the term ROPER (FEVR and ROP) [3].

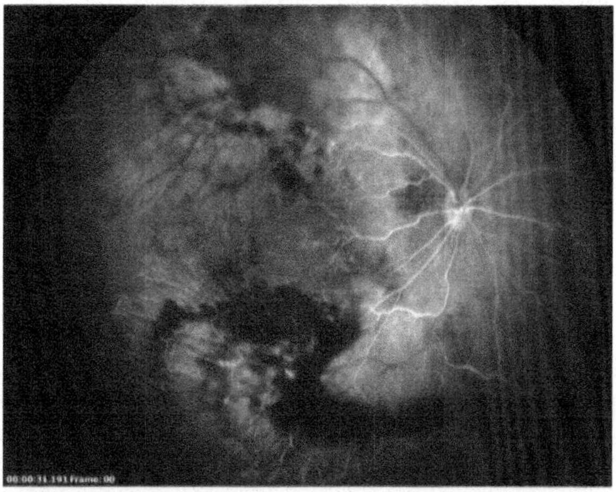

Fig. 8.17 The FA picture shows a very immature retina

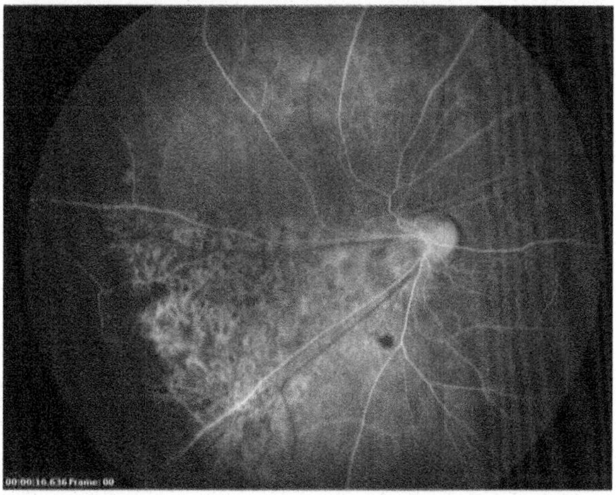

Fig. 8.18 Note the speckled hypo- and hyperfluorescence in the macular region. An avascular retina can be noted in the periphery

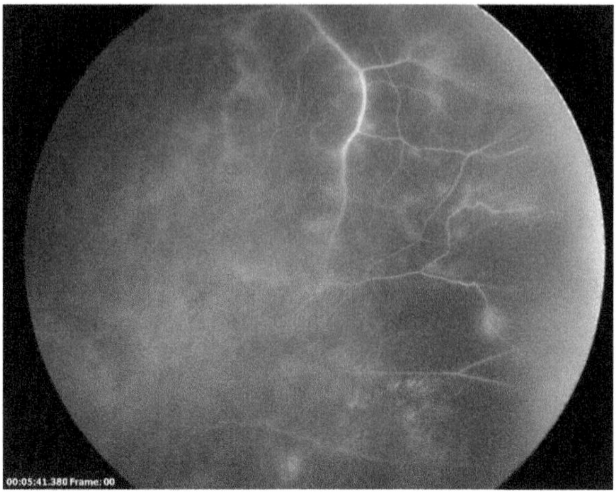

Fig. 8.19 Note the peripheral leakage and stretched retinal vessels

8.3 Optos Angiography Pictures

The Optos Californa allows to take wideangle pictures of the retina. The ultra-wide-angle imaging device captures more than 80% or 200 ° of the retina using laser scanning technology in a single image. An excellent autofluorescence function is available. Angiography allows visualization of the periphery of the retina. The Optos angiography can be used for older children without sedation [1, 5].

8.3.1 *Familial Exudative Vitreoretinopathy (FEVR)* (Figs. 8.20, 8.21, 8.22, and 8.23)

FEVR is a rather common congenital eye disease characterized of a peripheral retinal ischemia which can lead undetected to a retinal detachment. In this case an extensive retinal ischemia can be detected with angiography (Figs. 8.20, 8.21, 8.22, and 8.23). In order to obtain a view of the full extent of retinal ischemia a wide-field camera such as Optos with an angiography function is very helpful. For details see chapter "Diagnosis of familial exudative vitreoretinopathy".

8.3.2 *Morbus Coats* (Figs. 8.24, 8.25, and 8.26)

Coats disease is an idiopathic retinal vascular disorder characterized by retinal telangiectasia, exudation, and exudative retinal detachment. For details see chapter "Diagnosis of Coats disease". See Figs. 8.24, 8.25, and 8.26.

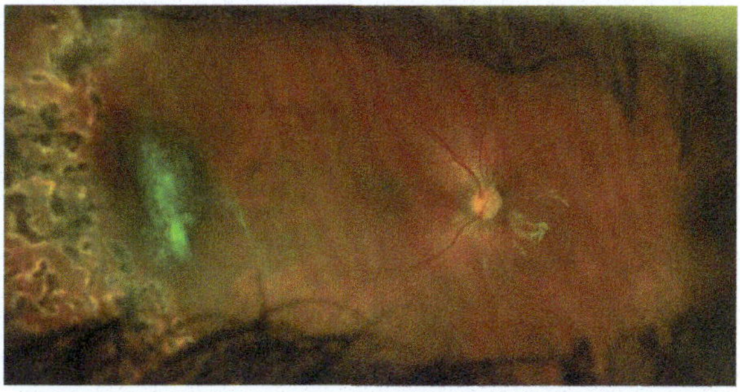

Fig. 8.20 A wide-angle colour picture of a young girl with FEVR

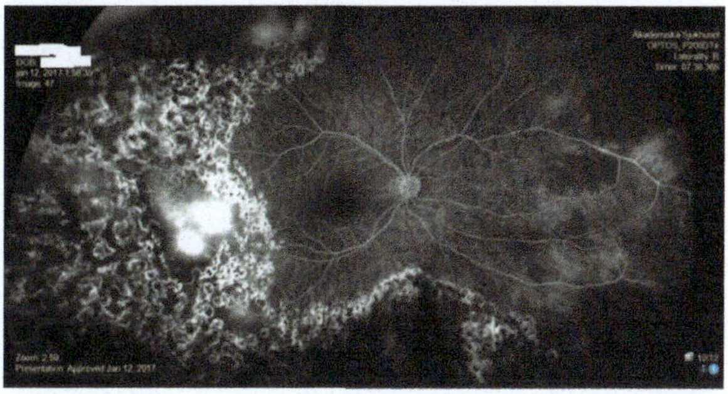

Fig. 8.21 FA angiography with an Optos camera shows the complete pathology from the nasal to the temporal periphery. The pathology is situated in the periphery and would be missed with a "normal" angiography camera

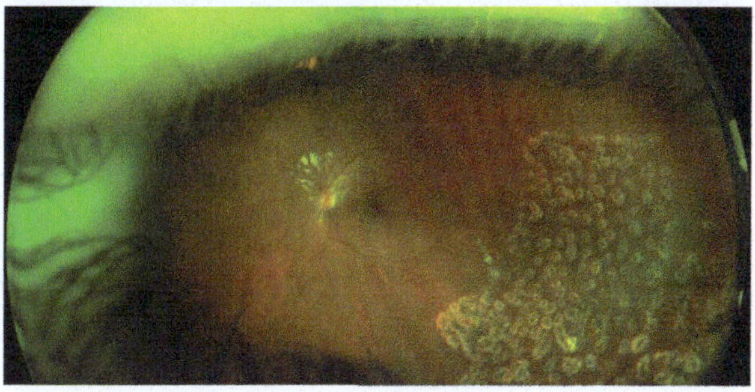

Fig. 8.22 A colour picture of the left eye. The left eye underwent a lenssparing vitrectomy due to a dense vitreous hemorrhage

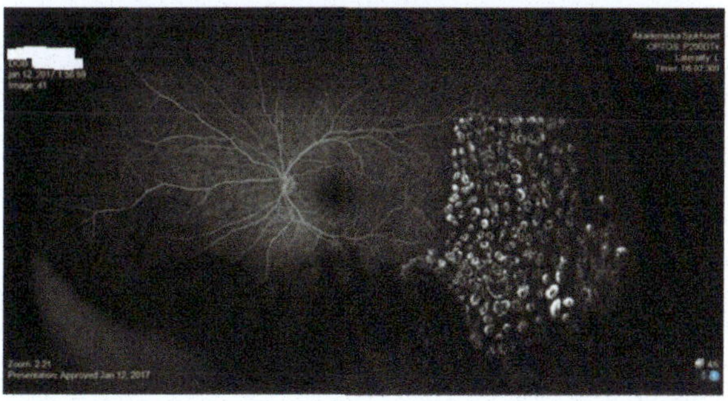

Fig. 8.23 A fluorescein angiography of the same eye. Note the ischemic retina in the temporal periphery which cannot be visualized with colour photography

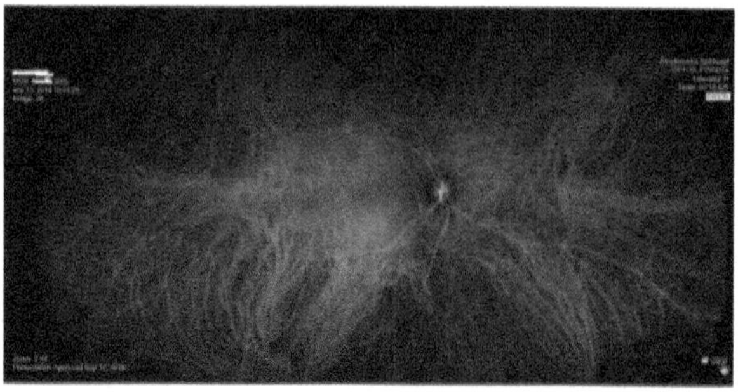

Fig. 8.24 ICG angiography of a 13 y/o male patient with Coats disease

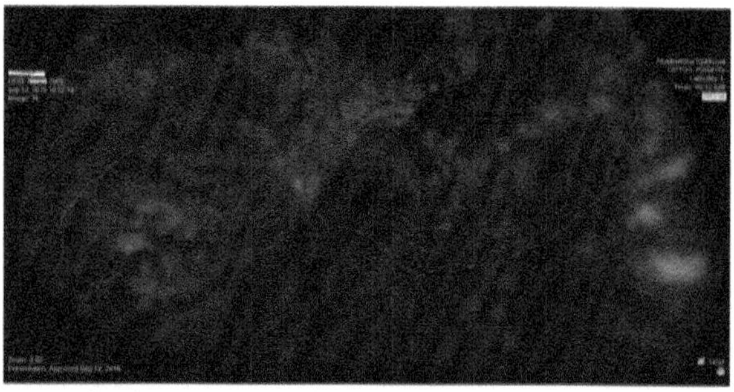

Fig. 8.25 Fluorescein angiography of a 13 y/o male patient with Coats disease. Observe the leakage from retinal vessels

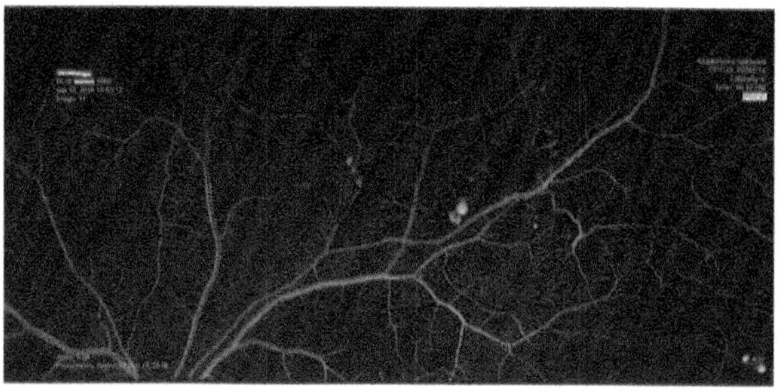

Fig. 8.26 Fluorescein angiography of a 13 y/o male patient with Coats disease. Observe the retinal teleangiectasia

References

1. Arnold RW, Grendahl RL, Kevin Winkle R, Jacob J. Outpatient, wide-field, digital imaging of infants with retinopathy of prematurity. Ophthalmic Surg Lasers Imaging Retina. 2017;48(6):494–7.
2. Chen CJ, Han IC, Tian J, Muñoz B, Goldberg MF. Extended follow-up of treated and untreated retinopathy in incontinentia pigmenti: analysis of peripheral vascular changes and incidence of retinal detachment. JAMA Ophthalmol. 2015;133(5):542–8.
3. John VJ, McClintic JI, Hess DJ, Berrocal AM. Retinopathy of prematurity versus familial exudative vitreoretinopathy: report on clinical and angiographic findings. Ophthalmic Surg Lasers Imaging Retina. 2016;47(1):14–9.
4. Miranda HA 2nd, Costa MC, Frazão MAM, Simão N, Franchischini S, Moshfeghi DM. Expanded spectrum of congenital ocular findings in microcephaly with presumed Zika infection. Ophthalmology. 2016;123(8):1788–94.

5. Patel CK, Fung TH, Muqit MM, Mordant DJ, Brett J, Smith L, Adams E. Non-contact ultra-widefield imaging of retinopathy of prematurity using the Optos dual wavelength scanning laser ophthalmoscope. Eye (Lond). 2013;27(5):589–96.
6. Swinney CC, Han DP, Karth PA. Incontinentia pigmenti: a comprehensive review and update. Ophthalmic Surg Lasers Imaging Retina. 2015;46(6):650–7.

Part III
Assessment

Chapter 9
Assessment of ROP Neonates

It is very important to be an experienced examiner of ROP disease before you start treating neonates. Why?

For several reasons:

1. To master binocular indirect ophthalmoscopy. You cannot perform laser coagulation otherwise.
2. To understand and to know the ROP disease. How does the disease develop in the course of time? You will treat too early or too late otherwise.
3. To develop a feeling for these very small patients. Their eyes are like raw eggs. Treat them like raw eggs.
4. A good screening and a good treatment necessitate each other. A good treatment does nor replace a poor screening and vice versa.

ROP disease develops slowly and then aggravates exponentially. In the beginning a weekly examination is sufficient but if ROP stage 3 is present then two examinations per week are required. If the right moment for treatment has come, you must succeed with the treatment. The first treatment decides about the fate of the eye. Why? Because the disease moves in an exponential function (Fig. 9.1). If the first treatment fails, then the disease progresses fast to stage 4 and 5, so that it is often too late for the second treatment.

As an examiner you must make *two important assessments* which determine the treatment. Is a (1) plus disease present and is (2) the disease located in zone I or zone II?

9.1 Assessment of Plus Disease

The most important diagnosis for an ophthalmologist treating ROP neonates, is to assess if plus disease is present or not. Plus disease means, that the central retinal vessels are thick and tortuous. Plus disease can be assessed by only examining the

U. Spandau, S. J. Kim, *Pediatric Retinal Vascular Diseases*,
https://doi.org/10.1007/978-3-030-13701-4_9

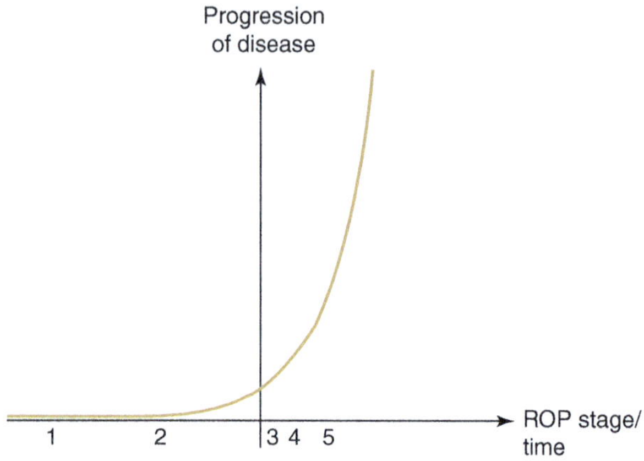

Fig. 9.1 The progression of ROP disease has an exponential function

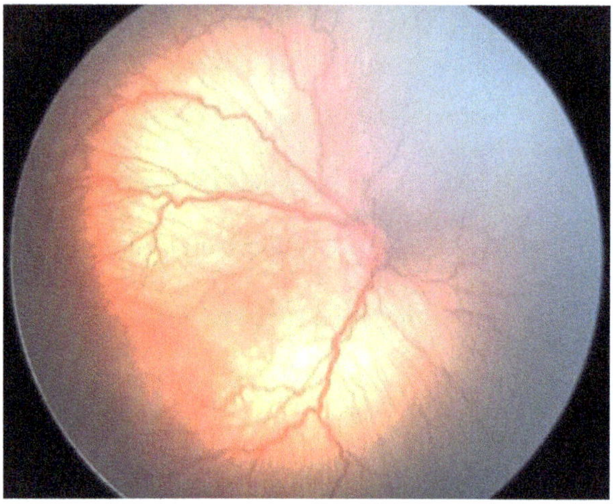

Fig. 9.2 Example for plus disease. Tortuous and thick vessels are typical for plus disease

posterior pole. It is, however, to some extent subjective how tortuous and how thick the vessels must be. The Figs. 9.2, 9.3, 9.4, 9.5, 9.6, and 9.7 show typical examples for plus disease.

Three tips, if you are insecure, if plus disease is present or not:

1. If the vessels are tortuous and thick in all 4 quadrants, then a plus disease is present (Fig. 9.5).
2. Examine the pictures of the previous follow-ups. If you see a progress, then a plus disease is likely (Figs. 9.6 and 9.7).
3. If you are still insecure, then schedule tight follow-ups (2x per week). If it is plus disease, then it will get worse within a short time (1–2 weeks).

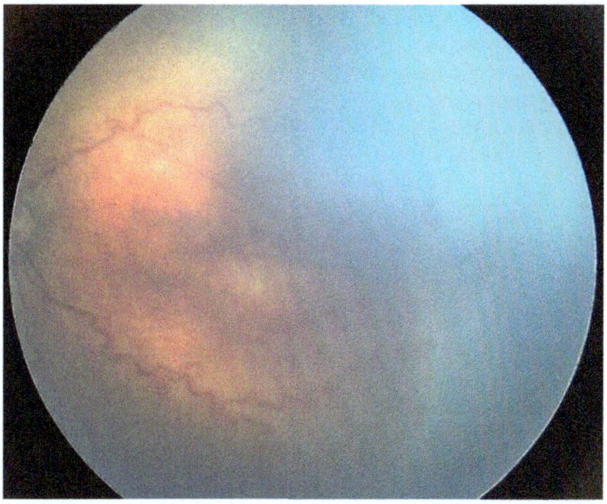

Fig. 9.3 Plus disease. Note the tortuous and thick vessels, which are typical for plus disease

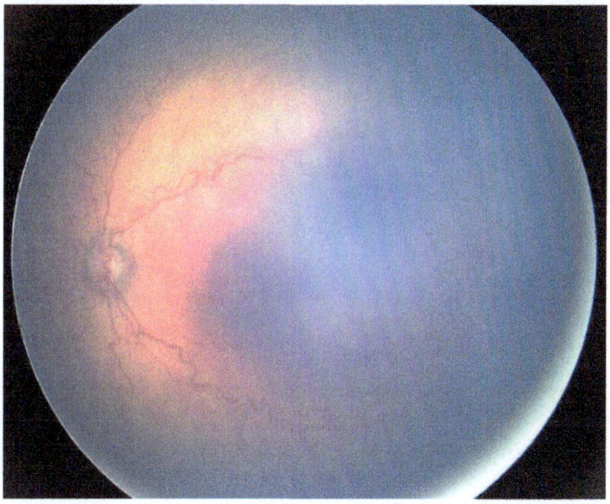

Fig. 9.4 Another example for plus disease. Note the tortuous and thick vessels

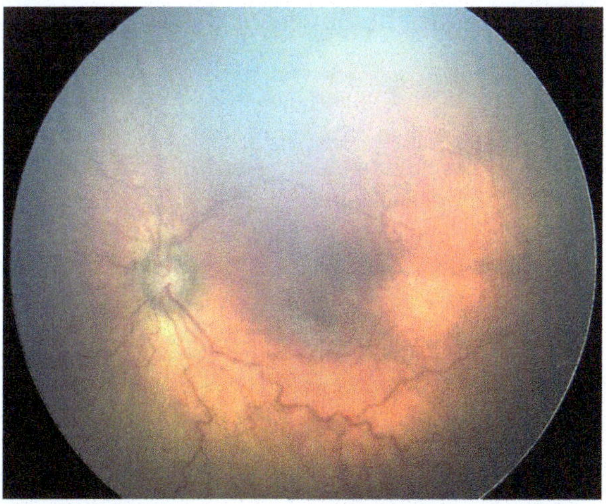

Fig. 9.5 One more example for plus disease. Note the tortuous and thick vessels in all 4 quadrants

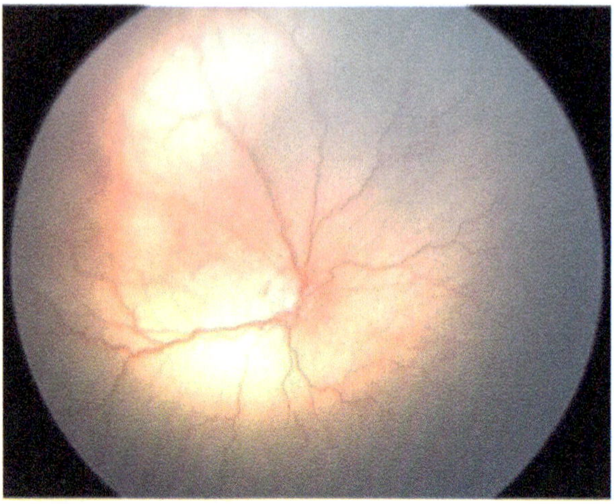

Fig. 9.6 Figures 9.6 and 9.7 are the same eye. Note the increase of plus disease during the screening. Figure 9.6 is preplus and Fig. 9.7 is a plus disease

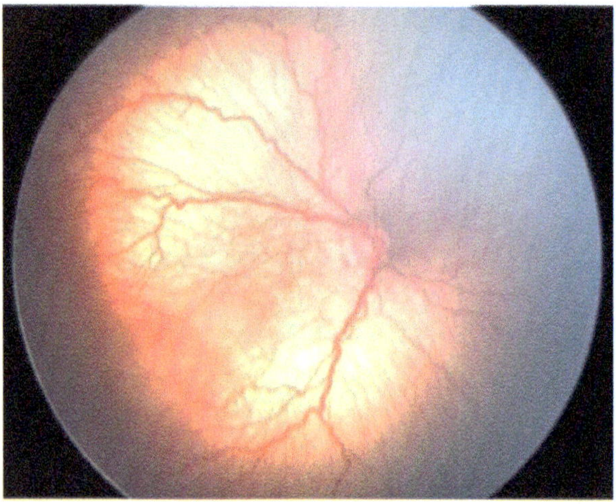

Fig. 9.7 One week later: The tortuosity increased centrally compared to Fig. 9.6. In all quadrants tortuous vessels are visible. This is a typical for plus disease

9.2 Assessment Zone I or Zone II

Why is it of utmost importance to determine prior to surgical treatment, if the retinopathy is present in zone I or in zone II? Because a retinopathy in zone I or in zone II requires different treatment modalities. In zone I anti-VEGF is superior to laser because laser coagulation in zone I has a high complication rate [3]. Where does zone II start? See Fig. 9.8. Zone II starts at 2 times the distance from the nasal part of the optic disc to the macula. Two examples are depicted in Figs. 9.9 and 9.10. Note that only a part of the temporal ischemia is located in zone I and the residual part is located in zone II. We define this nonetheless as zone I.

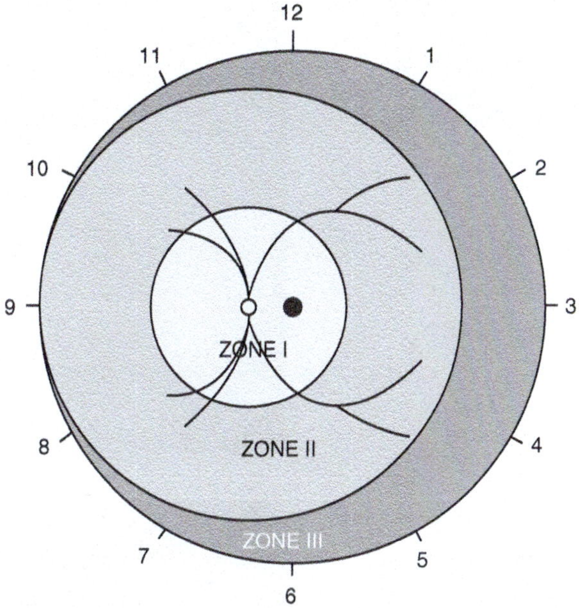

Fig. 9.8 Zone II starts at the distance 2x optic disc-macula

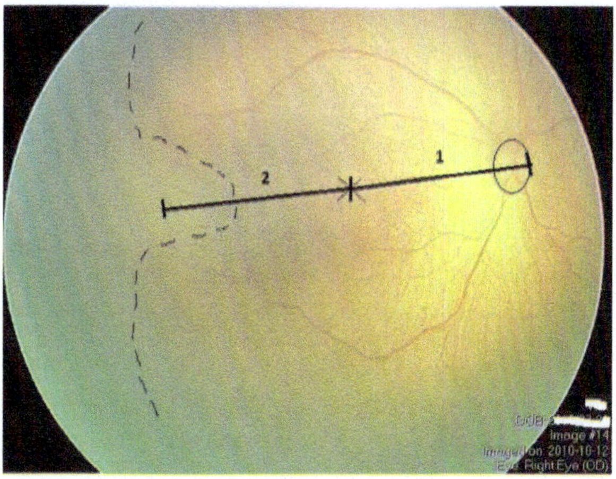

Fig. 9.9 Zone II starts two times the distance optic disc (small circle) to macula (X). The temporal retina is located in zone I. The inferior, nasal and superior retina is not located in zone II. We still define this eye as a zone I retinopathy and treat it with anti-VEGF

In a previous Swedish study of extremely preterm infants born before 27 weeks gestation age, a high incidence of ROP (73%) and a high frequency of treatment (20%) were reported [1]. With a continuous increase in the survival of very preterm neonates, the incidence of eyes with zone I will increase and consequently the necessity to treat with anti-VEGF and not with laser coagulation [2].

It is difficult to make this assessment without a Retcam device. One example: How would you decide in Fig. 9.11? Is this zone I or zone II. The neonate was born in week 23 and is now in week 32. The answer can be seen in Fig. 9.12. It is a zone I disease. The ischemia in the nasal periphery is also very pronounced (Fig. 9.13). Observe also the fellow eye (Fig. 9.14). Also here a ROP 3 plus disease is present.

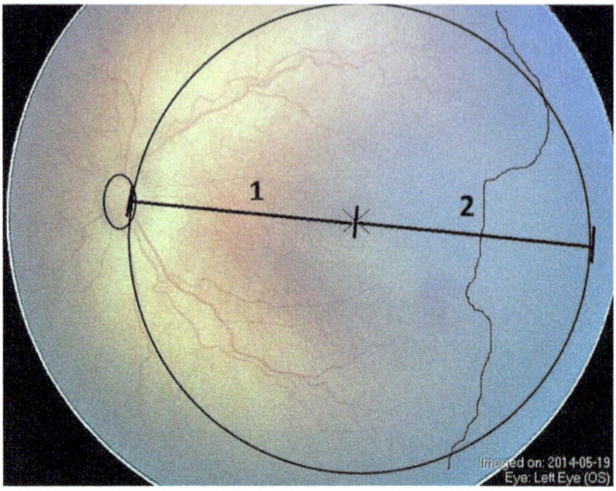

Fig. 9.10 Another example for zone II. The large circle shows the tissue which is inside zone I. Zone I starts two times the distance optic disc (small circle) to macula (X)

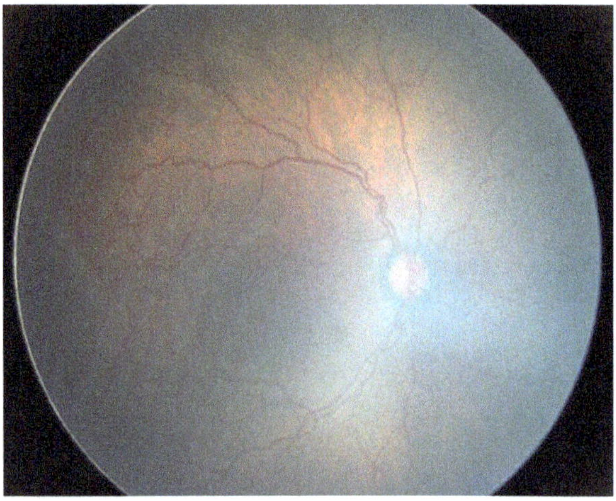

Fig. 9.11 Is this zone I or zone II?

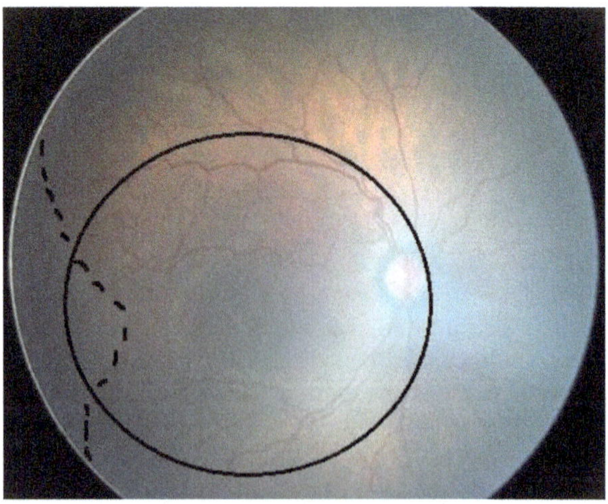

Fig. 9.12 The ischemia is within zone I. In this case an anti-VEGF treatment is advisable

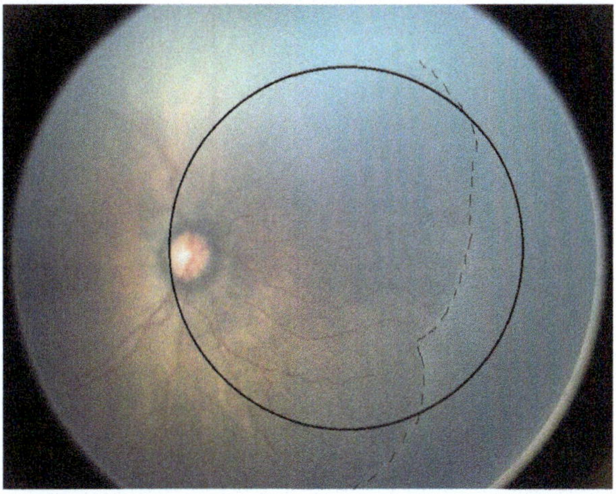

Fig. 9.13 Same eye as Fig. 9.11, note the pronounced ischemia in the *nasal* periphery. The circle demonstrates that the nasal side is also located in zone I

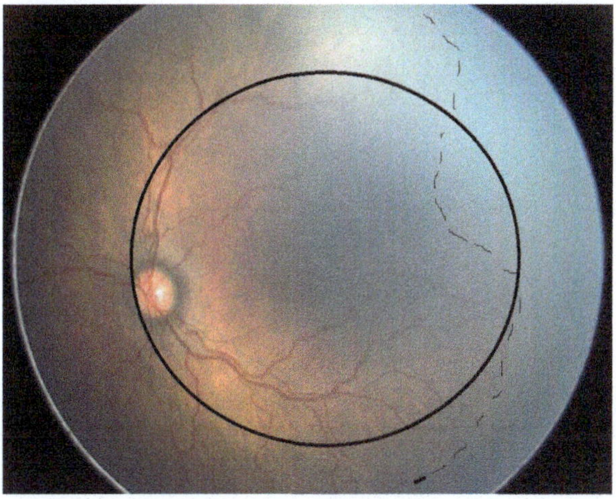

Fig. 9.14 Left eye of the same patient. Again, a ROP disease in zone I is present. Anti-VEGF treatment is advised

Key Points

1. Before treatment assess whether (1) plus disease is present and (2) in which zone it is located.
2. The assessment of plus disease is subjective. If you are insecure then observe the course of the disease. Did the plus symptoms increase compared with the previous examinations?
3. Zone I or zone II assessment is difficult with funduscopy but easy with a photograph. Zone II is two times the distance of optic disc to macula. Zone I diseases have a pronounced ischemia in the temporal and nasal retina.
4. If you are insecure if the ROP disease is on the border of zone I and zone II, then decide for an anti-VEGF treatment.
5. After the diagnosis has been made, the treatment must be carried out after 72 hours at the latest.

References

1. Austeng D, Källen KB, Ewald UW, Wallin A, Holmström GE. Treatment for retinopathy of prematurity in infants born before 27 weeks of gestation in Sweden. Br J Ophthalmol. 2010;94(9):1136–9.
2. Holmström G, Tornqvist K, Al-Hawasi A, Nilsson Å, Wallin A, Hellström A. Increased frequency of retinopathy of prematurity over the last decade and significant regional differences. Acta Ophthalmol. 2018 Mar;96(2):142–8.
3. Mintz-Hittner HA, Kennedy KA, Chuang AZ, BEAT-ROP Cooperative Group. Efficacy of intravitreal bevacizumab for stage 3+ retinopathy of prematurity. N Engl J Med. 2011;364:603–15.

Chapter 10
Lasercoagulation or Anti-VEGF: What Is the Better Treatment?

This chapter compares laser coagulation with anti-VEGF for ROP disease.

1. **Treatment success**
   For zone I anti-VEGF has a higher treatment success than laser coagulation. For zone II anti-VEGF and laser coagulation have an equal treatment success [7].
   Conclusion: anti-VEGF wins this race
2. **Surgical difficulty**
   Laser coagulation is technically more difficult than an injection
   Conclusion: anti-VEGF wins this race
3. **Complications**
   The BEAT-ROP study demonstrated a complication rate of 37% for laser coagulation and 3% for anti-VEGF [7, 8]
   Conclusion: anti-VEGF wins this race
4. **Recurrence and follow-up**
   Anti-VEGF has a higher recurrence rate than laser coagulation and requires a longer follow-up [1, 3, 4].
   Conclusion: Laser coagulation wins this race
5. **Lasercoagulation versus anti-VEGF regarding visual field**
   A major functional advantage of anti-VEGF treatment is the bigger visual field compared to laser photocoagulation. After anti-VEGF injection the retina can mature and vascularize resulting in a bigger visual field (Figs. 10.1 and 10.2) [7, 8].
   Conclusion: anti-VEGF wins this race
6. **Refractive outcome**
   The prevalence of high myopia is low in bevacizumab treated neonates and high in laser coagulation treated neonates. Regarding zone I the prevalence of high myopia (>8 diopters) is 4% after bevacizumab treatment und 51% after laser coagulation. Regarding zone II the prevalence for high myopia is 2% for bevacizumab and 36% for laser coagulation [2, 8].
   Conclusion: anti-VEGF wins this race

U. Spandau, S. J. Kim, *Pediatric Retinal Vascular Diseases*,
https://doi.org/10.1007/978-3-030-13701-4_10

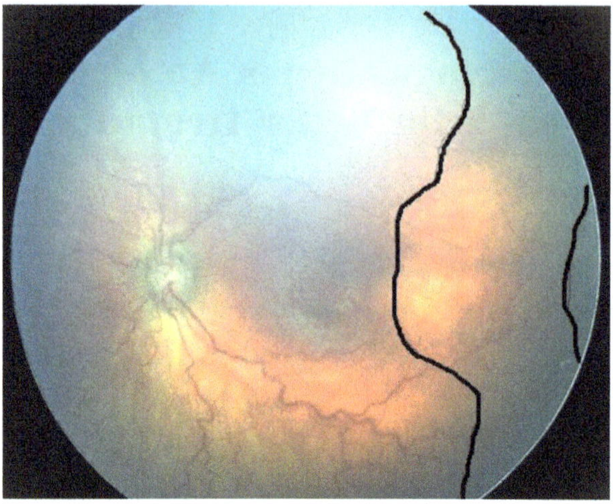

Fig. 10.1 This eye was first treated with Lucentis in zone I and then with laser photocoagulation in zone II. The first line (from left) shows the location of the ridge before anti-VEGF injection. The second line (from left) shows the location of the ridge before laser photocoagulation

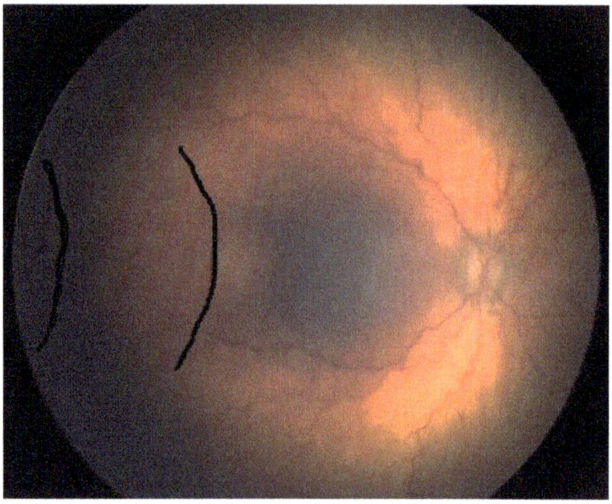

Fig. 10.2 Another example. This eye was first treated with Lucentis in zone I and 2 months later with laser photocoagulation in zone II. The first line (from right) shows the location of the ridge before anti-VEGF injection. The second line (from right) shows the location of the ridge before laser photocoagulation

7. **Retinal detachment**
   Regarding *short term data* the BEAT-ROP showed an equal rate of retinal detachment for both treatment modalities. Hu et al. report an increased rate of retinal detachment in the anti-VEGF group. There is, however, no *long-term data* available. Taking into consideration that the retina is not fully vascularized after a long follow-up, we presume that the risk for retinal detachment will be higher in the anti-VEGF group compared to the laser group [4, 7]
   Conclusion: Lasercoagulation wins this race
8. **Long term ocular effects**
   At 4 years of age bevacizumab-treated eyes showed abnormalities at the posterior pole and in the periphery. At the posterior pole an absence of foveal avascular zone was observed and in the periphery vessel leakage, avascular area and abnormal vessel branching was detected [6]. There are no known long term ocular effects for laser coagulation regarding the physiologic retina.
   Conclusion: Lasercoagulation wins this race

Table 10.1 Summary of a comparison of laser coagulation versus anti-VEGF

	Anti-VEGF	Laser coagulation
Treatment success	+	
Surgical difficulty	+	
Recurrence/follow-up		+
Complications	+	
Visual field	+	
Refractive outcome	+	
Retinal detachment		+
Long term ocular effect		+
Long term systemic effect		+

Anti-VEGF wins the *short-term* follow-up. It is unclear, who wins the *long-term* follow-up because the retinal detachment rate and the long-term ocular and systemic effects are not yet known

9. **Long term systemic effects**
   A 2-year follow-up evaluation of infants treated with bevacizumab versus laser for retinopathy of prematurity showed no adverse effects on medical or neurodevelopmental outcomes [5]. There are no known long term systemic effects of laser coagulation.
   Conclusion: Lasercoagulation wins (presumably) this race

The following table summarizes the results of the comparison of anti-VEGF versus laser coagulation (see Table 10.1). Anti-VEGF is the clear winner of this comparison. The main advantage of laser coagulation is the low recurrence rate and short follow-up. In all other aspects, especially in treatment success and surgical difficulty, anti-VEGF is superior to laser coagulation.

Key Points
- Anti-VEGF is not user dependent.
- Laser coagulation is user dependent
- Anti-VEGF achieves a larger visual field and results in less myopia
- Laser coagulation requires a short follow-up
- Anti-VEGF requires a long follow-up

References

1. Feng J, Qian J, Jiang Y, Zhao M, Liang J, Yin H, Chen Y, Yu W, Li X. Efficacy of primary intravitreal ranibizumab for retinopathy of prematurity in China. Ophthalmology. 2017;124(3):408–9.
2. Harder BC, Schlichtenbrede FC, von Baltz S, Jendritza W, Jendritza B, Jonas JB. Intravitreal bevacizumab for retinopathy of prematurity: refractive error results. Am J Ophthalmol. 2013;1555(6):1119–24.
3. Holmström G, Hellström A, Jakobsson P, Lundgren P, Tornqvist K, Wallin A. Five years of treatment for retinopathy of prematurity in Sweden: results from SWEDROP, a national quality register. Br J Ophthalmol. 2016;100(12):1656–61.

4. Hu J, Blair MP, Shapiro MJ, Lichetnstein SJ, Galasso JM, Kapur R. Reactivation of retinopathy of prematurity after bevacizumab injection. Arch Ophthalmol. 2012;130(8):1000–6.
5. Kennedy KA, Mintz-Hittner HA, BEAT-ROP Cooperative Group. Medical and developmental outcomes of bevacizumab versus laser for retinopathy of prematurity. J AAPOS. 2018;22(1):61–65.e1.
6. Lepore D, Quinn GE, Molle F, Orazi L, Baldascino A, Ji MH, Sammartino M, Sbaraglia F, Ricci D, Mercuri E. Follow-up to age 4 years of treatment of type 1 retinopathy of prematurity intravitreal bevacizumab injection versus laser: fluorescein angiographic findings. Ophthalmology. 2018;125(2):218–26.
7. Mintz-Hittner HA, Kennedy KA, Chuang AZ, BEAT-ROP Cooperative Group. Efficacy of intravitreal bevacizumab for stage 3+ retinopathy of prematurity. N Engl J Med. 2011;364:603–15.
8. Mintz-Hittner HA, Geloneck MM, Chuang AZ. Clinical management of recurrent retinopathy of prematurity after intravitreal bevacizumab monotherapy. Ophthalmology. 2016;123(9):1845–55.

Part IV
Laser Photocoagulation

Chapter 11
Technique of Lasercoagulation

In our experience laser coagulation is always successful for ROP 3+ in zone II. A failure or recurrence is very seldom. Successful laser coagulation is "normal" for clinical centers which treat many ROP newborn per year. The success rate in the ETROP study is 90% for zone II [2]. But the failure and recurrence rate for laser coagulation is much higher (30%) for clinics which treat only a handful newborn per year [1]. The most common reason for failure after laser coagulation is an incomplete laser treatment.

This is not the case for zone I. In zone I a recurrence may occur after a complete laser photocoagulation. It is therefore essential to distinguish between zone I and zone II eyes. This is only possible with an imaging device such as Retcam (Clarity Medical System Inc., USA).

The technique of lasercoagulation is difficult and requires much training. An eye with ROP 3+ requires a COMPLETE laser coagulation within ONE session. This is different to diabetes. Here a laser coagulation in many sessions is possible.

First you must learn to examine adults with the binocular indirect ophthalmoscope. If you master this technique fluently, then examine newborns on the weekly ROP examinations. This training requires at least 12 months. Then you can start with laser coagulation. You laser one eye and your mentor lasers the fellow eye. After approximately five laser treatments with your teacher you can start to treat alone.

One eye or both eyes? Sometimes ROP 3+ is not present in both eyes. One eye may have ROP 3+ and the other eye may have ROP 3 preplus. We laser treat always both eyes. Why? In the most cases the preplus eye will progress later on to a plus disease. Furthermore, an asymmetric treatment results in a grave anisometropia. The treated eye will become highly myopic and the fellow eye not. Finally, the newborn avoids a second general anaesthesia.

U. Spandau, S. J. Kim, *Pediatric Retinal Vascular Diseases*,
https://doi.org/10.1007/978-3-030-13701-4_11

11.1 Instruments for Laser Coagulation

1. Diode laser device (Fig. 11.1)
2. Binocular indirect ophthalmoscope (Fig. 11.2)
3. Volk 25D lens (Fig. 11.3)
4. Scleral depressor (Fig. 11.4)
5. Lid speculum (Fig. 11.5)

Laser device (Fig. 11.1) We use always a diode laser (Iridex, CA). An alternative is an Argon laser. The initial settings of the laser device are 100/100/300: Power: 100 ms, Duration: 100 ms, Interval: 300 ms.

Laser indirect ophthalmoscope (LIO) (Fig. 11.2) The laser indirect ophthalmoscope is a helmet which contains a light source and a laser device. The laser indirect ophthalmoscope is connected to the diode laser (Iridex, CA).

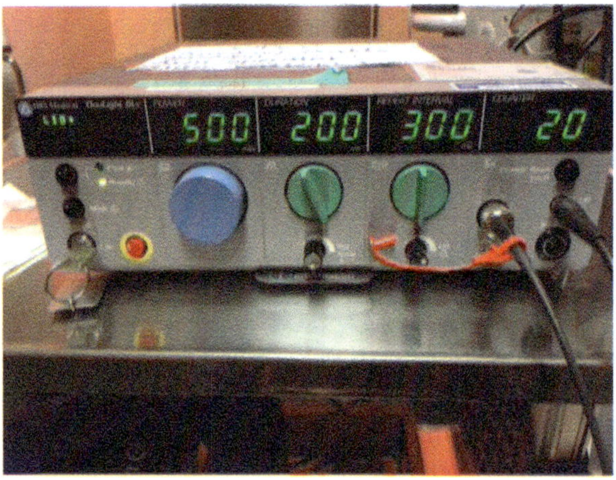

Fig. 11.1 A diode laser (Iridex) and two attached cables from binocular laser ophthalmoscope for laser and light

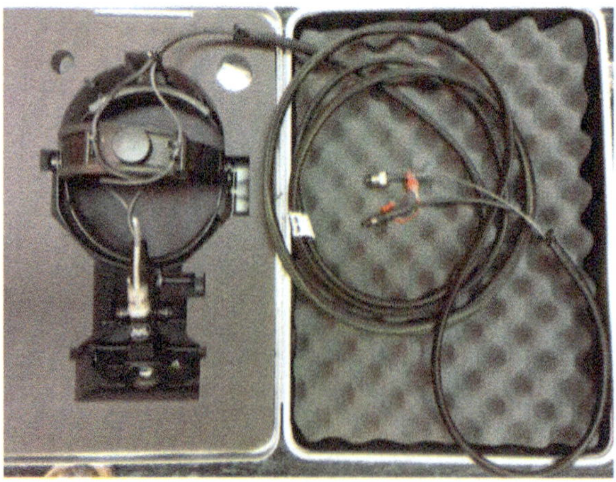

Fig. 11.2 A binocular indirect laser ophthalmoscope (LIO) (Iridex, Iridex). The two cables are attached to the laser device (Fig. 11.1)

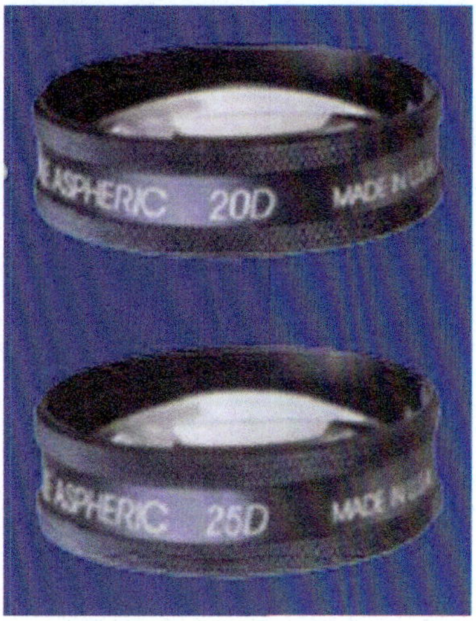

Fig. 11.3 20D and 25D lens from Volk. Both lenses are suitable for laser. We use preferably the 25D lens

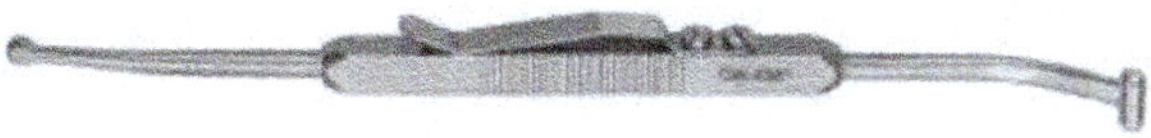

Fig. 11.4 Sclera depressor with small and large indentor (Geuder, Germany)

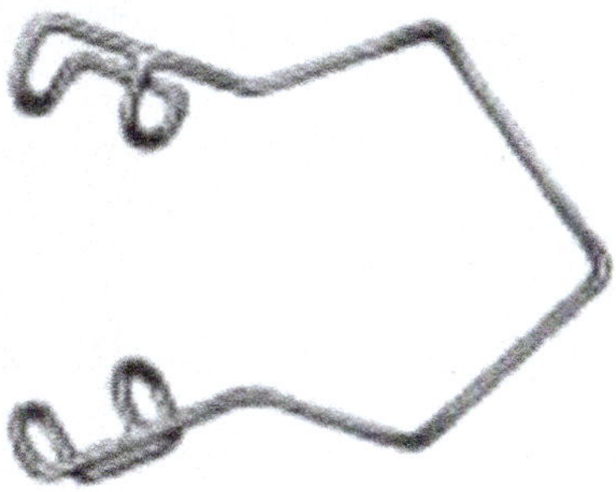

Fig. 11.5 Lid speculum for ROP newborns (Geuder No. 17023, Germany)

Volk 25D lens (Fig. 11.3) We use usually the 25D lens from Volk. An alternative is the 20D lens which is better for the ridge but not so good for ora serrata. Another alternative is the 30D lens which may give a too small image.

Scleral depressor (Fig. 11.4) A scleral depressor is very important for laser coagulation. You can only reach the ora serrata with a scleral depressor. If possible, we laser with the big indentor because it enables treating more tissue at once. At the ora serrata we prefer the small indentor. Alternatively, you can use a cotton wool swab or a strabismus hook.

Lid speculum (Fig. 11.5) We recommend a small lid speculum for newborns.

The laser treatment of newborn with ROP is very different because the eyes are very small and because the pathology is located in the periphery of the eye. If you laser treat the temporal periphery and the central ridge it is best to laser in a standing position (Fig. 11.6). If you laser treat the nasal, superior and inferior retina you may need to laser in a sitting position (Fig. 11.7).

We use usually a diode laser. Alternatively, you can use an Argon laser. The *normal amount* of laser effects is 1200–1800 laser spots (minimum: 1000 laser spots, maximum: 2500 laser spots).

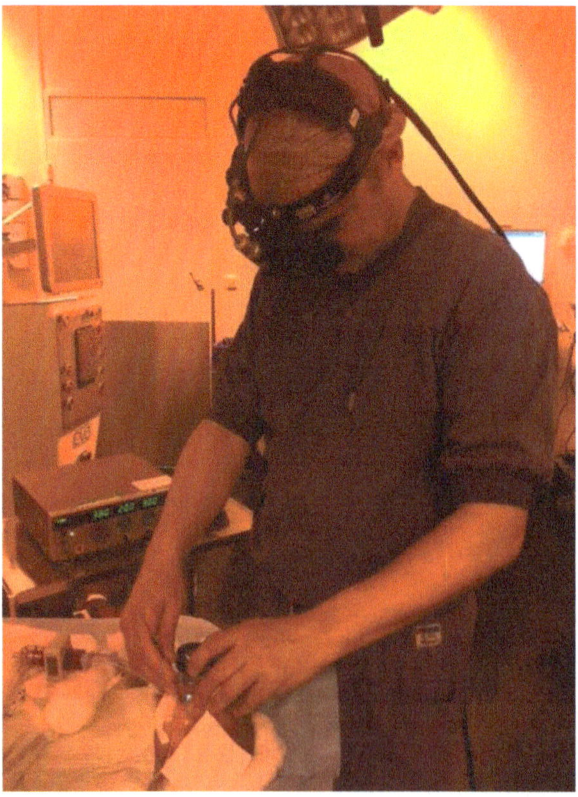

Fig. 11.6 A standing position is fine for the temporal ischemic retina. Note the sclera depressor

The normal settings for a diode laser are: 500 m (power), 200 ms (duration) and 300 ms (interval) (Fig. 11.8).

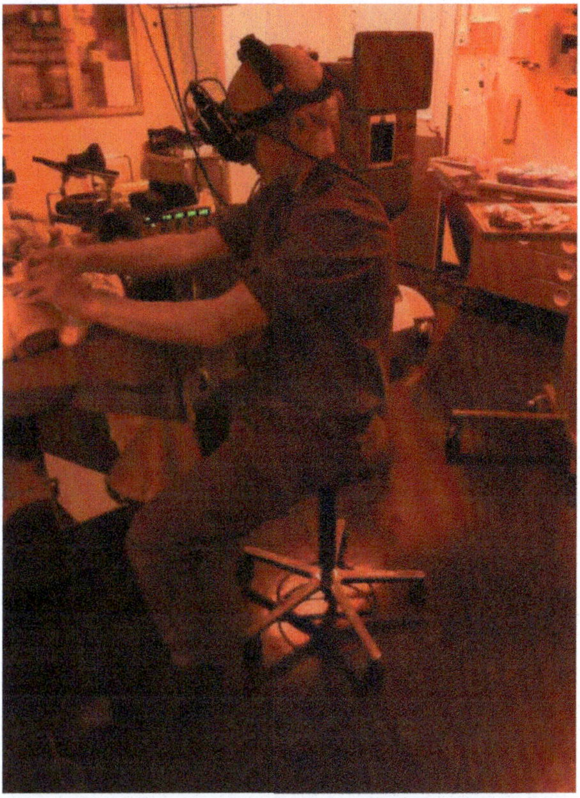

Fig. 11.7 A sitting position is sometimes required to reach the nasal, superior and inferior ischemic retina

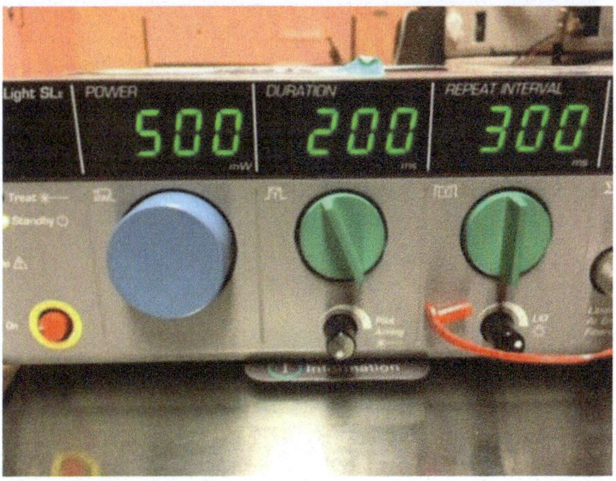

Fig. 11.8 A diode laser (Iridex, CA). Normal laser settings for laser coagulation of a ROP newborn

11.2 Laser Treatment Step-by-Step (Figs. 11.9, 11.10, 11.11, 11.12, 11.13, 11.14, 11.14, 11.15, 11.16, 11.17, 11.18, and 11.19)

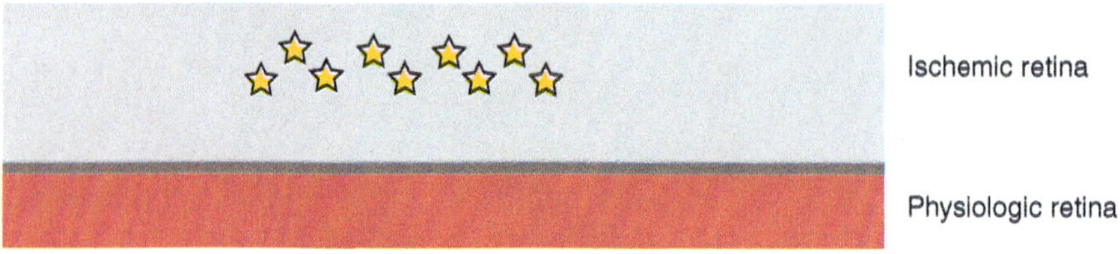

Fig. 11.9 Start at the temporal quadrant and find the appropriate laser settings

Fig. 11.10 Laser photocoagulation of the temporal pole from ora serrata almost to the ridge

Fig. 11.11 Avoid overtreatment when moving from temporal to inferior and superior retina

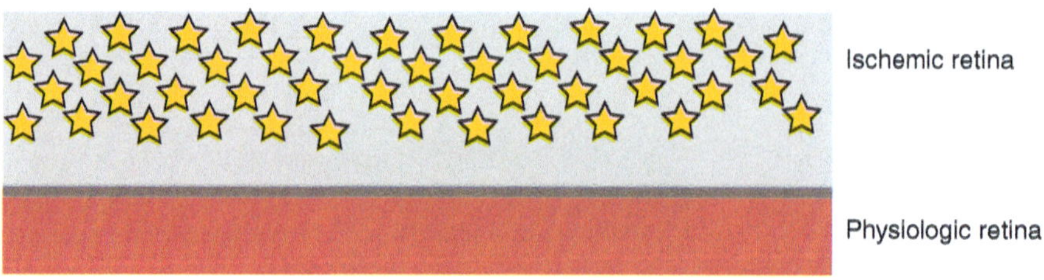

Fig. 11.12 Treat from the ora serrata until close to the ridge

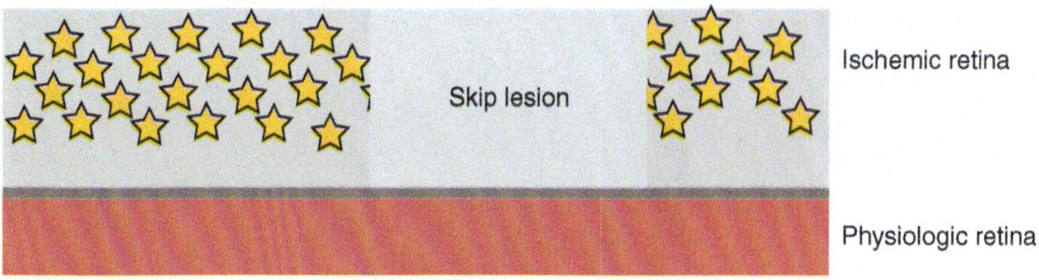

Fig. 11.13 When moving from one treated area to the next avoid creating a skip lesion

Fig. 11.14 Now treat the ridge. Increase power and work without scleral depressor

Fig. 11.15 For peripheral laser coagulation use the scleral depressor to indent the ora serrata

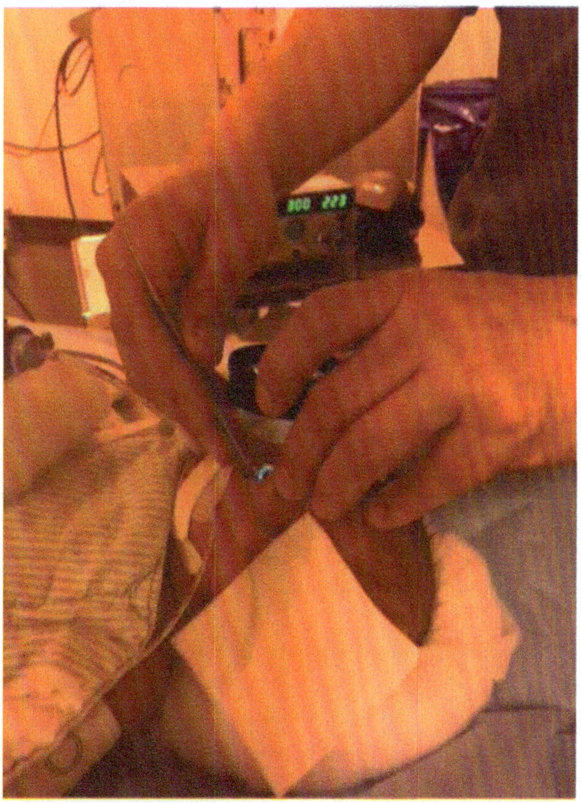

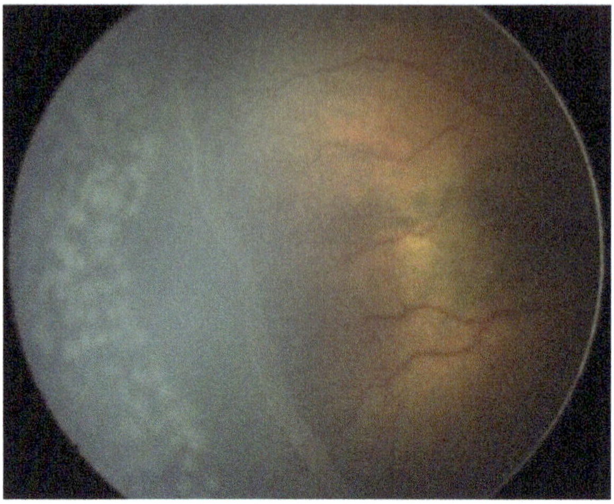

Fig. 11.16 Laser treat from the ora serrata almost to the ridge

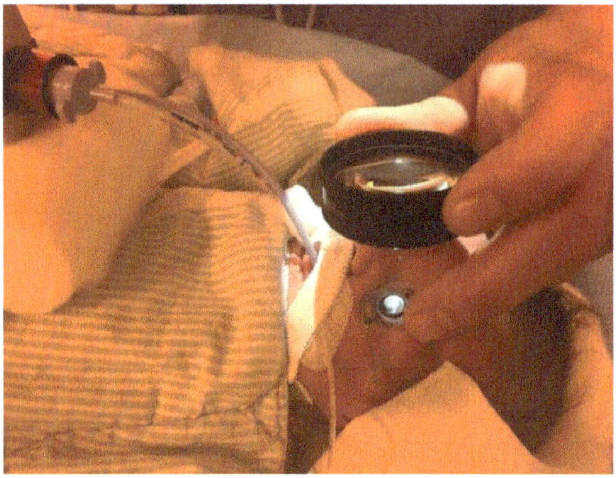

Fig. 11.17 For central laser treatment of the ridge work without scleral depressor

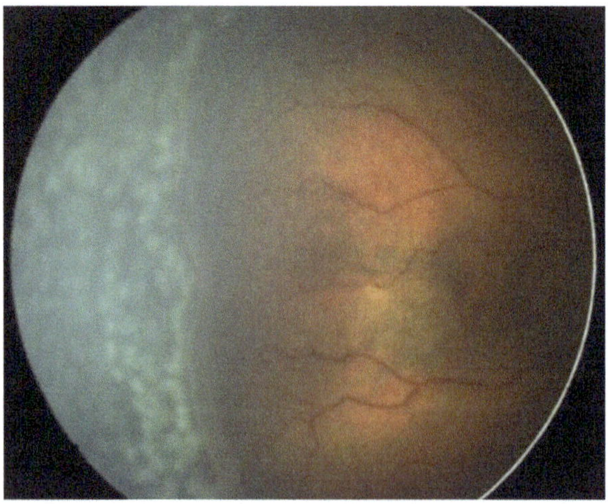

Fig. 11.18 Laser treat the ridge. Usually a higher laser power is required

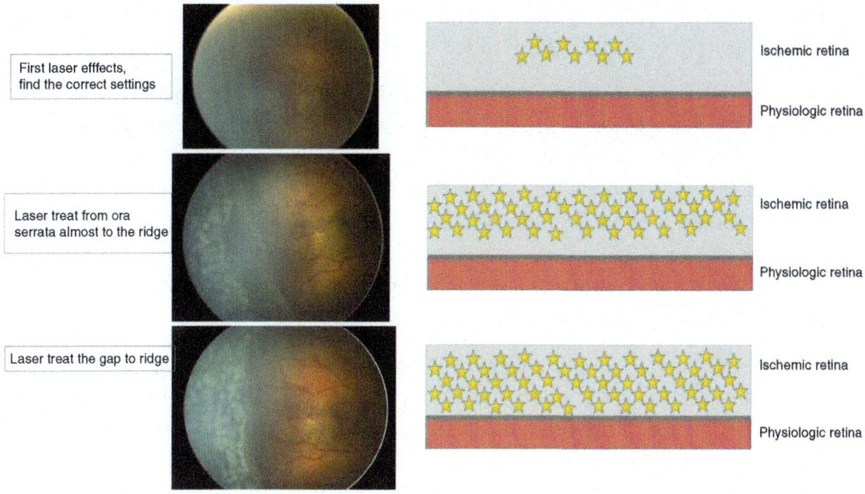

Fig. 11.19 A brief overview of the laser coagulation of ROP newborn

1. **Start with the temporal retina. Find the correct laser power.**
2. **Laser treat the temporal retina from ora serrata almost to the ridge**
3. **Laser treat the superior, nasal and inferior retina.**
4. **Treat the ridge.**
5. **Inspect the retina for skip lesions and incomplete laser.**

The surgery in detail:

1. **Start with the temporal retina. Find the correct laser power** (Figs. 11.5, 11.15, and 11.16)

The pupil must be well dilated, a small pupil is not sufficient for laser photocoagulation. See chapter pupil dilatation.

Laser coagulation of the newborns eye is best performed in two 360° rounds. The first round treats the ischemic retina from the ora serrata almost to the ridge. In the second round the ridge is laser treated.

We start always with the temporal retina. Why? The temporal retina has the biggest ischemic area. Therefore, the visualization of the temporal ischemic retina is the best of all quadrants and the ridge is well visible.

Indent the retina with the broad side of the sclera depressor and place a few laser spots on the indented retina (Fig. 11.9). If you do not see a laser effect, then increase **power** to 200 ms and try again. If you see no laser effect increase power to 300 ms and continue like this until you reach 1000 ms. If you still do not see a laser effect, then increase **duration** to 200 ms and reduce power to 100 ms. Then increase power again in 100 ms steps to 1000 ms.

You should achieve a laser effect with approximately 300–600 ms power and 200 ms duration. A laser duration of 300 ms is too high and never necessary in our experience. A normal laser setting with our (old) laser device (Iridex, CA) is power: 400–700 ms, duration: 200 ms and interval: 300 ms.

If the retina bleaches very much or you see a burst in the retina with a bleeding, then the laser power is too high. Reduce power by 100 ms and try again.

Important If you laser the eye with too high laser energy it may happen that within 1 week the ROP progresses so much that the "eye tilts". Too aggressive laser coagulation aggravates the intraocular VEGF expression. This may happen if you use a duration of 300 ms for laser. Use a maximal duration of 200 ms. Otherwise, a rubeotic iris and finally a retinal detachment develops.

2. **Laser treat the temporal retina from ora serrata almost to the ridge** (Figs. 11.10, 11.11, and 11.16)

If you achieve laser spots on the retina then the first difficult step is achieved. Continue now with laser coagulation of the temporal ischemic retina. Treat with a density of a distance of maximal one laser spot between two spots (Fig. 11.10). Use the scleral depressor to reach the ora serrata (Figs. 11.15 and 11.16). Do not treat the ridge yet.

By moving the 25D or 20D lens forwards or backwards you can increase or decrease the size of the laser spots. Large laser spots save time. Large laser spots are advisable for the periphery and small laser spots for the ridge.

3. **Laser treat the superior, nasal and inferior retina** (Figs. 11.12, 11.13, and 11.14)

If you continue from the temporal to the superior or inferior retina be aware that the size of ischemic retina reduces very much. The ischemic retina becomes a thin strip inferior and superior and a bit broader nasally. This circumstance may easily lead to overtreatment into the physiologic retina (Fig. 11.11).

If you treat the inferior, superior and nasal retina it is easier to start with the small indentor of the scleral depressor. Place the scleral depressor at the limbus and move it slowly towards the equator. As soon as you see the ora serrata, start with laser treatment. Continue with laser treatment almost to the ridge (Fig. 11.12).

If you are done with one area, then place the depressor again at the limbus and continue with the next area. But do not lose contact to the old treatment area in order to prevent a skip lesion (Fig. 11.13). The inferior and superior retina is difficult to assess. You often have to move like a monkey to find a suitable position for laser coagulation. Remember that the ischemic retina decreases substantially in size outside the temporal pole. It is a thin strip of ischemic retina.

4. **Treat the ridge** (Figs. 11.14, 11.17, 11.18)

In the second round you treat the ridge (Fig. 11.14). The lasercoagulation is easier without scleral depressor. Here you need an increased laser power because the retina is thicker. You need approximately 200 ms extra power. The duration remains unchanged at 200 ms.

5. **Inspect the retina for skip lesions and incomplete laser**

If you have completed laser, double check that the complete retina 360° from the ora serrata to the ridge is treated. You can do this with:

1. 25D Volk lens
2. Retcam

Look for untreated areas, examine the retina up to the ora serrata and ascertain yourself that the complete ridge is treated. Do not close the case before you are really certain that you treated the complete ischemic retina because undertreatment may result in a progression of the disease and finally end in a retinal detachment.

Pits & Pearls
Visualization of the ischemic retina is difficult: The ischemic retina is a thin strip superior and inferior, a broader strip nasal and a broad tongue temporal. The ischemic retina is grey and has no vessels. The demarcation line is the border between ischemic and physiologic retina. The physiologic retina is light red and has vessels.

Follow-up We prescribe the eye drops Dexamethasone 1 mg/ml 2xd and Atropine 0.1% 2x/d for 2 weeks. The eyes require a weekly follow-up. On the first follow-up the retinopathy should be stable or less but not worse. If the retinopathy is worse, then perform a thorough examination in order to exclude an undertreatment. If you do not find an undertreatment then examine the newborn again after 3 days. If the retinopathy has worsened, we recommend an immediate examination in general anaesthesia to exclude skip lesions. We recommend also an immediate anti-VEGF injection.

On the second week follow-up, the retinopathy should have further regressed. After 4 weeks laser scars have formed, and the retinopathy has resolved.

11.3 In Conclusion

Laser coagulation of a newborn is technically a very difficult procedure which requires much training. See Fig. 11.19. An optimal laser coagulation within ONE session is however required to achieve a regression of the retinopathy. An undertreatment results within a few weeks in progression of the retinopathy.

If a progression occurs, we recommend an immediate intravitreal anti-VEGF injection.

References

1. Holmström G, Tornqvist K, Al-Hawasi A, Nilsson Å, Wallin A, Hellström A. Increased frequency of retinopathy of prematurity over the last decade and significant regional differences. Acta Ophthalmol. 2018;96(2):142–8.
2. Repka MX, Tung B, Good WV, Capone A Jr, Shapiro MJ. Outcome of eyes developing retinal detachment during the Early Treatment for Retinopathy of Prematurity study. Arch Ophthalmol. 2011;129(9):1175–9.

Chapter 12
Angiography Assisted Laser Photocoagulation for Newborn and Children

Laser photocoagulation of a ROP newborn may be difficult due to poor visualization. Especially the border between physiologic and ischemic retina is sometimes difficult to determine.

In other pediatric retinal diseases such as familial exudative vitreoretinopathy (FEVR) or incontinentia pigmenti (IP) the border between ischemic and physiologic retina cannot be discerned with ophthalmoscopy. Only angiography can tell us where exactly the border between physiologic and ischemic retina is localized. In these cases, an angiography is required before laser coagulation.

We developed therefore an angiography assisted laser photocoagulation (Fig. 12.1). Within one session, several laser coagulations and Retcam angiographies are performed until the complete ischemic retina is laser treated.

12.1 The Technique Step-by-Step (Fig. 12.1)

1. Fluorescein is injected, and the first angiography is performed. The border between physiologic and ischemic retina is determined (Figs. 12.1 and 12.2).
2. The first laser photocoagulation is performed.
3. No fluorescein is reinjected. The second first angiography is performed. The skip lesions are determined.
4. A second laser photocoagulation is performed.
5. No fluorescein is reinjected. The third angiography is performed. The skip lesions are determined.
6. A third laser photocoagulation is performed.
7. No fluorescein is reinjected. The fourth angiography is performed. Now, laser coagulation is usually completed (Fig. 12.3).

We demonstrate the technique with a case report. A full-term newborn with incontinentia pigmenti was laser treated before due to a peripheral ischemia. In this

U. Spandau, S. J. Kim, *Pediatric Retinal Vascular Diseases*,
https://doi.org/10.1007/978-3-030-13701-4_12

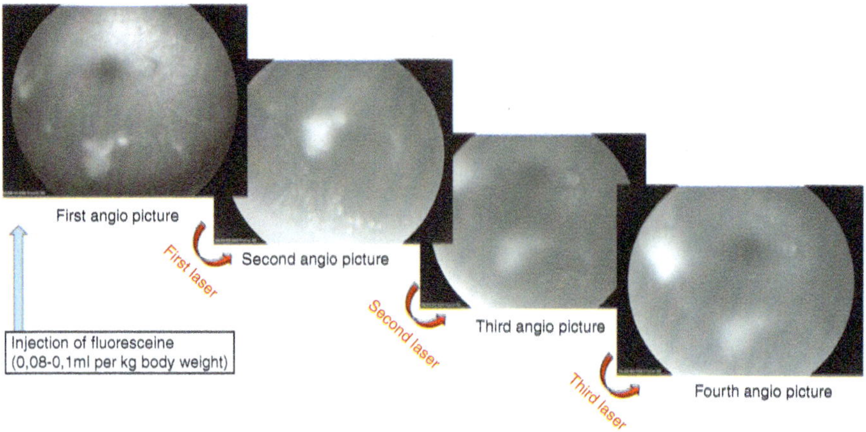

Fig. 12.1 Fluorescein is injected once. After the first angiography pictures a laser photocoagulation is performed. Then the second angiography picture is taken and so on

Fig. 12.2 First angiography: Note the inferior ischemia

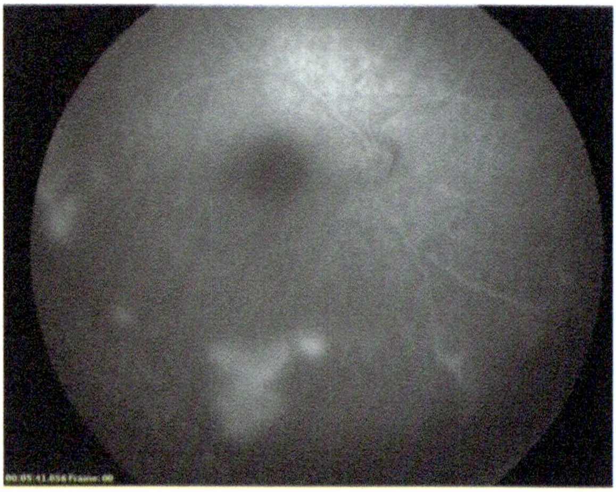

Fig. 12.3 Last angiography: After 3 laser photocoagulations the inferior ischemia is filled up with laser

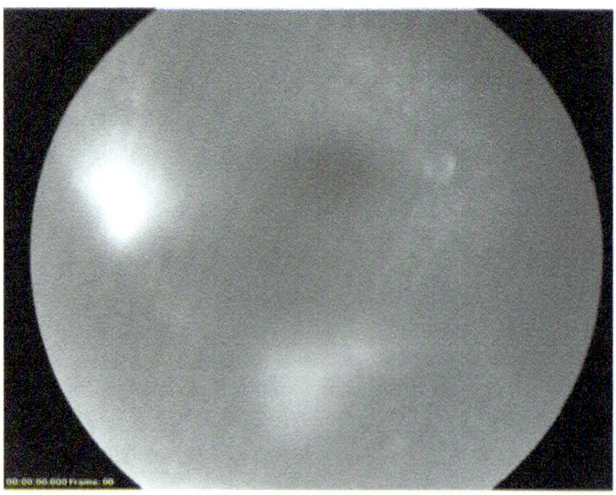

session the old laser coagulation is assessed with angiography and an additional laser coagulation planned if necessary. The Retcam angiography shows a residual ischemia which has not yet been laser treated (Fig. 12.4). A laser photocoagulation with binocular ophthalmoscope is performed. Then a second angiography is performed. A small residual ischemia is still visible (Fig. 12.5). Two additional rows of laser are added. The ischemia is now filled up with laser (Fig. 12.6).

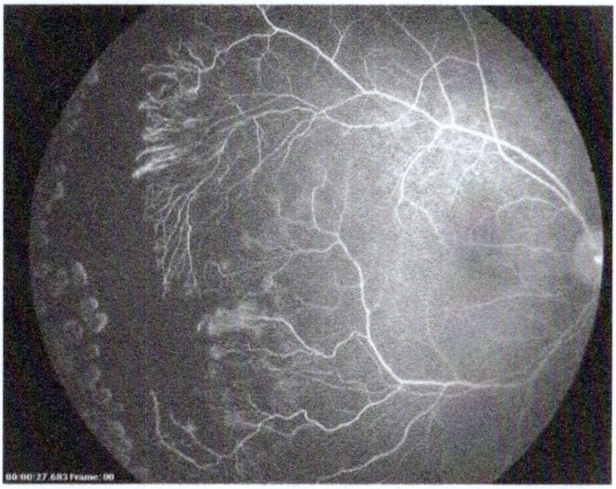

Fig. 12.4 The first angiography. A newborn with Incontinentia pigmenti. Note the irregular vascular sprouting, vascular pruning and the ischemic retina. In the periphery old laser effects are visible

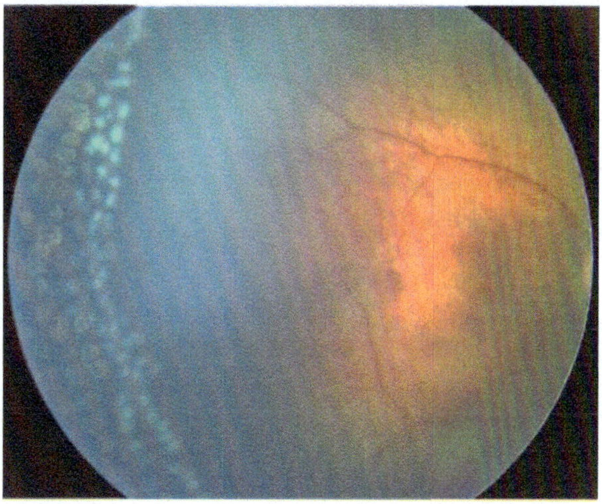

Fig. 12.5 New laser effects have been added. A visualization of the ischemic retina is not possible

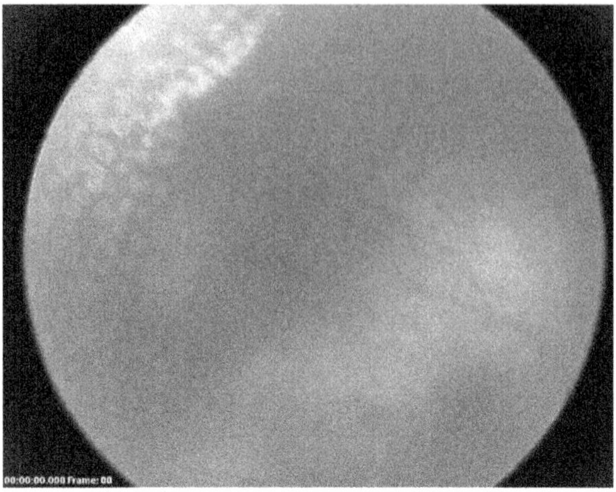

Fig. 12.6 The third angiography. Note the old and fresh laser effects

Chapter 13
Inadequate Laser Coagulation

A laser treatment in zone II has a 90% success rate. In our experience, a clinical center for ROP treatment has a 100% success rate for laser coagulation. We had no recurrence after laser coagulation since 10 years. This is only true for zone II. This is not true for zone I because this very aggressive retinopathy may progress even if the retina is 100% treated. For more details see chapter "**Recurrence of ROP after laser coagulation in zone I**".

Coming back to zone II laser treatment: In our experience a complete laser coagulation in zone II leads to a regression of the retinopathy. But if a progression occurs, then it is most likely caused by an incomplete laser treatment. We will show colour and angiography pictures proving this notion. All these eyes progressed to a retinal detachment.

It is therefore essential to perform a complete laser coagulation from the beginning OR to initiate a second laser treatment as soon as possible.

13.1 Case Series Report

Case 1 (Figs. 13.1, 13.2, 13.3, 13.4, and 13.5) A premature neonate developed ROP 3+ in zone II in a hospital elsewhere. Laser photocoagulation was performed. The retinopathy did not regress and 3 weeks later the neonate was referred to us for examination and additional treatment.

An examination with Retcam showed an under-treated ischemic retina and an over-treated physiologic retina (Figs. 13.1 and 13.2). The Retcam angiography confirms the under-treatment because it visualizes the ischemic retina very well (Figs. 13.3 and 13.4). A strong leakage from the retinal proliferations at the ridge corresponds to the ischemic retina. In addition, an overtreatment can be observed on the temporal side from 4–5 o'clock (Figs. 13.3 and 13.4) and on the nasal side (Fig. 13.5). Remark: A mild overtreatment as shown is this case has no negative effect.

U. Spandau, S. J. Kim, *Pediatric Retinal Vascular Diseases*,
https://doi.org/10.1007/978-3-030-13701-4_13

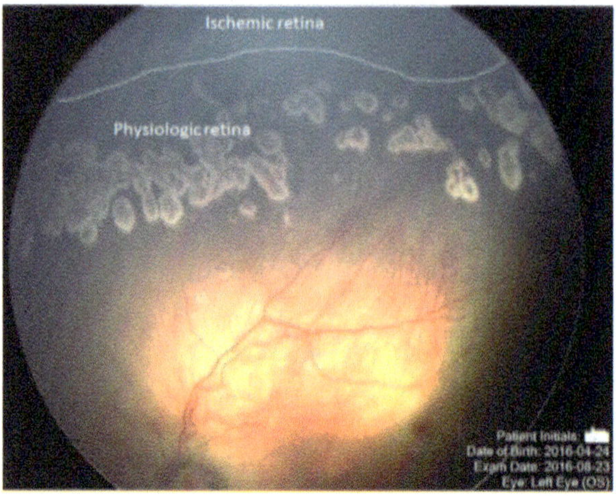

Fig. 13.1 Undertreated ischemic retina and over treated physiologic retina

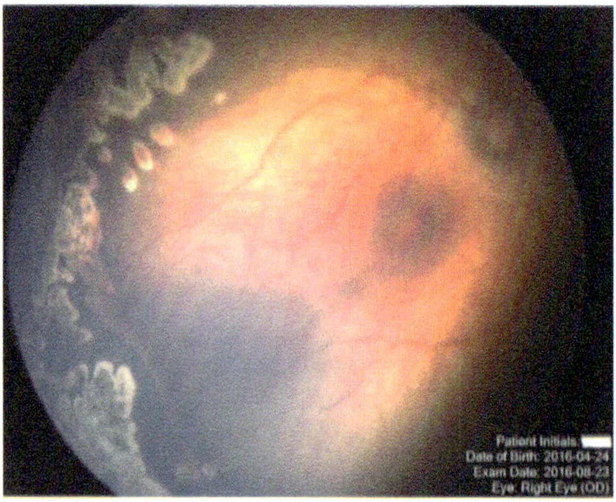

Fig. 13.2 The undertreated ischemic retina can be seen on the temporal ridge

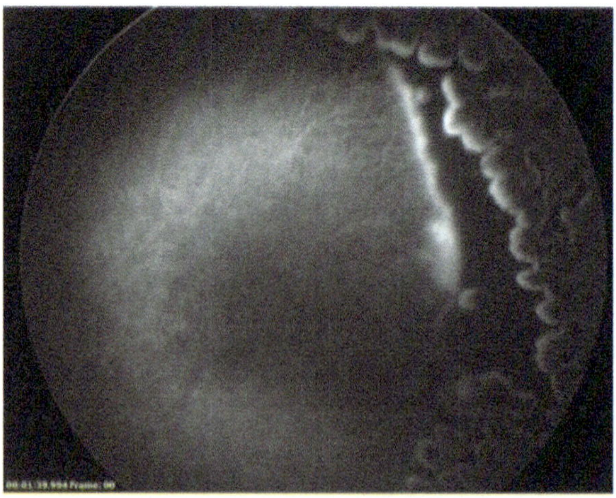

Fig. 13.3 The angiography reveals not treated ischemic retina and the proliferations at the ridge

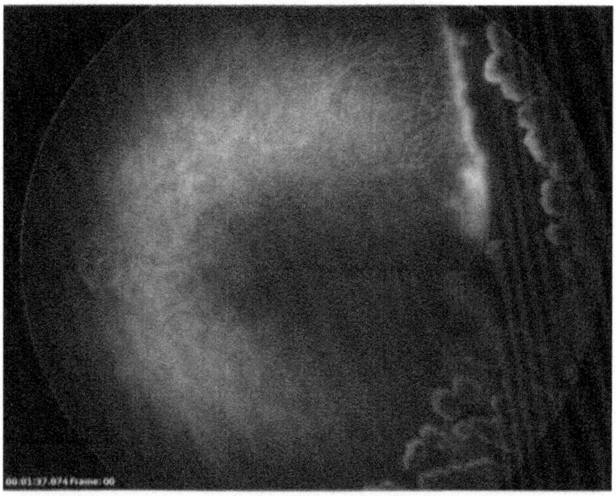

Fig. 13.4 Observe also the overtreatment at 4–5 o'clock

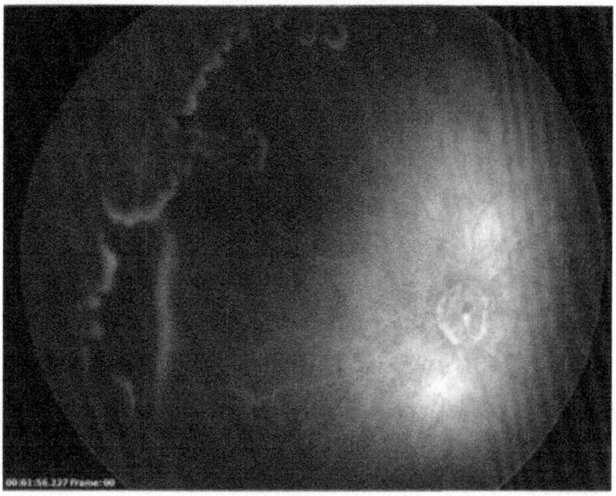

Fig. 13.5 An untreated ischemic retina on the nasal side. Observe also the overtreatment from 9 to 11 o'clock

Case 2 This newborn was diagnosed for ROP 3+ at a hospital elsewhere (Figs. 13.6 and 13.7). A laser photocoagulation was performed. The retinopathy progressed and 8 days later intravitreal Lucentis was injected. The retinopathy progressed to stage 4A and a cerclage was placed. The retinopathy persisted and the newborn was referred to us. An examination with Retcam angiography revealed a big skip lesion on the temporal side and many subretinal exudates in the periphery. We performed a lens sparing vitrectomy and laser coagulation. The retinopathy regressed, and the retina reattached.

Conclusion An incomplete laser treatment may lead to a progression of the retinopathy and is the most common cause for failure of laser treatment. An undertreatment must be detected as early as possible and be counter treated as fast as possible. Perform weekly follow-ups after laser treatment. If the retinopathy worsens within

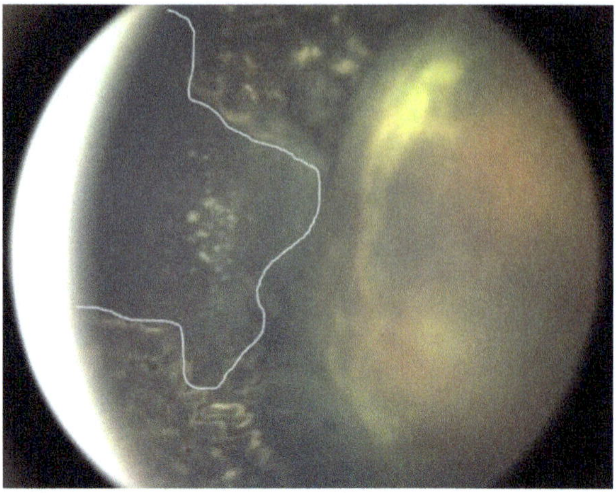

Fig. 13.6 A big skip lesion is present in otherwise well treated retina. Note also the exudates

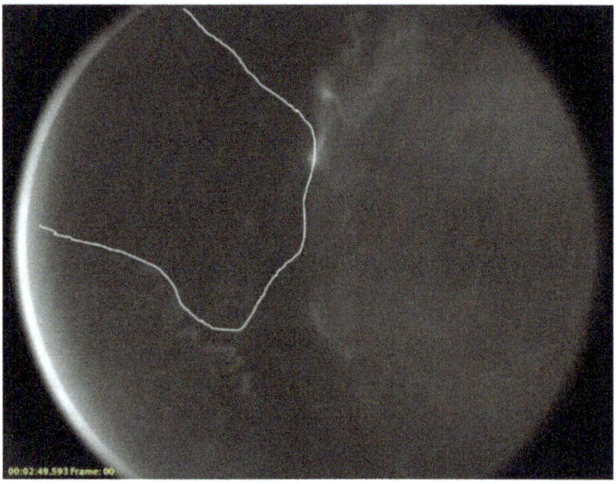

Fig. 13.7 The angiography shows clearly the untreated ischemic retina

2 weeks after laser coagulation, schedule immediately a laser retreatment through an experienced surgeon or perform an anti-VEGF injection. In contrast, a mild overtreatment with laser has no negative effect on the retinopathy. If the retinopathy progresses and you do not find skip lesions then we recommend placing two rows of laser spots in the physiologic retina (posterior to the ridge).

Remark If you are not experienced with indirect laser coagulation then do always combined treatments: Laser coagulation and anti-VEGF in the same sitting.

Part V
Anti-VEGF Injection

Chapter 14
Size of a Newborn Eye

More and more clinics use intravitreal anti-VEGF for the treatment of retinopathy of prematurity (ROP). There are many concerns regarding the possible ocular and systemic side effects of this medication. In the BEAT-ROP study, a dosage of 0.625 mg was recommended, but a rationale for this dosage was not given [7].

In case of a bilateral injection of 0.65 mg Avastin, a newborn with a weight of 1.5 kg receives the same dose as an adult person with a weight of 75 kg after one unilateral injection. It is known, that one unilateral bevacizumab injection in an adult can suppress systemic VEGF levels for several weeks [6].

What is the advantage of a lower dose of anti-VEGF medication? A lower dose of bevacizumab might decrease the risk of possible ocular and systemic side effects of anti-VEGF therapy.

What are the *systemic* side effects? Anti-VEGF enters the blood stream and may influence the vascular development of lungs, kidneys and brain.

What are the *ocular* side effects? If you inject anti-VEGF in a newborn with ROP then you achieve two pathophysiologic effects:

1. Reduction of *pathologic* neovascularization
2. Reduction of *physiologic* vascularization of the peripheral retina

It is therefore important that the dose of the anti-VEGF medication is *so high* that the pathologic proliferations disappear and *so low* that the physiologic vascularization is not inhibited [10].

To find a rationale for an optimal dosage for intravitreal injection of bevacizumab in ROP neonate, we performed two calculations of the size of the newborn eye.

First calculation The axial length of a neonate with a gestational age of 34 weeks is 16 mm [1]. Using the formula 4/3*p*r3, the result is that the neonates eye is 3.12 times smaller than the adults eye.

U. Spandau, S. J. Kim, *Pediatric Retinal Vascular Diseases*,
https://doi.org/10.1007/978-3-030-13701-4_14

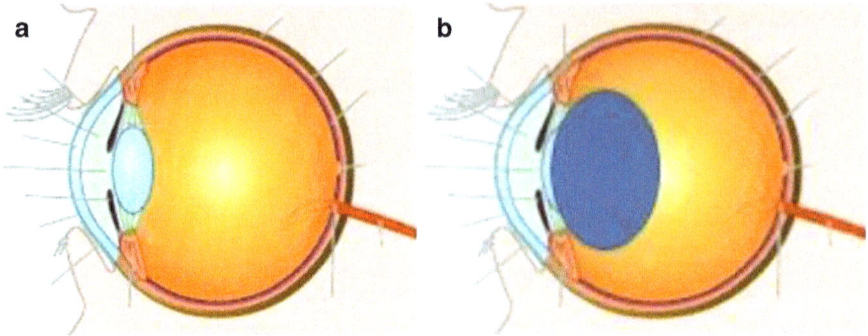

Fig. 14.1 (**a**) Adult's eye with an axial length of 23.5 mm and a volume of 5.4 ml. (**b**) Neonate's eye with an axial length of 16 mm and a volume of 1.7 ml

Second calculation The length of the vitreous of a newborn is 10.48 mm, and the length of the vitreous of an adult is 15.0 mm [4].

Using the same formula, the neonate eye is calculated to be 2.91 times smaller than the adult's eye.

Taken both calculations together, the neonate's eye is approximately three times smaller than the adult's eye (Fig. 14.1). The volume of the neonate's vitreous may be even smaller than calculated because of the big size of the neonate's lens.

New calculated dose The usual bevacizumab dosage of an adult is 1.25 mg. The recommended dosage for ROP newborn is 0.625 mg [7]. According to our calculations, however, the size-adjusted dosage of a neonate should be not higher than 1.25 mg/3 = 0.4 mg.

This rationale is confirmed by studies which demonstrate that a dosage of 0.312 mg showed good anatomical and functional results in ROP neonates [2, 5, 9].

Recent studies demonstrated that an ultra-low dose of 0.031 mg Avastin is effective to treat ROP plus disease [3, 8, 10]. This dose corresponds to 5% of the normal dose. The regress of the retinopathy is slower, but the vascularization of the immature retina is faster.

The practical disadvantage of the small doses is that they have to be diluted, in contrast to the 0.625 mg dose that requires no dilution. This problem can be solved, if the hospital pharmacy prepares the medication with the required dose.

Conclusion Recent studies indicate that a much lower dosage than recommended in the BEAT-ROP study may be sufficient to treat ROP. The following chapter will introduce these dosage dependency studies demonstrating that a much lower dose of bevacizumab and ranibizumab is sufficient to treat ROP.

References

1. Ehlers N, Mathiesen ME, Andersen H. The prenatal growth of the human eye. Acta Ophthalmol (Kbh). 1968;46:329–49.
2. Harder BC, Baltz SV, Jonas JB, Schlichtenbrede FC. Intravitreal bevacizumab for retinopathy of prematurity. J Ocul Pharmacol Ther. 2011;27:623–7.
3. Hillier RJ, Connor AJ, Shafiq AE. Ultra-low-dose intravitreal bevacizumab for the treatment of retinopathy of prematurity: a case series. Br J Ophthalmol. 2018;102(2):260–4. https://doi.org/10.1136/bjophthalmol-2017-310408. Epub 2017 June 27
4. Larsen JS. The sagittal growth of the eye. Acta Ophthalmol. 1971;49:441–4.
5. Lorenz B. Kommentar: anti-VEGF-Einsatz gut abwägen. Klin Monatsbl Augenheilkd. 2011;225:488–90.
6. Matsuyama K, Ogata N, Matsuoka M, Takahashi K, Nishimura T. Plasma levels of vascular endothelial growth factor and pigment epithelium-derived factor before and after intravitreal injection of bevacizumab. Br J Ophthalmol. 2010;94(9):1215–8.
7. Mintz-Hittner HA, Kennedy KA, Chuang AZ, BEAT-ROP Cooperative Group. Efficacy of intravitreal bevacizumab for salyage 3+ retinopathy of prematurity. N Engl J Med. 2011;364:603–15.
8. Şahin A, Gürsel-Özkurt Z, Şahin M, Türkcü FM, Yıldırım A, Yüksel H. Ultra-low dose of intravitreal bevacizumab in retinopathy of prematurity. Ir J Med Sci. 2018;187:417–21.
9. Spandau U. What is the optimal dosage for intravitreal bevacizumab for retinopathy of prematurity? Acta Ophthalmol. 2013;91(2):e154.
10. Wallace DK, Kraker RT, Freedman SF, Crouch ER, Hutchinson AK, Bhatt AR, Rogers DL, Yang MB, Haider KM, VanderVeen DK, Siatkowski RM, Dean TW, Beck RW, Repka MX, Smith LE, Good WV, Hartnett ME, Kong L, Holmes JM, Pediatric Eye Disease Investigator Group (PEDIG). Assessment of lower doses of intravitreous bevacizumab for retinopathy of prematurity: a phase 1 dosing study. JAMA Ophthalmol. 2017;135:654–6.

Chapter 15
Dose of Anti-VEGF Injection in Infants

Although anti-VEGF agents such as bevacizumab have been widely used for the treatment of ROP throughout the world, there has been few dose-response relationship studies in ROP. In initial period of bevacizumab use in ROP, a half of adult dose was the most commonly used as in the BEAT-ROP study (0.625 mg in 0.025 ml of solution) [1]. Recently, there are growing number of studies on use of lower dose of bevacizumab.

15.1 Comparison of Intraocular Volume Between Infant Versus Adult Eyes

If we assume that eyeball is a ball filled with vitreous fluid, the volume will be 4/3 × π × (axial length/2). Previous studies on axial length of premature infants showed that the axial length ranges from 15 to 17 mm at the PMA of 32 to 40 weeks [2]. Therefore, compared to average adult eyes (the axial length is about 23 mm), the intraocular volume of infant eyes may range from 27% to 40% of adult eyes (Table 15.1). In other words, the maximal concentration of an injected agent in infant eyes will be 2.5–3.6 folds of that in adult eyes. Thus, theoretically, the injection dose should be about 1/3–1/4 of adult dose. Moreover, if your goal of anti-VEGF injection for ROP is not a long-term suppression of VEGF as a monotherapy and you prefer adding laser treatment after some time, lower dose can be tried.

U. Spandau, S. J. Kim, *Pediatric Retinal Vascular Diseases*,
https://doi.org/10.1007/978-3-030-13701-4_15

Table 15.1 Estimated vitreous volume and maximum intravitreal concentration in infant eyes compared to those of adult eyes

Axial length (mm)	Volume	% adult vol.	Maximal concentration after injecting 0.625 mg of bevacizumab (mg/ml)	x adult conc.
15	1.77	27.7	0.35	3.6
16	2.14	33.7	0.29	3.0
17	2.57	40.4	0.24	2.5
23	6.37	100	0.10	1.0

15.2 Dose of Intravitreal Bevacizumab (Avastin) for ROP

15.2.1 Dose of Bevacizumab in Case Series Studies

In the BEAT-ROP study, a prospective randomized study comparing laser versus bevacizumab in stage 3+ ROP and in many other studies, 0.625 mg of bevacizumab in 0.025 ml solution was intravitreally administered [1]. Recent studies have reported the outcome of lower dose of bevacizumab. In Kim et al., study in 2014 [3] and Yoon et al. study in 2016 [4] in South Korea, 0.25 mg (1/5 of adult dose for AMD) of bevacizumab was effective as a combined therapy with laser treatment for zone I+ ROP. Hiller et al. study in United Kingdom in 2018 retrospectively reviewed outcome of 0.16 mg (about 1/8 of adult dose for age-related macular degeneration) in 29 eyes of 15 patients with treatment-requiring ROP [5]. The 'treatment success' was defined as complete regression of retinopathy and vascularisation into (or laser ablation of) zone 3. Primary success (in response to IVB 0.16 mg alone) was observed in 79.3% and secondary success (where additional treatment was required) was observed in 93.1%. Retreatment was done in **Recurrence of ROP** 6/29 eyes (20.6%).

It should be noted that the definition of treatment success and recurrence of ROP after injection is not consistent among the studies. So, comparison between studies is not straightforward.

15.2.2 Results of a Phase 1 Dosing Study by Pediatric Eye Disease Investigator Group (PEDIG)

Recently, the short-term results of a dosing study of intravitreal bevacizumab in ROP by Pediatric Eye Disease Investigator Group (PEDIG) were published [6, 7]. This study enrolled preterm infants with treatment-requiring ROP (type 1 ROP) in 1 or both eyes and no previous treatment. In this study, an intravitreal injection of bevacizumab in 10 μL was given to the study eye using a 300-μL syringe (Fig. 15.1) with a 5/16-inch, 30-gauge fixed needle.

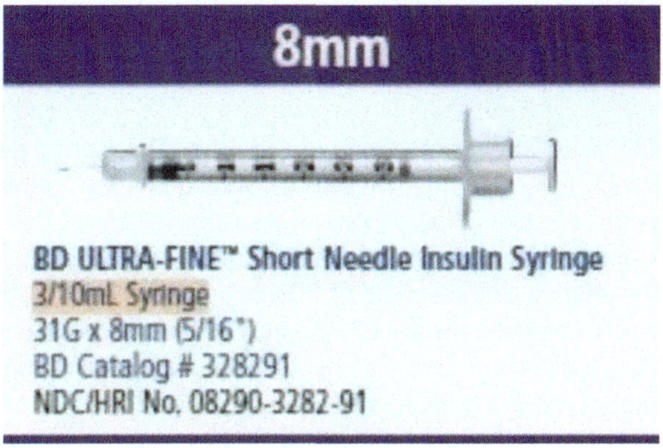

Fig. 15.1 0.3 ml insulin syringe with an 8 mm needle. The 8 mm needle is safer for the short eyes of neonates. (BD USA, Photocourtesy BD)

The primary outcome measure was "successful treatment of ROP" defined as improvement by 4 days or sooner and no recurrence of type 1 ROP or severe neovascularization requiring additional treatment within 4 weeks. For infants with plus disease, improvement by the 4-day post-injection exam is defined as plus disease no longer being present. For infants with type 1 ROP without plus disease (i.e., zone I, stage 3), improvement by the 4-day post-injection exam is defined as: (1) a significant reduction in severity and/or extent of extraretinal neovascularization, and, (2) if pre-plus was present pre-injection, reduction in the degree of abnormal vascular dilation and/or tortuosity.

A dose was considered effective if it successfully treated at least 80% of subjects. An independent committee reviewed the outcomes and determined the next bevacizumab dose to test in 10–14 infants based on the success proportion: dose reduced for 80% or greater success, dose repeated for 70% to less than 80% success, and dose increased, or the study ended for less than 70% success. Three dose reductions were evaluated, with each one-half the previous dose concentration (0.125 mg, 0.063 mg, and 0.031 mg each in 10 μL, diluted with normal saline).

Secondary outcome measures include plasma levels of Avastin and VEGF before injection, and at 2 and 4 weeks post-injection, number of eyes requiring additional treatment/s for ROP, any adverse events or complications, assessment of vision at 12 month corrected age, and so on.

The results of this study showed that success was achieved in 11 of 11 eyes at 0.25 mg, 14 of 14 eyes at 0.125 mg, 21 of 24 eyes at 0.063 mg, and 9 of 9 eyes at 0.031 mg, which is about 5% of the dose used in the BEAT-ROP study and about 1/40 of adult dose for age-related macular degeneration.

Although further long-term investigation is warranted to determine the optimal dose and systemic safety, the short-term results of this study suggest that much lower dose than that commonly used may be effective at least for 4 weeks. If there's a risk for neurodevelopmental disability by intravitreal bevacizumab (so far there are conflicting results on this issue), lower dose may reduce the risk and/or other possible systemic adverse effects.

15.2.3 Practical Problems for Using Lower Dose of Bevacizumab

In PEDIG study, bevacizumab was diluted with normal saline to achieve the dose of 0.125 mg, 0.063 mg, and 0.031 mg each in 10 μL. However, the vehicle of Avastin is not normal saline. A vial of Avastin has 25 mg/ml of bevacizumab in aqueous solution with sodium phosphonate, trehalose dehydrate, and polysorbate. Although the pharmaceutical grade of PBS or solutions having similar components cannot be easily obtained, the use of PBS may be considered instead of normal saline. In addition, the dilution process might increase the risk of contamination. Therefore, dilution of Avastin with normal saline should be tried carefully.

15.3 Dose of Ranibizumab (Lucentis) for ROP

15.3.1 Comparing Alternative Ranibizumab Dosages for Safety and Efficacy in Retinopathy of Prematurity (CARE-ROP) Study [8]

The recent CARE-ROP pilot study in Germany demonstrated that ranibizumab is effective in controlling acute phase ROP and that 24% of the standard adult dose (0.12 mg) appears equally effective as 40% (0.20 mg). In addition, superior vascularization of the peripheral retina with 0.12 mg of ranibizumab indicates that the lower dose may be favorable. Moreover, the VEGF plasma levels were not systematically altered in either group, suggesting that systemic VEGF suppression might be less prevalent after ranibizumab than it is after bevacizumab. In fact, Bakri and colleagues showed that Ranibizumab has a much lower serum half-life than Bevacizumab (20 days versus 2 hours) [9].

Key Points

1. In case of a bilateral Avastin injection with a 0.625 mg dose a neonate with 1–2 kg weight receives the same dose as an adult patient with 60–80 kg weight.
2. The PEDIG study demonstrates that a dose of 0.031 mg is sufficient to treat ROP. This dose is 5% of the adult's dose.
3. An anti-VEGF injection is not user-dependent. A laser treatment, however, is user dependent.
4. Ranibizumab (Lucentis®) does not suppress VEGF levels in the serum (Stahl et al. 2018)
5. The optimal dose is 0.2 μl or even 0.1 μl ranibizumab.

References

1. Mintz-Hittner HA, Kennedy KA, Chuang AZ, BEAT-ROP Cooperative Group. Efficacy of intravitreal bevacizumab for stage 3+ retinopathy of prematurity. N Engl J Med. 2011;364:603–15.
2. Laws DE, Haslett R, Ashby D, O'Brien C, Clark D. Axial length biometry in infants with retinopathy of prematurity. Eye (Lond). 1994;8:427–30.
3. Kim J, Kim SJ, Chang YS, Park WS. Combined intravitreal bevacizumab injection and zone I sparing laser photocoagulation in patients with zone I retinopathy of prematurity. Retina. 2014;34:77–82.
4. Yoon JM, Shin DH, Kim SJ, Ham DI, Kang SW, Chang YS, Park WS. Outcomes after laser versus combined laser and bevacizumab treatment for type 1 retinopathy of prematurity in zone I. Retina. 2017;37:88–96.
5. Hillier RJ, Connor AJ, Shafiq AE. Ultra-low-dose intravitreal bevacizumab for the treatment of retinopathy of prematurity: a case series. Br J Ophthalmol. 2018;102:260–4.
6. Wallace DK, Kraker RT, Freedman SF, Crouch ER, Hutchinson AK, Bhatt AR, Rogers DL, Yang MB, Haider KM, VanderVeen DK, Siatkowski RM, Dean TW, Beck RW, Repka MX, Smith LE, Good WV, Hartnett ME, Kong L, Holmes JM, Pediatric Eye Disease Investigator Group (PEDIG). Assessment of lower doses of intravitreous bevacizumab for retinopathy of prematurity: a phase 1 dosing study. JAMA Ophthalmol. 2017;135:654–6.
7. Wallace DK, Dean TW, Hartnett ME, Kong L, Smith LE, Hubbard GB, McGregor ML, Jordan CO, Mantagos IS, Bell EF, Kraker RT, Pediatric Eye Disease Investigator Group. A dosing Study of bevacizumab for retinopathy of prematurity: late recurrences and additional treatments. Ophthalmology. 2018;125:1961–6. https://doi.org/10.1016/j.ophtha.2018.05.001.
8. Stahl A, Krohne TU, Eter N, Oberacher-Velten I, Guthoff R, Meltendorf S, Ehrt O, Aisenbrey S, Roider J, Gerding H, Jandeck C, Smith LEH, Walz JM, Comparing Alternative Ranibizumab Dosages for Safety and Efficacy in Retinopathy of Prematurity (CARE-ROP) Study Group. Comparing alternative ranibizumab dosages for safety and efficacy in retinopathy of prematurity: a randomized clinical trial. JAMA Pediatr. 2018;172:278–86.
9. Bakri SJ, Snyder MR, Reid JM, et al. Pharmacokinetics of intravitreal ranibizumab (Lucentis). Ophthalmology. 2007;114:2179–82.

Chapter 16
Technique of Anti-VEGF Injection

16.1 General Guidelines for Intravitreal Injection

Several points make intravitreal injections of a newborn more difficult than of an adult. (1) The anatomy of the neonate eye. An absent pars plana requires an injection site 1–1.5 mm behind the limbus. The presence of a big lens increases the risk of a lens injury during an intravitreal injection (2) The drug volume is very small. If you inject a small drug volume then the distance the plunger has to travel is short. It is, therefore, difficult to assess whether the medication left the syringe. (3) The latter problem can be solved by using a microscope. You can only verify a successful injection with a surgical microscope. You have a high pressure to succeed with the first injection because a failure will result in a progression of the ROP disease. This pressure does not exist in adult's diseases such as AMD or diabetic macular edema.

16.2 Considerations Before Injection

16.2.1 Clinical Setting

In infants and children, intravitreal injections may be performed in a neonatal intensive care unit (NICU) or in an operating room. In the NICU, injection can be done at the bedside. The *advantages of bedside injections* are: (1) No general anaesthesia is required, (2) The burden for the newborn is very low (3) Less burden for the pediatric ward. The *disadvantages* are: (1) Surgically more difficult, (2) Non-sterile conditions (3) Higher complication risk such as lens injury due to lack of microscope.

Electronic Supplementary Material The online version of this chapter (https://doi.org/10.1007/978-3-030-13701-4_16) contains supplementary material, which is available to authorized users.
The videos can be accessed under http://extras.springer.com/Search. Enter the ISBN number of your book and download the videos.

U. Spandau, S. J. Kim, *Pediatric Retinal Vascular Diseases*,
https://doi.org/10.1007/978-3-030-13701-4_16

The *advantages of an injection in the OR* are: (1) General anaesthesia (2) Excellent sterile conditions (3) Low infection risk (4) Quiet head (5) Use of microscope (6) Reduced complication profile (lens injury) (7) Visualization of medication inside vitreous cavity, the *disadvantages* are: (1) This setup may only be possible in tertiary centers such as University hospitals.

16.2.2 Bilateral Injections

When bilateral intravitreal injections are necessary, the injection for each eye should be performed as a separate procedure, using separate preparation for each eye.

16.2.3 Sedation

Intravitreal injections can be performed on awake infants at the bedside in the NICU. Injections may also be performed on infants with intravenous sedation or general anesthesia. Age, body weight, general conditions, systemic co-morbidities, and accompanying procedures such as retinal imaging using fundus camera and OCT or laser photocoagulation should be considered before deciding the appropriate sedation method. Benefits, risks, and possible complications related to sedation can be discussed with attending pediatricians and informed consent should be obtained from the patient's *parent* or legal *guardian*.

16.2.4 Pre-existing Systemic/Ocular Conditions

Bleeding tendency, ocular hypertension/glaucoma, and active external infection such as viral keratoconjunctivitis should be checked. There are limited studies on the incidence of adverse events in eyes with active external infection in infants. A recent study in Turkey showed that 9 eyes with active adenoviral keratoconjunctivitis showed no adverse events after intravitreal injections for ROP [1].

16.3 Intravitreal Injection Technique in Infants

16.3.1 Pupil Dilation

Pupil dilation is necessary for assessment whether the medication entered the eye. Pupil dilation is also necessary for fundus examinations before and right after injection.

16.3.2 Anesthesia

Topical anesthesia (e.g. proparacaine topical eyedrops) is recommended. Subconjunctival anesthesia is not recommended because a conjunctival chemosis makes the injection more difficult.

16.3.3 Anti-sepsis

Wearing sterile gloves and surgical masks is recommended. Lid retraction using a sterile speculum is also recommended. There is no evidence to support the routine use of a sterile drape, but many doctors prefer using sterile drape for infants in NICU. Povidone-Iodine should be applied to the ocular surface and eyelids. According to the US guideline for intravitreal injection, povidone-iodine should be the last agent applied to the injection site [2]. Using pre-, peri-, and post-operative (topical) antibiotics is generally not recommended.

16.3.4 Needle and Syringe

30-gauge or thinner needles are generally recommended. A ½ inch needle (12.7 mm) is commonly used for adult patients. However, this may be too long for newborns. The axial length of a ROP eye at 36 weeks PMA is 15.2 mm and 1 mm shorter than a healthy eye of the same age (Fig. 16.1) [3]. Thus, if a ½ inch needle is inserted into the hub at 1 mm from corneal limbus, it might make a retinal damage. A recent report on a at 56-week PMA postmortem enucleated eye measured 20 mm in axial

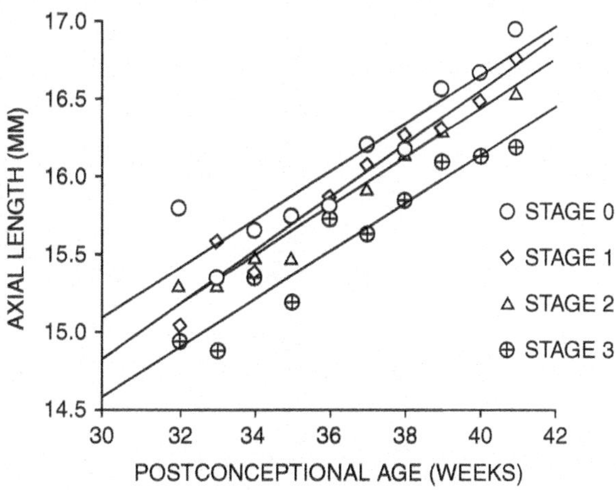

Fig. 16.1 Mean axial length and maximum acute stage of ROP (right eye), with linear regression. Axial length was reduced in infants with higher stages of ROP but the rates of growth during the study period did not differ significantly with stage of ROP. (Reprinted by permission from Springer Nature, Eye, Laws et al. [3] Copyright (1994))

length and a standard 30 G ½ inch needle was shown to cause posterior pole perforation if inserted into the hub [4]. Therefore, especially for premature infant, a shorter needle such as 5/16 inch needle may be safer. As syringe we recommend an insulin syringe in order to inject small volumes (Fig. 16.2).

16.3.5 Volume of Medication

We inject 0.02 ml ranibizumab or bevacizumab with the depicted insulin syringe in Fig. 16.2. An even better dose is the injection volume of 0.01 ml. The latter dose requires the usage of a surgical microscope in order to see this minimal amount of medication entering the eye (Fig. 16.3).

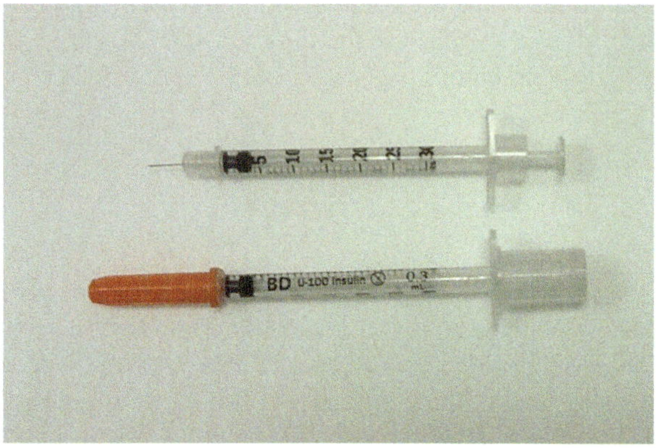

Fig. 16.2 Insulin syringe with a 31G, 8 mm needle. The 8 mm needle may be safer for the short eyes of neonates

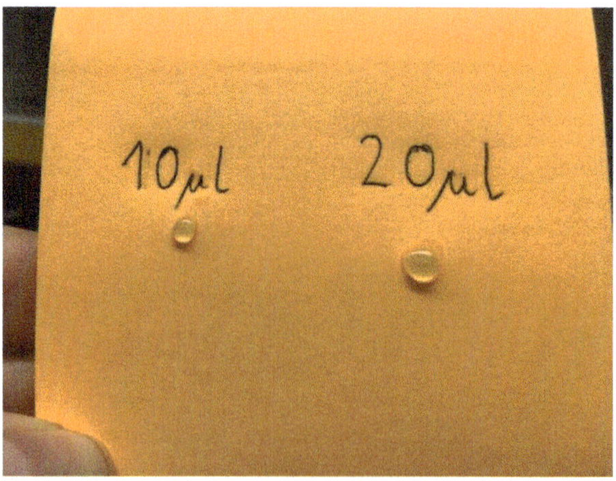

Fig. 16.3 0.01 ml (10 µl) and 0.02 ml (20 µl) volume of a fluid

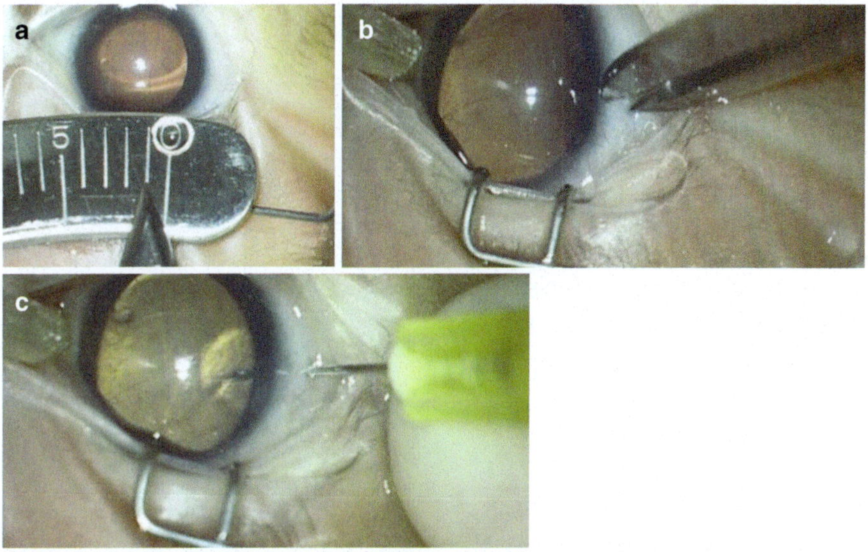

Fig. 16.4 (**a**) Intravitreal injection in an infant with treatment-requiring ROP. The distance from the limbus is 1 mm. (**b**) Measure the injection site with the caliper (**c**) Observe that the medication enters the vitreous. Only if you have seen that the medication was injected into the vitreous, you know that the treatment was successful. This is the big advantage in using a surgical microscope

16.3.6 Location of Injection

In premature infants with treatment-requiring ROP, intravitreal injection may safely be performed 1.0–1.5 mm posterior to the limbus (Fig. 16.4). It should be noted that in the BEAT-ROP study, injections were done 2.5 mm posterior to the limbus [5]. However, this poses a substantial risk for retinal damage in the infant eye.

16.3.7 How to Inject at the Bedside

After applying povidone-Iodine solution to the ocular surface and eyelids, eyelid retraction with sterile speculum, and marking injection site with a caliper, injection can be done with or without an assistant. If injection is done without an assistant, hold eyeball with forceps or an eyeball rotator in one hand and hold the syringe in the other hand. Then, push the plunger with the index finger. If injection is done with an assistant, hold eyeball with forceps or an eyeball rotator in one hand and hold the syringe in the other hand. And then, the assistant pushes the plunger.

16.3.8 How to Inject in the Operation Room with the Microscope

We recommend that the surgeon holds the syringe and the scrub nurse pushes the plunger. Mark the sclera 1.0–1.5 mm behind the limbus. Pierce the sclera with the 30G needle and move the needle slowly towards the optic nerve. The lens of a neonate is very big compared to the globe. A lens injury of a neonate lens is easier done than in an adult's lens. Focus the microscope image behind the lens. After a while the needle appears. Now the assistant pushes slowly the plunger. You see that the medication enters the vitreous cavity. Remove the syringe and close the sclerotomy wound with a cotton wool swab.

16.3.9 After Injection

The intraocular pressure can rise. Thus, after injection, central retinal arterial/venous perfusion should therefore be confirmed, although there has been no report on central arterial occlusion after intravitreal injection in infants, to the best of my knowledge. Also, during fundus examination, any new bleeding or lens damage can be inspected.

16.3.10 Follow-Up Examinations

Follow-up examinations are done at 2–4 days after injection to exclude an endophthalmitis. The next follow-up is 7 days post injection to examine the fundus. Then weekly examinations are recommended. The positive effect of the injection should be clearly visible after 2 weeks. After 1 week we expect a stable or slightly improved fundus but no deterioration. If a deterioration is present, then re-examine the neonate 3 days later. If the deterioration persists, then reinject immediately anti-VEGF.

Key Points for Anti-VEGF Injection

- The optimal dose for ranibizumab and bevacizumab has not been found yet.
- The best medication may be ranibizumab because it may not suppress systemic VEGF as much as bevacizumab
- The usual dose for ranibizumab is 0.02 ml (0.2 mg) or 0.01 ml (0.1 mg).
- The best syringe to use is an insulin syringe with a 30G needle

References

1. Koçluk Y, Alyamaç Sukgen E. Intravitreal anti-VEGF treatment for retinopathy of prematurity in infants with active adenoviral keratoconjunctivitis. Cutan Ocul Toxicol. 2018;37:15–8.
2. Avery RL, Bakri SJ, Blumenkranz MS, Brucker AJ, Cunningham ET Jr, D'Amico DJ, Dugel PU, Flynn HW Jr, Freund KB, Haller JA, Jumper JM, Liebmann JM, McCannel CA, Mieler WF, Ta CN, Williams GA. Intravitreal injection technique and monitoring: updated guidelines of an expert panel. Retina. 2014;34:S1–S18.
3. Laws DE, Haslett R, Ashby D, O'Brien C, Clark D. Axial length biometry in infants with retinopathy of prematurity. Eye (Lond). 1994;8:427–30.
4. Wright LM, Vrcek IM, Scribbick FW 3rd, Chang EY, Harper CA 3rd. Technique for infant intravitreal injection in treatment of retinopathy of prematurity. Retina. 2017;37:2188–90.
5. Mintz-Hittner HA, Kennedy KA, Chuang AZ, BEAT-ROP Cooperative Group. Efficacy of intravitreal bevacizumab for stage 3+ retinopathy of prematurity. N Engl J Med. 2011;364:603–15.

Part VI
Failure, Recurrence and Follow-Up

Chapter 17
Recurrence and Complications After Laser Coagulation and Anti-VEGF Treatment

The definition of a successful anti-VEGF treatment for ROP plus disease is somewhat unclear. In the BEAT-ROP study "recurrence" was the primary outcome measure [1]. Recurrence is a known effect of anti-VEGF treatment in diseases such as neovascular AMD, CRVO, diabetic maculopathy and so on. These diseases require repeated anti-VEGF injections and we do not regard a recurrence of a macular edema as a treatment failure. What does "recurrence" mean for an anti-VEGF treatment for ROP plus disease? If an anti-VEGF injection results in a disappearance (regression) of ROP plus disease, then a treatment **success** has occurred. If during the further follow-up a reactivation develops, i.e. the ROP plus disease reappears then a recurrence has occurred. But this recurrence is not a treatment failure. However, if despite an anti-VEGF injection, the ROP plus disease did not disappear but persisted, then a treatment failure has occurred. But this treatment **failure** is not a recurrence but a persistence.

Recurrence implies, therefore, reactivation after a period of regression while *persistence*, on the other hand, is defined as lack of adequate **regression** after treatment. Sometimes it is difficult to distinguish recurrence from **persistence**. An ongoing activation after treatment is defined as persistence but a complete disappearance of plus disease is defined as regression and a delayed reactivation as recurrence. A regression is a success, a persistence is a failure. We define arbitrary a treatment failure within the first month a s persistence and after 1 month as recurrence (see Fig. 17.1).

Another important outcome measure for successful ROP treatment is the complication rate. The BEAT-ROP study reported that the complication rate for anti-VEGF is much lower (3%) compared to laser photocoagulation (37%) [2]. In the laser coagulation group a huge amount of macular dragging occurred. For details see Table 17.1. Other studies report a higher incidence of retinal detachments after anti-VEGF treatment compared to laser photocoagulation [4].

The before mentioned outcome parameters measure only the structural or anatomical outcome. But the most important parameter for us is the final visual acuity outcome. A good functional outcome parameter as used in the ongoing Rainbow

U. Spandau, S. J. Kim, *Pediatric Retinal Vascular Diseases*,
https://doi.org/10.1007/978-3-030-13701-4_17

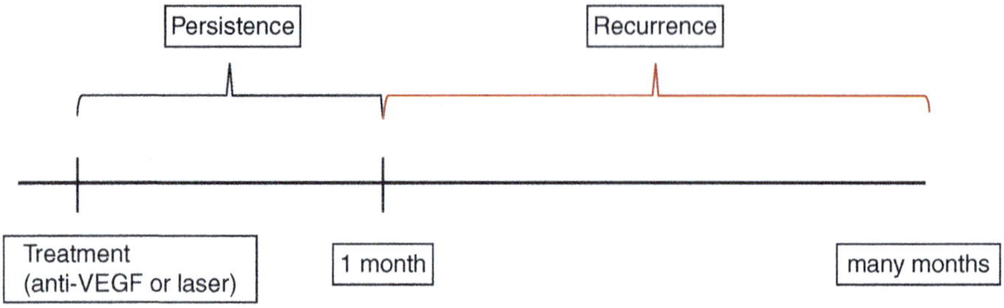

Fig. 17.1 Persistence versus recurrence. If ROP 3+ persists for 1 month after treatment, then it is defined as persistence. If ROP 3+ recurs after 1 month then we define it as recurrence

Table 17.1 A comparison of the complication rate for bevacizumab and laser coagulation

Complications [2, 3]		
	Bevacizumab injection	Laser coagulation
Macular dragging	1	22
Retinal detachment	2	2
Corneal opacity		1 requiring corneal transplant
lens opacity		3 requiring lens removal
Total	**3%**	**37%**

study (Lucentis for ROP zone I and II) is the "visual acuity at 6 years of age". This data is, however, missing and the following years will give us more insight.

In summary: The main parameters describing ROP treatment are (1) failure or success, (2) complication and (3) recurrence. Recurrence is a less important outcome parameter for ROP disease. An important outcome parameter for ROP treatment is failure (or success). This parameter can be measured as a favourable anatomical outcome or as a functional parameter such as visual acuity with 6 years of age [5]. Another important outcome parameter is a low complication rate (macular dragging, retinal detachment).

The recurrence rate of anti-VEGF is higher than of laser coagulation
The BEAT-ROP study reports a lower recurrence rate for anti-VEGF than for laser photocoagulation [2]. For details see Table 17.2. But we know today that anti-VEGF treatment has a higher recurrence rate than laser photocoagulation [1, 4].

Regarding anti-VEGF treatment, many studies demonstrate a recurrence rate of approximately 50% [2, 3, 6, 8]. The recurrence rate of laser coagulation is low with approximately 10% [9].

Timing of recurrence for laser coagulation and anti-VEGF treatment
(Table 17.3)
The recurrence of laser coagulation occurs much earlier than the recurrence for anti-VEGF. In eyes with zone I disease the time to recurrence is 6 weeks after laser coagulation and 19 weeks after anti-VEGF treatment [2, 4]. For details see Table 17.3. There is one crucial difference between recurrence for anti-VEGF and

Table 17.2 The recurrence rate for laser coagulation, bevacizumab and ranibizumab

Recurrence rate		
	Zone I	Zone II
Laser coagulation	42% [2]	12% [2]
	26% [2] 30% [6]	
Bevacizumab (Avastin®)	31,6% [1] 50% [7]	5% [2]
Ranibizumab (Lucentis®)	61% [3] 67% [8]	31% [3]

Table 17.3 The Recurrence time for Bevacizumab and Ranibizumab

Recurrence time	
Bevacizumab (Avastin®)	11–21 (peak at 16) weeks, maximal 65 [1] 4–35 (peak at 1.4), maximal 69 [4]
Ranibizumab (Lucentis®)	4-29 (peak 8.6) weeks [3]

laser coagulation. A recurrence for laser coagulation is in the most cases a persistence because a complete laser coagulation results in a disappearance of the plus disease. And only an incomplete laser coagulation results in a persistence. In contrast, after anti-VEGF treatment the ROP plus disease disappears and later on a recurrence takes place (See Fig. 17.1).

Risk factors for Recurrence

Low gestational age and low weight are risk factors for recurrence. The average gestational age is significantly lower in recurrent ROP group (23.9 weeks) compared to non-recurrent ROP infants (24.8 weeks). In addition, the average birth weight is significantly lower in the recurrent APROP infants (512 grams) than the ROP stage 3+ infants (638 grams) [1].

Ranibizumab (Lucentis®) has an earlier recurrence than Bevacizumab (Avastin®)

There is a growing body of evidence that Ranibizumab has a higher recurrence rate than Bevacizumab [3, 10, 11]. Recent studies showed a recurrence rate of 31–50% for Bevacizumab and 66% for Ranibizumab.

Bevacizumab: Studies report a mean recurrence at 14.4–16 weeks [2, 4].

Ranibizumab: Feng J observed a main recurrence at 8.5 weeks GA [3]. For details see Table 17.3.

Usual injection time for first anti-VEGF treatment

The usual injection time for the first anti-VEGF treatment is 33.8 weeks for zone I ROP and 35.5 weeks for zone II ROP weeks [2, 4]. See Fig. 17.2.

Usual injection time for second anti-VEGF treatment

For Ranibizumab, the mean injection time for the second anti-VEGF treatment is 8 weeks after the first injection. For Bevacizumab the mean time for the second injection is 16 weeks; this is double as late compared to Ranibizumab [1, 3]. See Fig. 17.2.

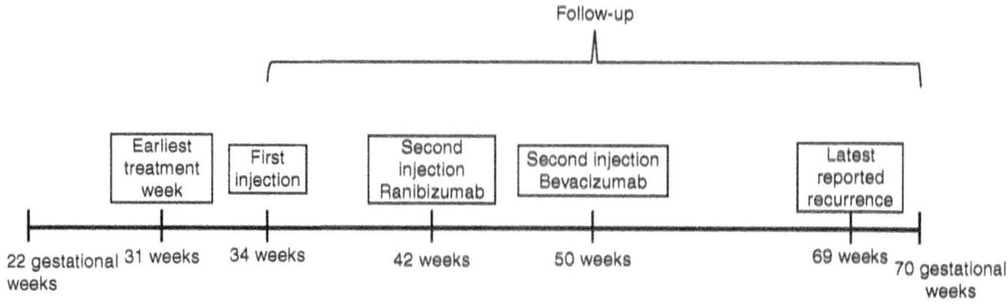

Fig. 17.2 The usual timing of anti-VEGF treatment for ROP newborn [1–4, 7]

Third anti-VEGF injection

In the most cases only one or a second injection is required. A third injection is very seldom [3]. For zone I, one injection is sufficient in 40% of eyes and 60% require a second injection. For zone II, one injection is sufficient in 70% of cases and 30% require a second injection [3].

17.1 Recurrence/Reactivation After Laser Coagulation

A recurrence in zone I may happen despite complete laser coagulation. A newborn eye does not tolerate a too central laser coagulation and may react with a progression. 42% of newborns with zone I have a recurrence after laser coagulation according to the BEAT-ROP study [2].

A recurrence in zone II occurs in 10% of the neonates according to the ETROP Study and 12% according to the BEAT ROP study. The main cause for reactivation in zone II is an incomplete laser coagulation. For details see Table 17.2.

Taking zone I and zone II together the recurrence rate for laser coagulation is 26% [2]. The BEAT-ROP study was criticized for the high recurrence rate for laser coagulation but this number is confirmed by a national study from Sweden. A national survey of all treatment centers in Sweden showed an overall recurrence rate of 30% for laser coagulation (zone I and zone II). Treatment centers with big patient numbers had a low recurrence rate and treatment centers with small patient numbers had a high recurrence rate [6].

17.2 Complication Rate for Laser Coagulation

In the BEAT-ROP study, the complication rate for laser coagulation was really high: 22 eyes had a macular dragging, two eyes a retinal detachment, three cataracts requiring lens removal and one corneal opacity requiring a corneal transplant [2]. For details see Table 17.1.

Key points
1. A recurrence is not a failure
2. A favourable anatomical outcome or a disappearance of plus disease are a treatment success.
3. Anti-VEGF has a *high* recurrence rate and a *low* complication rate
4. Anti-VEGF has a late recurrence window and requires a long fellow up
5. Ranibizumab has a short recurrence time of approximately 8 weeks and Bevacizumab a long recurrence time of approximately 16 weeks.
6. Lasercoagulation has a *rather low (10–30%)* recurrence rate and a *high* complication rate
7. Lasercoagulation has a much higher complication rate than anti-VEGF
8. Lasercoagulation has an early recurrence and requires a short follow-up
9. Important: If you are not experienced with indirect laser coagulation then do always combined treatments: Laser coagulation and anti-VEGF in the same sitting.

References

1. Mintz-Hittner HA, Geloneck MM, Chuang AZ. Clinical management of recurrent retinopathy of prematurity after Intravitreal Bevacizumab monotherapy. Ophthalmology. 2016;123(9):1845–55.
2. Mintz-Hittner HA, Kennedy KA, Chuang AZ, BEAT-ROP Cooperative Group. Efficacy of intravitreal bevacizumab for stage 3+ retinopathy of prematurity. N Engl J Med. 2011;364:603–15.
3. Feng J, Qian J, Jiang Y, Zhao M, Liang J, Yin H, Chen Y, Yu W, Li X. Efficacy of primary Intravitreal Ranibizumab for retinopathy of prematurity in China. Ophthalmology. 2017;124(3):408–9.
4. Hu J, Blair MP, Shapiro MJ, Lichetnstein SJ, Galasso JM, Kapur R. Reactivation of retinopathy of prematurity after Bevacizumab injection. Arch Ophthalmol. 2012;130(8):1000–6.
5. Early Treatment for Retinopathy of Prematurity Cooperative Group, Good WV, Hardy RJ, Dobson V, Palmer EA, Phelps DL, Tung B, Redford M. Final visual acuity results in the early treatment for retinopathy of prematurity study. Arch Ophthalmol. 2010;128(6):663–71.
6. Holmström G, Hellström A, Jakobsson P, Lundgren P, Tornqvist K, Wallin A. Five years of treatment for retinopathy of prematurity in Sweden: results from SWEDROP, a national quality register. Br J Ophthalmol. 2016;100(12):1656–61.
7. Garcia Gonzalez JM, Snyder L, Blair M, Rohr A, Shapiro M, Greenwald M. Prophylactic peripheral laser and fluorescein angiography after bevacizumab for retinopathy of prematurity. Retina. 2018;38(4):764–72.
8. Holmström G, Tornqvist K, Al-Hawasi A, Nilsson Å, Wallin A, Hellström A. Increased frequency of retinopathy of prematurity over the last decade and significant regional differences. Acta Ophthalmol. 2018;96(2):142–8.
9. Repka MX, Tung B, Good WV, Shapiro M, Capone A Jr, Baker JD, Barr CC, Phelps DL. van. Thomas BJ, Yonekawa Y, Trese MT. Complete resolution of large retinal fold after transection of retrolental membrane during lens-sparing vitrectomy for retinopathy of prematurity: a 15-year follow-up. Retin Cases Brief Rep. 2016;10(1):93–5.
10. Bakri SJ, Snyder MR, Reid JM, et al. Pharmacokinetics of intravitreal bevacizumab (Avastin). Ophthalmology. 2007;114:855–9.
11. Hu Q, Bai Y, Chen X, Huang L, Chen Y, Li X. Recurrence of retinopathy of prematurity in Zone II Stage 3+ after Ranibizumab treatment: a retropspective study. Ophthalmol. 2017;2017:5078565. Published online 2017 Apr 9. https://doi.org/10.1155/2017/5078565.

Chapter 18
Combined Laser and Anti-VEGF Treatment for Zone I ROP

Although the overall outcomes of ROP treatment have improved, the treatment for zone I ROP, especially AP-ROP is still challenging. A considerable number of eyes with zone I ROP develop macular dragging, retinal detachment, or retrolental membrane after laser treatment. In addition, laser-treated eyes with zone I ROP may develop visual field constriction and significant refractive errors, such as high myopia. During the last 10 years, intravitreal anti-VEGF treatment has shown promising anatomical outcome, especially for zone I ROP [1]. Also, intravitreal anti-VEGF monotherapy has been associated with less refractive errors [2]. However, the optimal dose, influences on other organs, and follow-up protocol including retreatment indications are not known yet.

To overcome those disadvantages of conventional laser and anti-VEGF monotherapy, combined treatments have been investigated in several studies. Combined laser and anti-VEGF treatment can be done in several ways: (1) concomitant laser and anti-VEGF injection; (2) concomitant laser not covering whole peripheral avascular retina and anti-VEGF injection; and (3) laser first and then anti-VEGF injection in several weeks.

Kim and colleagues investigated the anatomical and refractive outcomes of combined intravitreal bevacizumab (IVB; 0.01 ml) and zone I sparing laser photocoagulation and IVB with deferred laser photocoagulation compared to conventional laser treatment in infants with Type 1 ROP in Zone I [3, 4]. In this study, 101 eyes from 51 infants with Type 1 ROP in zone I were analysed. Group I consisted of 44 eyes that received laser treatment only; Group II consisted of 30 eyes that received combined IVB and zone I sparing laser ablation; and Group III consisted of 27 eyes that underwent IVB with deferred laser photocoagulation (Fig. 18.1) [4]. The mean GA and the birth weight were 24.3 ± 1.1 weeks and 646 ± 143 g, respectively [4].

This study showed that IVB with both concomitant laser and deferred laser therapy showed a significantly better anatomical outcome than conventional laser therapy alone [4]. A normal posterior pole was observed in 77.3% in Group I and 100% in Group II and III ($P < 0.001$) [4]. Unfavorable anatomical outcomes were observed only in Group I [4]. Moreover, IVB with deferred laser treatment resulted

U. Spandau, S. J. Kim, *Pediatric Retinal Vascular Diseases*,
https://doi.org/10.1007/978-3-030-13701-4_18

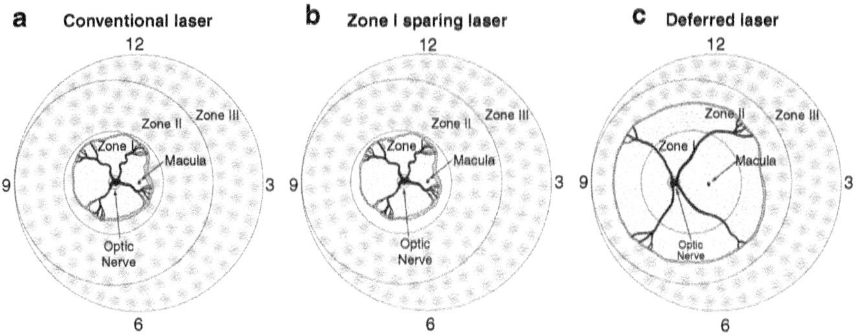

Fig. 18.1 Diagrams showing the 3 methods of laser treatment. The conventional laser treatment, near-confluent laser photocoagulation, was performed on the whole area of the avascular retina extending to the ora serrata laser treatment in Group I (**a**). Near-confluent laser photocoagulation was performed on the avascular retina anterior to the margin of Zone I extending to the ora serrata in Group II. Avascular retina posterior to the margin of Zone I was left without laser ablation (**b**). After IVB injection, the retina was more vascularized. Then, laser photocoagulation was performed on the avascular retina extending to the ora serrata in Group III (**c**). Gray circles indicate the laser-treated areas. (Reprinted from Yoon et al. [4] https://journals.lww.com/retinajournal/Abstract/2017/01000/OUTCOMES_AFTER_LASER_VERSUS_COMBINED_LASER_AND.12.aspx Copyright (2017), with permission from Wolters Kluwer Health, Inc.)

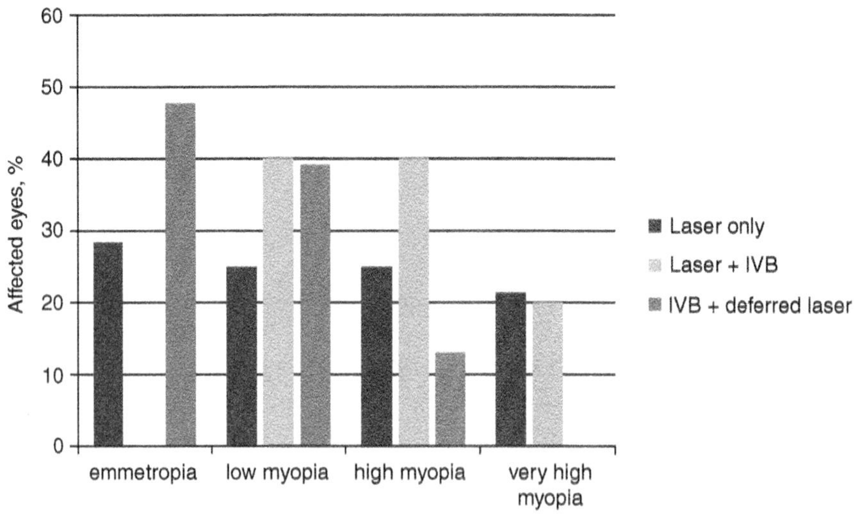

Fig. 18.2 Distribution of refractive errors among the 3 groups. Distribution of spherical equivalent refractive error among the 3 groups at the age of 12 months to 18 months. Each category is defined as follows: emmetropia (<−1 to 1.0 D), low myopia (<−5.0 to −1.0 D), and high myopia (<−8.0 to −5.0 D), very high myopia (≥ − 8.0 D). (Reprinted from Yoon et al. [4] https://journals.lww.com/retinajournal/Abstract/2017/01000/OUTCOMES_AFTER_LASER_VERSUS_COMBINED_LASER_AND.12.aspx Copyright (2017), with permission from Wolters Kluwer Health, Inc.)

in less myopic refractive error than the other two methods did (Fig. 18.2) [4]. The average refractive errors of patients at 12–18 months of age in Groups I, II, and III were −4.62 ± 4.00 D, −5.53 ± 2.21 D, and −1.40 ± +2.19 D, respectively ($P < 0.001$) [4].

Although this study has several limitations, including its retrospective (a historical comparison) and nonrandomized nature, this case series included consecutive patients with zone I ROP over a 10-year period at a single center [4].

In conclusion, this study showed that in zone I ROP, anti-VEGF with concomitant or deferred laser therapy may show more favorable anatomic outcomes than conventional laser treatment alone [4]. In addition, anti-VEGF with deferred laser treatment may result in less myopic refractive error [4]. Moreover, anti-VEGF with deferred laser treatment has potential advantages including lower possibility of late reactivation, lower number of examinations after treatment, and preservation of larger unlasered retinal areas.

References

1. Mintz-Hittner HA, Kennedy KA, Chuang AZ, BEAT-ROP Cooperative Group. Efficacy of intravitreal bevacizumab for stage 3+ retinopathy of prematurity. N Engl J Med. 2011;364:603–15.
2. Geloneck MM, Chuang AZ, Clark WL, Hunt MG, Norman AA, Packwood EA, Tawansy KA, Mintz-Hittner HA, BEAT-ROP Cooperative Group. Refractive outcomes following bevacizumab monotherapy compared with conventional laser treatment: a randomized clinical trial. JAMA Ophthalmol. 2014;132:1327–33.
3. Kim J, Kim SJ, Chang YS, Park WS. Combined intravitreal bevacizumab injection and zone I sparing laser photocoagulation in patients with zone I retinopathy of prematurity. Retina. 2014;34:77–82.
4. Yoon JM, Shin DH, Kim SJ, Ham DI, Kang SW, Chang YS, Park WS. Outcomes after laser versus combined laser and Bevacizumab treatment for Type 1 retinopathy of prematurity in zone I. Retina. 2017;37:88–96.

Chapter 19
Recurrence of ROP After Anti-VEGF Treatment

19.1 Introduction

Potential advantages of anti-VEGF treatment over laser ablation in ROP include better anatomical outcome (especially in zone I ROP), treatment administration even in eyes with corneal opacity or small pupil, faster improvement in plus disease, more preservation of retina (with subsequent larger visual field), and less refractive error [1]. However, there are also potential risks of recurrence, abrupt progression of tractional retinal detachment and systemic adverse effects. Many studies reported that some eyes showed early or late reactivation, which necessitated additional treatment or extended follow-up.

19.2 Clinical Course Following Anti-VEGF Treatment

Usual clinical course after anti-VEGF treatment for the treatment of type I ROP is as follows: plus disease usually starts to regress within 1 week (often as early as 1 day) and extraretinal fibrovascular proliferation regresses by 2–4 weeks. And then, the eye looks quiet for the next few weeks. In some eyes, recurrence occurs 2~3 months after initial treatment. The first sign of recurrence is development of pre-plus-like vascular abnormalities or formation of new demarcation line. Recurrence of neovascularization may occur at the advancing edge and at the initial ridge/EFP [2]. Some eyes may have a late reactivation despite a long period of quiescence (as late as 3 years) [3, 4].

U. Spandau, S. J. Kim, *Pediatric Retinal Vascular Diseases*,
https://doi.org/10.1007/978-3-030-13701-4_19

19.3 Incidence of Recurrence

Incidences of recurrence after anti-VEGF treatment from major clinical studies are shown in Table 19.1. The recurrence rate is not low but is variable. The baseline characteristics of included eyes, definition of recurrence, and re-treatment criteria are variable between studies, which limits comparison of recurrence rate between studies.

BEAT-ROP study in 2011 [5] showed significantly lower recurrence rate for eyes with zone I, stage 3+ ROP that received bevacizumab than eyes that received laser ablation. However, there are some criticisms on relatively short follow-up duration (until 54 weeks' PMA) and unusually high recurrence rate (higher than 40%) of laser-treated eyes in zone I ROP. In their retrospective study in 2016 [2], they investigated recurrence rate until at least 65 weeks' PMA. The incidence of recurrence (needing re-treatment) was 7.2%. Interestingly, eyes with AP-ROP showed high recurrence rate (31.6%).

In Wallace et al. dosing study in 2018 [6], there was no relationship between lower dose of bevacizumab and need for re-treatment. However, the sample size is not adequate to test this hypothesis. Overall recurrence rate is higher than that of BEAT-ROP study, which used higher dose of bevacizumab (0.625 mg).

Recurrence rate in eyes with ranibizumab treatment might be higher than that in eyes with bevacizumab treatment, possible because of shorter half-life of ranibizumab. However, in a comparative case series studies by Chen et al. [7] and Gunay et al. [8], re-treatment rates were not different between ranibizumab- and bevacizumab-treated eyes. In 2 other small case series, recurrence rate was higher in ranibizumab-treated eyes. Further investigation is warranted to compare recurrence rates and safety profiles among anti-VEGF agents.

19.4 Timing of Recurrence

In Mintz-Hittner et al. study in 2016, intravitreal bevacizumab monotherapy in 471 eyes of 241 infants (including patients included in BEAT-ROP study) was retrospectively reviewed [2]. Recurrence incidence was 8.3% (20/241) for infants and 7.2% (34/471) for eyes. Recurrence risk period was between approximately 45 and 55 weeks PMA, with mean recurrence of 51.2 ± 4.6 weeks PMA and mean interval of 16.2 ± 4.4 weeks between treatments.

In CARE-ROP study in 2018 [9], mean (± SD) time between initial treatment and retreatment was 87 ± 18 days in the 0.12-mg ranibizumab group and 53 ± 3 days in the 0.20-mg group. One infant in the 0.20-mg group required a second retreatment 71 days after the first treatment.

Table 19.1 Incidence of recurrence after anti-VEGF treatment for ROP from major clinical studies

Authors and publication year	Study design	Anti-VEGF agent, dose	Number of eyes	Indication for anti-VEGF treatment	Follow-up duration	Incidence of recurrence (%)	Definition of recurrence
Wallace et al. 2018 (PEDIG) [6]	A masked, dose de-escalation study	Bevacizumab,0.250 mg	11	Type I ROP	Until 6 months corrected age	18[a]	"Early failure" was defined as no improvement 3–5 days after injection or recurrence of type 1 ROP or severe neovascularization requiring additional treatment within 4 weeks. "Late recurrence" was defined as recurrence of plus disease or neo- vascularization that prompted investigators to give additional treatment after 4 weeks.
		0.125 mg	16			25[a]	
		0.063 mg	24			33[a]	
		0.031 mg	10			0[a]	
		Total	61			23[a]	
Mintz-Hittner et al. 2011 (BEAT-ROP study) [5]	Randomized controlled trial	Bevacizumab,0.625 mg	31	Zone I, stage 3+ ROP	54 weeks' PMA	6	the recurrence of neovascularization in one or both eyes arising from the retinal vessels and requiring retreatment
			39	Posterior zone II, stage 3+ ROP		5	
Mintz-Hittner et al. 2016 [2]	Retrospective case series (including patients of BEAT-ROP)	Bevacizumab,0.625 mg	471	Type I ROP	65 weeks' PMA	7.2(31.6% in AP-ROP)	Recurrence of type I ROP
Stahl et al. 2018 (CARE-ROP) [9]	Randomized, double-blind IIT	Ranibizumab, 0.12 mg	18	Type I ROP (including AP-ROP) in zone I or stage 3+ ROP in posterior zone II	Until 24 weeks after initial treatment	22.2	recurrences that were severe enough to warrant retreatment
		0.20 mg	14			28.6	

[a]Eyes with "recurrence" included eyes with "early failure" and "late recurrence"

References

1. Darwish D, Chee RI, Patel SN, Jonas K, Ostmo S, Campbell JP, Chiang MF, Chan RVP. Anti-Vascular endothelial growth factor and the evolving management paradigm for retinopathy of prematurity. Asia Pac J Ophthalmol (Phila). 2018;7:136–44.
2. Mintz-Hittner HA, Geloneck MM, Chuang AZ. Clinical management of recurrent retinopathy of prematurity after Intravitreal Bevacizumab monotherapy. Ophthalmology. 2016;123:1845–55.
3. Snyder LL, Garcia-Gonzalez JM, Shapiro MJ, Blair MP. Very late reactivation of retinopathy of prematurity after monotherapy with Intravitreal Bevacizumab. Ophthalmic Surg Lasers Imaging Retina. 2016;47:280–3.
4. Hajrasouliha AR, Garcia-Gonzales JM, Shapiro MJ, Yoon H, Blair MP. Reactivation of retinopathy of prematurity three years after treatment with Bevacizumab. Ophthalmic Surg Lasers Imaging Retina. 2017;48:255–9.
5. Mintz-Hittner HA, Kennedy KA, Chuang AZ, BEAT-ROP Cooperative Group. Efficacy of intravitreal bevacizumab for stage 3+ retinopathy of prematurity. N Engl J Med. 2011;364:603–15.
6. Wallace DK, Dean TW, Hartnett ME, Kong L, Smith LE, Hubbard GB, McGregor ML, Jordan CO, Mantagos IS, Bell EF, Kraker RT, Pediatric Eye Disease Investigator Group. A dosing study of Bevacizumab for retinopathy of prematurity: late recurrences and additional treatments. Ophthalmology. 2018;7 https://doi.org/10.1016/j.ophtha.2018.05.001.
7. Chen SN, Lian I, Hwang YC, Chen YH, Chang YC, Lee KH, Chuang CC, Wu WC. Intravitreal anti-vascular endothelial growth factor treatment for retinopathy of prematurity: comparison between Ranibizumab and Bevacizumab. Retina. 2015;35:667–74.
8. Gunay M, Sukgen EA, Celik G, Kocluk Y. Comparison of Bevacizumab, Ranibizumab, and laser photocoagulation in the treatment of retinopathy of prematurity in Turkey. Curr Eye Res. 2017;42:462–9.
9. Stahl A, Krohne TU, Eter N, Oberacher-Velten I, Guthoff R, Meltendorf S, Ehrt O, Aisenbrey S, Roider J, Gerding H, Jandeck C, Smith LEH, Walz JM, Comparing Alternative Ranibizumab Dosages for Safety and Efficacy in Retinopathy of Prematurity (CARE-ROP) Study Group. Comparing alternative Ranibizumab dosages for safety and efficacy in retinopathy of prematurity: a randomized clinical trial. JAMA Pediatr. 2018;172:278–86.

Chapter 20
Persistence of ROP Disease After Laser Coagulation or Anti-VEGF: What to Do?

One week after laser coagulation or anti-VEGF treatment the retinopathy may be unchanged or improved but not worse. Two weeks later the retinopathy should be improved.

If this is not the case, then a persistence is present. Schedule 3 days later a thorough examination, if necessary in general anaesthesia. It is important to reach an assessment. What stage of ROP is present? Is a detachment present? The next questions are: Why is a persistence present? Is this a failed primary therapy? In case of an anti-VEGF treatment: Did the medication not enter the eye? In case of a laser coagulation: Is an undertreatment present? Are skip lesions present?

What to do? If you are not a clinical center for ROP then refer the neonate immediately to a clinical center for assessment and further treatment. If you are a clinical center, then schedule a treatment in general anaesthesia. If you find skip lesions, then perform a completing laser coagulation and/or inject intravitreal anti-VEGF. If you do not find skip lesions, then add two rows of laser posterior to the temporal ridge. If a focal detachment is present on the temporal ridge, then add laser and inject anti-VEGF. Our treatment algorithm is depicted in Fig. 20.1.

After 2 weeks the retinopathy should have regressed. If the retinopathy persists or progresses, then schedule immediately an examination in general anaesthesia. If the retina is attached perform a completing laser coagulation and inject anti-VEGF. If the focal detachment persists (stage 4A) then perform a lens sparing vitrectomy or place an encircling band. Our complete follow-up and treatment algorithm for stage 4A is depicted in Fig. 20.2.

U. Spandau, S. J. Kim, *Pediatric Retinal Vascular Diseases*,
https://doi.org/10.1007/978-3-030-13701-4_20

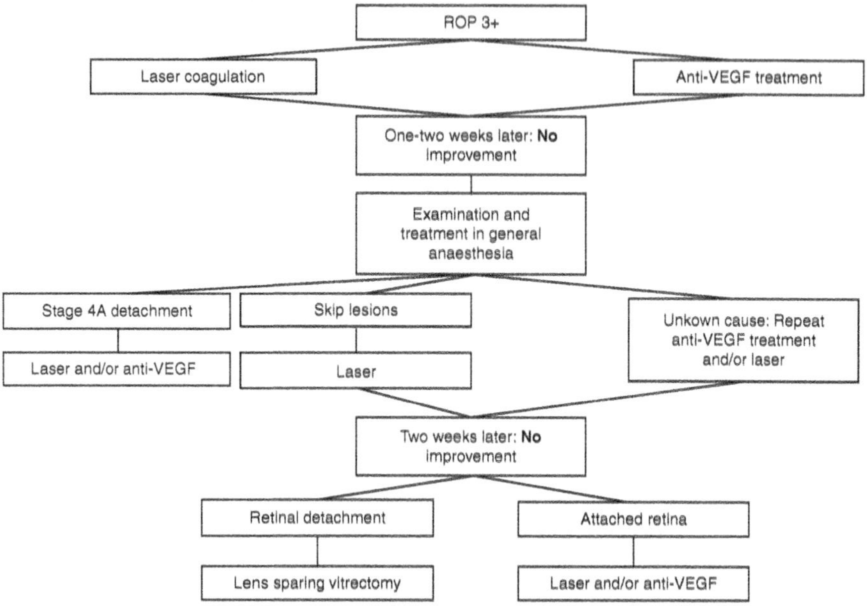

Fig. 20.1 Our algorithm for follow-up after primary treatment

20.1 Treatment Algorithm for ROP 3+ Disease for Treatment Centers and Non-treatment Centers

Laser coagulation is technically very difficult. The quality of laser coagulation is poor at non-treatment centers. This notion is confirmed by a high recurrence rate of 30% of laser in non-treatment centers [1, 2]. If 30% of neonates have to be lasered a second time, then not all will regress but some will progress to a macular dragging or retinal detachment. The BEAT-ROP study showed a high complication rate for laser coagulation of 37% [3]. In contrast, there is a minimal recurrence rate and consequently minimal complications for laser coagulation at treatment centers.

This is not true for intravitreal injections. The complication rate for injections is very low in a treatment center as well as in non-treatment centers ([1]; Retrospective study, unpublished results). The reason for this is, that intravitreal injections are technically easy. Laser coagulation is user-dependent, whereas intravitreal injection is not user-dependent.

We propose therefore two different treatment algorithms depending, if you work at a treatment center for ROP or not. Laser coagulation should only be performed at a treatment center because it is technically difficult and requires much training. In contrast, non-treatment centers should only perform injections but no laser coagulation. If an eye requires a laser coagulation, the patient can be referred to a treatment center.

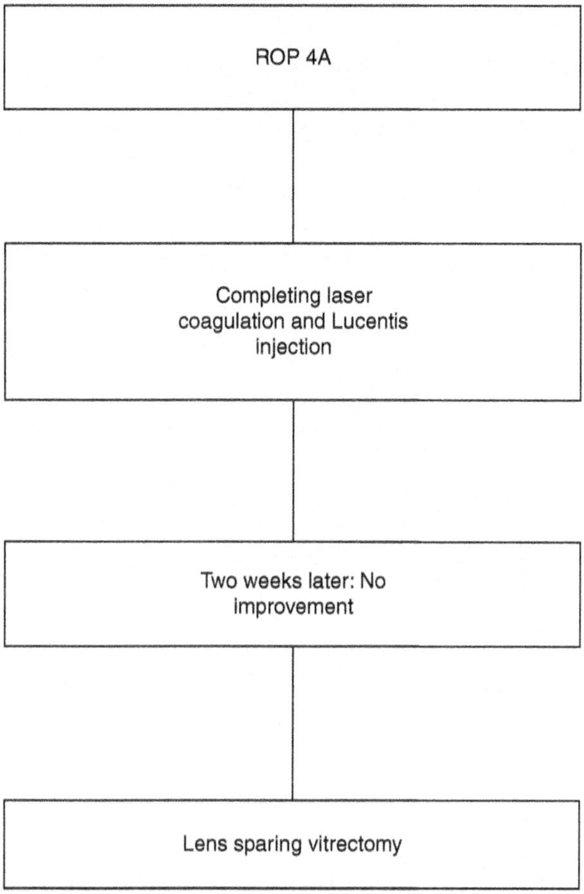

Fig. 20.2 Treatment algorithm for stage 4A disease

For *non-treatment centers* we recommend the following treatment algorithm (Fig. 20.3):

For *treatment centers* we recommend the following treatment algorithm (Fig. 20.4):

Figure 20.4 depicts the treatment algorithm of the University of Uppsala. We perform an anti-VEGF injection for plus disease in zone I and laser coagulation for zone II. If a recurrence occurs after anti-VEGF injection we treat with a laser coagulation. Other treatment centers would reinject anti-VEGF if a recurrence occurs. We perform a laser coagulation in zone II since this treatment modality has been established in the ETROP study.

The following *case report* is a typical example for our treatment algorithm:

- *General history:*

  A pregnant woman performed an amniocentesis in week 21 to exclude a Down syndrome. One week later she got contractions and gave birth to 22 + 0 week born neonate.

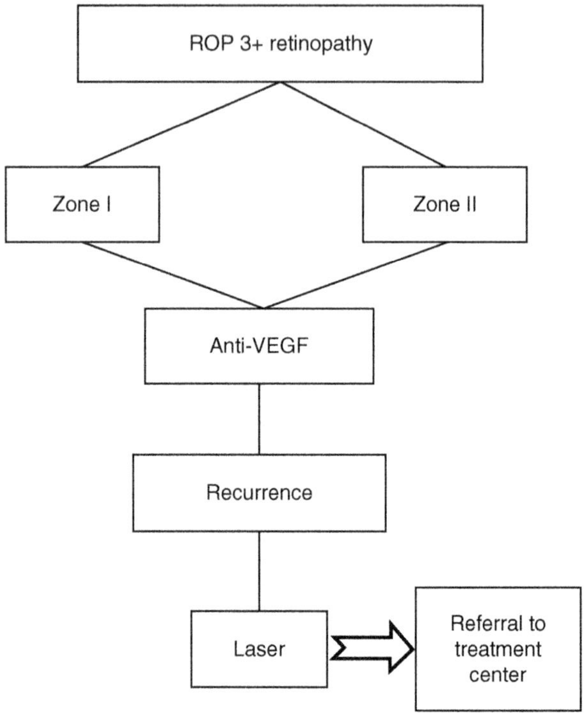

Fig. 20.3 Treatment algorithm for non-treatment centers. Only injections are performed here and are done for zone I and zone II retinopathies. A laser coagulation is referred to a treatment center

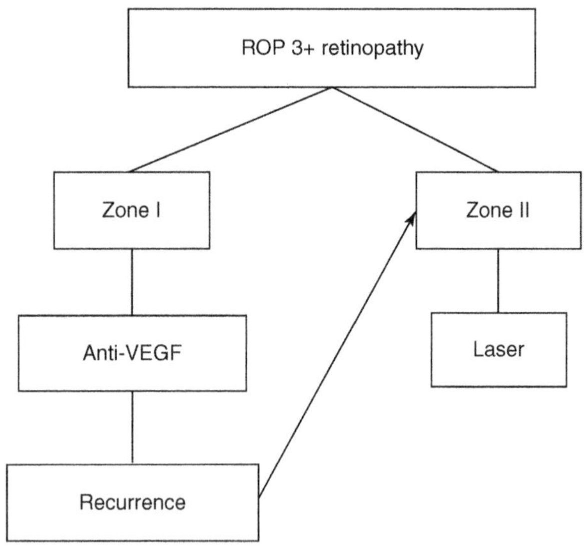

Fig. 20.4 Treatment algorithm for treatment centers. Treatment centers perform injections as well as laser coagulations. For zone I an anti-VEGF injection is performed and for zone II a laser coagulation is recommended

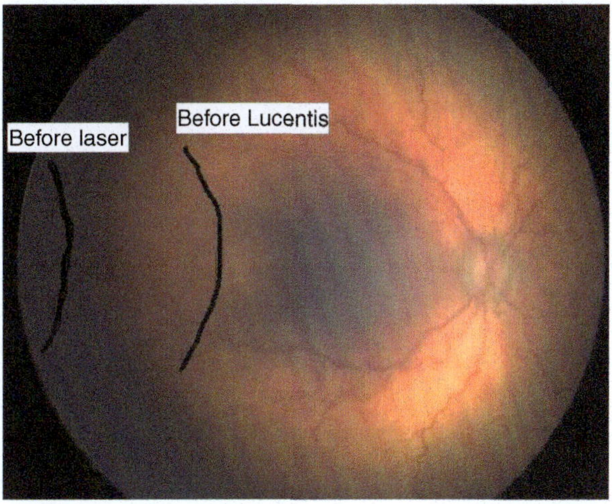

Fig. 20.5 RE: Week 43. A recurrence in zone II. The location of the ridge before Lucentis injection and now before laser coagulation is marked

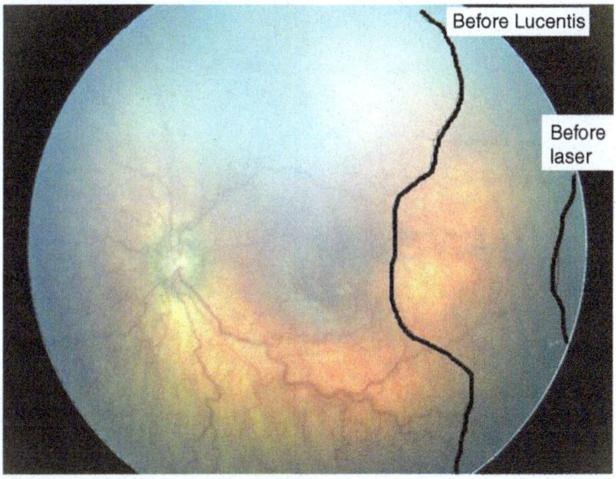

Fig. 20.6 LE: Week 43. A recurrence in zone II. The location of the ridge before Lucentis injection and now before laser coagulation is marked

- *Ocular history:*

  The neonate was screened from week 31. In week 33 a ROP plus disease in zone I was diagnosed. Intravitreal Lucentis was injected in both eyes. Post injection there was a rapid improvement in both eyes and the plus disease, the proliferations and the hemorrhages disappeared. In week 43 a recurrence was detected (Figs. 20.5, 20.6, and 20.7). In the meantime, the retina had matured from zone I to zone 2 (Figs. 20.5 and 20.6). A laser treatment of both eyes was performed (Fig. 20.8). Within 2–3 weeks the plus disease disappeared (Figs. 20.8 and 20.9).
- Remark: If you are not experienced with indirect laser coagulation then do always combined treatments: Laser coagulation and anti-VEGF in the same sitting. You will avoid many complications.

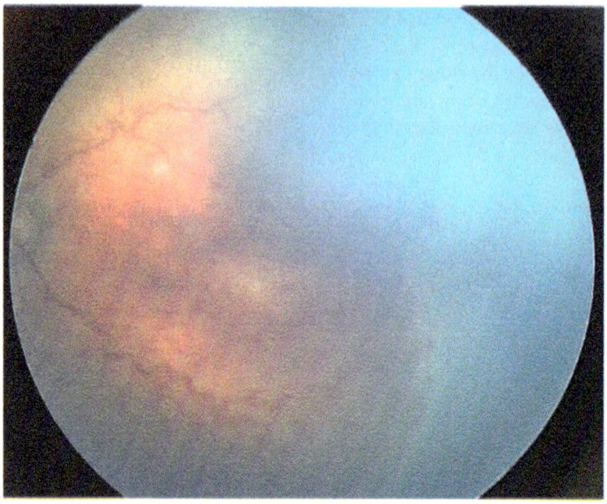

Fig. 20.7 LE: Week 43: The ridge in zone II is clearly visible

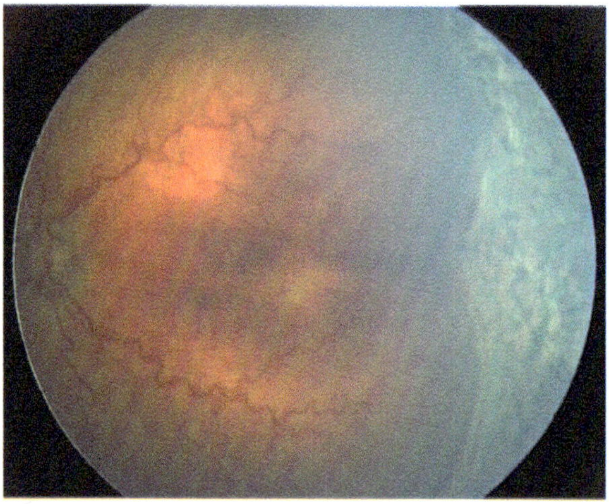

Fig. 20.8 LE: Week 45: The ischemic area is completely laser treated. Plus disease is still present but no deterioration was visible. We were discussing to inject anti-VEGF intravitreal but in the following week the plus disease was markedly reduced

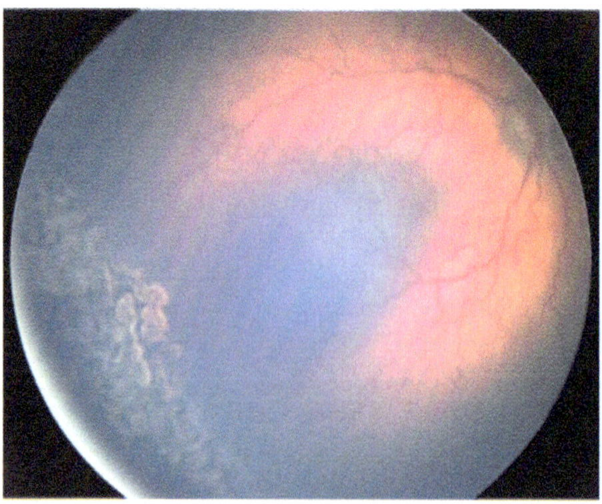

Fig. 20.9 RE: Week 45: The ischemic area is completely laser treated. Plus disease has disappeared

References

1. Holmström G, Hellström A, Jakobsson P, Lundgren P, Tornqvist K, Wallin A. Five years of treatment for retinopathy of prematurity in Sweden: results from SWEDROP, a national quality register. Br J Ophthalmol. 2016;100(12):1656–61.
2. Mintz-Hittner HA, Kennedy KA, Chuang AZ, BEAT-ROP Cooperative Group. Efficacy of intravitreal bevacizumab for stage 3+ retinopathy of prematurity. N Engl J Med. 2011;364:603–15.
3. Mintz-Hittner HA, Geloneck MM, Chuang AZ. Clinical management of recurrent retinopathy of prematurity after intravitreal bevacizumab monotherapy. Ophthalmology. 2016;123(9):1845–55.

Part VII
Surgery

Chapter 21
Lens-Sparing Vitrectomy (LSV) for ROP Stage 4A and B

Surgical treatment for cases of retinopathy of prematurity that develop retinal detachment (RD) was significantly advanced by the adoption of lens-sparing vitrectomy (LSV). A lens sparing vitrectomy is always the method of choice because a lens removal in the pediatric population is associated with inhibition of visual development and development of aphakic glaucoma.

If, however, extensive anterior fibrovascular membranes are present then a lens removal is necessary to prevent induction of a retinal break (see Chap. 24).

We operate all children eyes with 27G. 27G has the smallest sclerotomies and the sclera of young eyes is soft and leaks more easily than an adult eye. We perform a perpendicular and not a lamellar insertion of trocars due to the risk of damaging the lens. If you perform a perpendicular insertion with 23G or 25G trocars you need to suture the sclerotomies. In 27G a suture is not necessary and the sutureless vitrectomy allows a fast-postoperative recovery.

21.1 Physiology of a Neonate Eye

In the neonatal eye, the pars plana region is incompletely developed and almost not existent. The axial length of a newborn eye is 16 mm in the 34th gestational week and 17 mm in the 40th gestational week. The anterior retina lies just behind the pars plicata. A pars plana does not exist. The site of sclerotomy is therefore much closer to the limbus. The sclerotomy should be performed 1.0–1.5 mm behind the limbus. See Table 21.1. The newborn eye has a huge lens compared to the globe. A big lens and a short sclerotomy site allow only a small canal to insert and manoeuvre the instruments. Utmost care is

---

Electronic Supplementary Material The online version of this chapter (https://doi.org/10.1007/978-3-030-13701-4_21) contains supplementary material, which is available to authorized users.
The videos can be accessed under http://extras.springer.com/Search. Enter the ISBN number of your book and download the videos.

U. Spandau, S. J. Kim, *Pediatric Retinal Vascular Diseases*,
https://doi.org/10.1007/978-3-030-13701-4_21

needed in inserting a vitreoretinal instrument or in administering an injection, because it may cause inadvertent lens touching, traction on the vitreous base, and retinal damage. The vitreous body of a newborn is completely intact. No degeneration of the vitreous body is present. The vitreous body is very firmly attached to the retina; a PVD is virtually not possible. If you try to induce a PVD you risk creating a retinal tear.

21.2 Retinal Detachment Secondary to ROP

Retinal detachment secondary to ROP is a tractive retinal detachment and not a rhegmatogenous retinal detachment (Fig. 21.1). Due to the fact that a retinal break is not present, there is no need for a tamponade or even postoperative posture. The aim of surgery is to remove the vitreous body in order to relieve retinal traction. The

Table 21.1 Site of sclerotomy in relation to the age

Age	0	1–6 mts	6–12 mts	1–3 yrs	3–6 yrs	6–18 yrs	Adult phakic	Adult pseudophakic
Site of sclerotomy (mm)	1.0	1.5	2.0	2.5	3.0	3.5	4.0	3.5

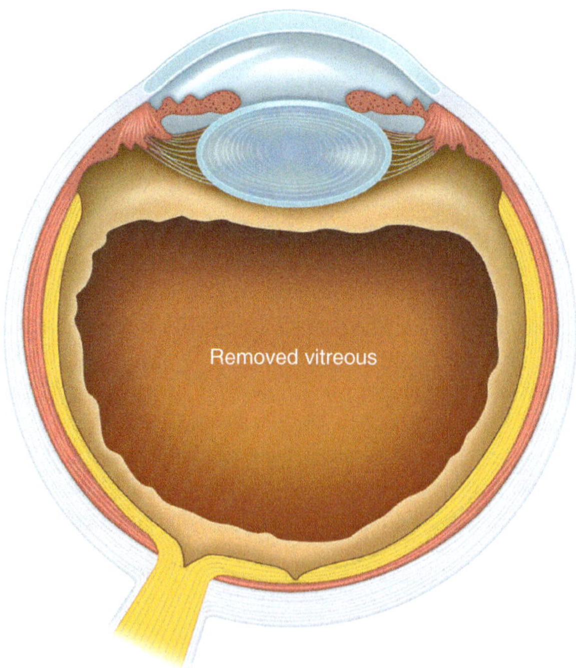

Fig. 21.1 A retinal detachment secondary to ROP is a tractive detachment. If you remove the core vitreous the retina will reattach

retina will reattach in a few days after surgery. In addition, an anti-VEGF injection is needed to reduce the vascular activity and remove the pathologic cause of the tractive detachment. We use ranibizumab (Lucentis®) because the half-life in serum is lower compared to bevacizumab (Avastin ®).

A lensectomy should be avoided if possible because it results in severe amblyopia.

21.3 Timing of Surgery

Timing of surgery is of utmost importance. In retinopathy of prematurity a vigilant screening is of vital importance in order to avoid advanced retinopathies. We only operate ROP stage 4A (retinal detachment with attached macula) and 4B (retinal detachment with detached macula). Our treatment algorithm is depicted in Fig. 21.2. In case of stage 4B detachment we operate immediately. In case of stage 4A we treat first with intravitreal anti-VEGF injection. If the detachment deteriorates, we proceed with a lens sparing vitrectomy. We do no operate stage 5 ROP because the outcome is very poor. Do not operate too late. The risk that you will not succeed is high and the risk that you will have complications is even higher. Try to operate in stage 4A.

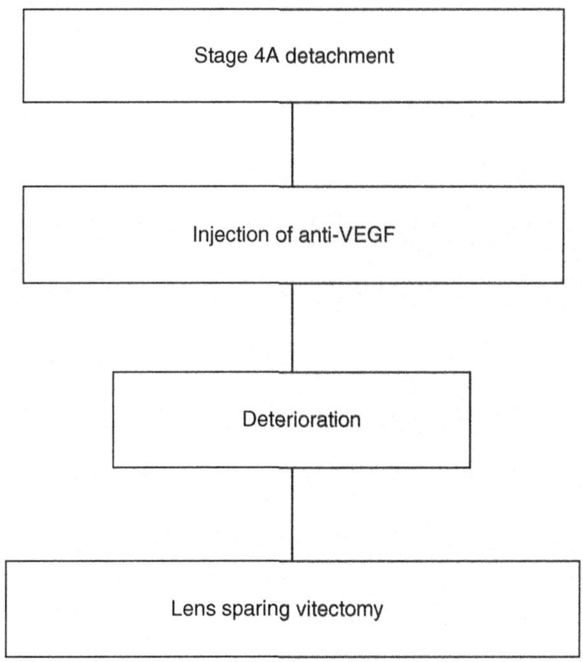

Fig. 21.2 Our treatment algorithm for treatment of stage 4A detachment. In case of stage 4B detachment, we operate immediately

21.4 Anatomical and Functional Outcome of Surgery for 4A and 4B Detachment

The outcome of retinal detachment surgery for newborns is very disillusioning. The anatomical outcome is poor, and the functional outcome is even poorer. The six-year follow-up of the ETROP study showed that only 10% of stage 4A detachments had a favourable visual acuity outcome but none of stage 4B and none of stage 5.

The ETROP study included 401 patients (802 eyes). 89 eyes (11%) developed a retinal detachment. 70 eyes were examined at a 6-year follow-up. Of these eyes, 28 eyes (40%) had a stage 4A, 14 eyes (20%) a stage 4B and 13 eyes (19%) a stage 5 detachment. 50 eyes (71%) were operated with vitrectomy and at the 6-year follow-up 17 eyes (34%) had an attached macula. Nine eyes (12%) were operated with encircling band and after 6 years 6 eyes (67%) had an attached macula. Eleven eyes (15%) were not operated and only observed and after 6 years 2 eyes (8%) had an attached macula. Regarding the stage of retinal detachment, 31% with stage 4A had an attached macula, 60% of stage 4B and 0% of stage 5. Regarding the functional outcome only eyes with a stage 4A detachment had a favorable visual acuity outcome: 10% of stage 4A eyes had a visual acuity >0.1 [12].

Conclusion If a retinal detachment occurs, the best chance for a favorable outcome is when a stage 4A detachment with attached macula is present. As soon as the macula is detached (stage 4B detachment) the prognosis is poor. Therefore, the therapeutic window of a stage 4A detachment must not be missed.

21.5 Surgery

The surgery is difficult, and you have to operate absolutely without complications: No lens touch, no retina touch and NO retinal tear. A lens touch will result in a lensectomy and amblyopia. A retinal touch with retinal tear will result in retinal detachment and blindness. Be careful when inserting the trocars and instruments. Insert the trocars perpendicular. Aim towards the optic nerve. Perform a central and peripheral vitrectomy. Do not induce a PVD; it is impossible in newborn. Do not come too close to the retina, you may induce a retinal tear. A tamponade is not necessary.

Surgery step-by-step (Table 21.1 and Figs. 21.1, 21.2, 21.3, and 21.4)

<u>**Instruments**</u>

1. 3-port 27G trocar system
2. 120D lens

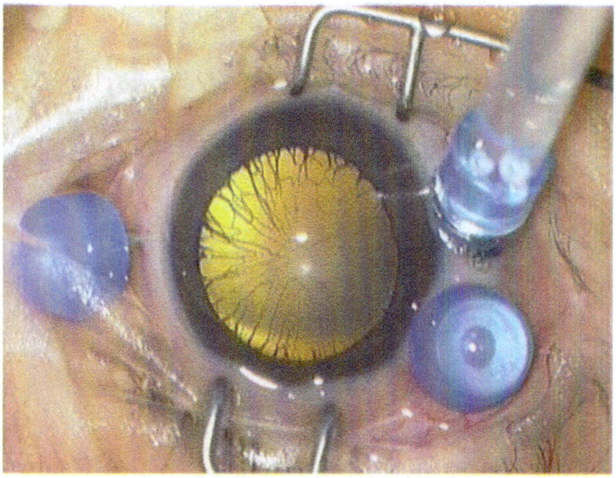

Fig. 21.3 A 27G lens sparing vitrectomy (DORC) in a newborn eye in 34th gestational week. Note the tunica vasculosa lentis

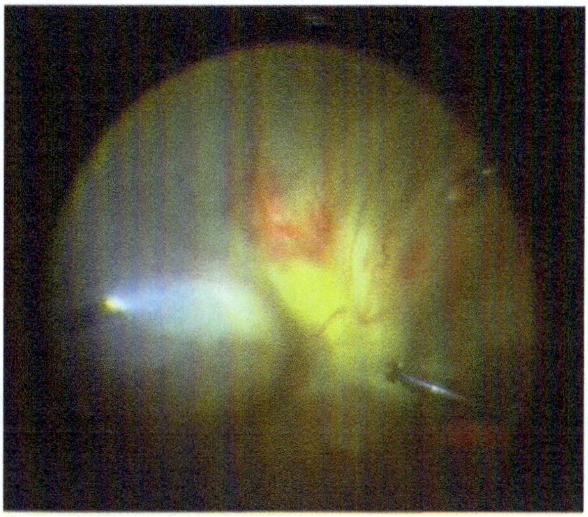

Fig. 21.4 A stage 4B detachment

Medication

- Lucentis®, alternatively Avastin®

Tamponade

- None

Individual steps

1. **3-port 27G trocar system**
2. **Core vitrectomy**

3. **Peripheral vitrectomy**
4. **Maybe air Tamponade**
5. **Removal of two trocars and infusion line**
6. **Injection of 0.05 ml Lucentis**
7. **Removal of instrument trocar**

The surgery step-by-step: (Figs. 21.3, 21.4, 21.5, 21.6, and 21.7)

1. **3-port 27G trocar system**

   Insert the trocar cannulas 1.0–1.5 mm behind the limbus. Aim with the trocar cannulas towards the optic nerve. We insert the trocars straight (perpendicular) into the eye due to the risk of damaging the lens (Fig. 21.3). The sclerotomies will remain watertight. Then attach the infusion line to the infusion trocar and double check that the infusion trocar is located inside the vitreous body.

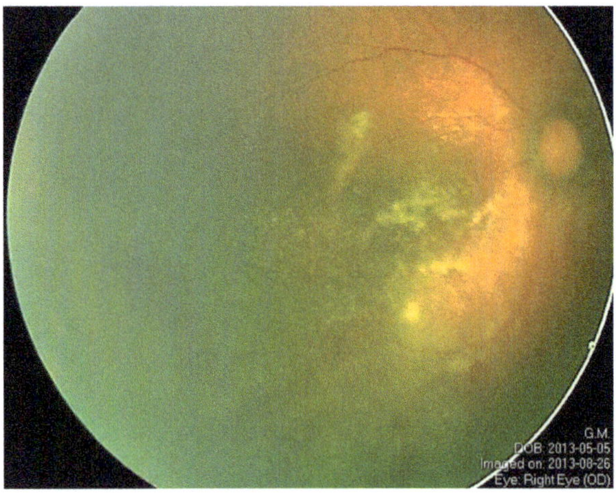

Fig. 21.5 The same eye with a 14-days follow up. The retina is reattached

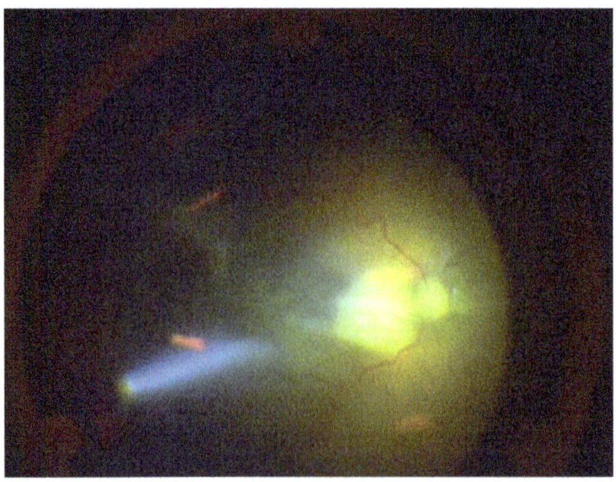

Fig. 21.6 A stage 4A detachment

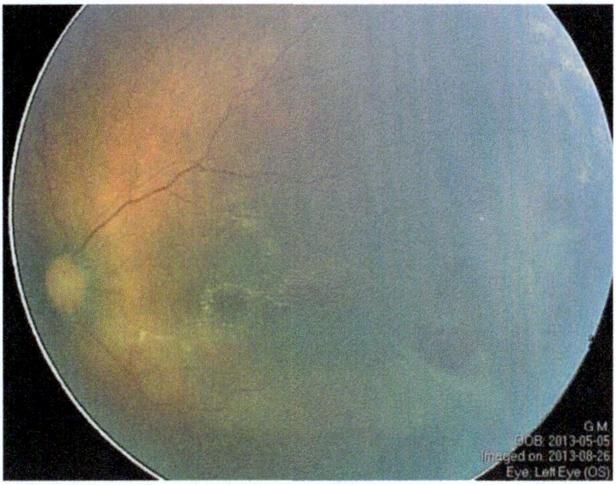

Fig. 21.7 The same eye with a 14-days follow up. The retina is reattached

Surgical pearls no. 73

Location of infusion cannula in pediatric vitrectomy: The infusion cannula tends to turn towards the lens resulting in a blockage of the infusion. The dangerous consequence of this event is a bulbar hypotony with choroidal detachment. Observe therefore constantly the position of the infusion trocar during surgery.

2. **Core vitrectomy**
3. **Peripheral vitrectomy**

   Insert the instruments carefully by aiming them towards the optic nerve. Remember: The lens of a newborn is much larger than the lens of an adult (ratio lens/globe). Begin with a core vitrectomy and continue then with a peripheral vitrectomy. Remove the vitreous only up to the equator. (Figs. 21.1, 21.4, and 21.6). Hold a secure distance to the retina. Caution: Avoid a retinal touch. If you induce an iatrogenic hole you can close the case.
4. **Tamponade**

   A tamponade is usually not necessary because a retinal break is not present. In case of a vitreous hemorrhage we recommend an air tamponade.
5. **Removal of two trocars**

   Remove first one instrument trocar. Remove then the infusion line with trocar. A suture is not necessary even if you performed a perpendicular incision!
6. **Injection of 0.05 ml Lucentis**

   Attach a 27G backflush cannula to the Lucentis syringe. Inject 0.05 ml Lucentis through the second instrument trocar into the vitreous cavity.

   Surgical pearls no. 74

   Anti-VEGF dose for ROP: We inject the adult dose of Lucentis. The reasoning for this is that a medication in an eye without vitreous body has a shorter half-life than in an eye with vitreous body. Alternatively inject 0.1 ml Avastin.
7. **Removal of instrument trocar**

   Remove finally second instrument trocar. Doing the injection this way ensures that no medication leaves the eye through the infusion line.

21.6 Complications

1. The infusion trocar may rotate towards the lens and block the infusion resulting in a choroidal detachment.
2. A retinal tear will lead inevitably to a retinal detachment which cannot be cured.
3. A lens touch will result in lensectomy and consequently amblyopia.

21.7 FAQ

Does the retina reattach after removal of the vitreous?
Yes. The vitreous body in newborns is completely intact. The vascular activity of the retina causes an inflammatory contraction of the vitreous resulting in retinal traction and detachment. If you remove the vitreous body and reduce the vascular activity with anti-VEGF, the retina will reattach within a few days.

21.8 Case Report No. 1: ROP Stage 4 (Figs. 21.3, 21.4, 21.5, 21.6, and 21.7)

The neonate was laser treated in the 36th gestational week because of ROP stage 3+. One week later the retina on both eyes was detached. The right eye presented with a stage 4B detachment, retinal exudates at the posterior pole and a big subretinal hemorrhage. The left eye had a stage 4A detachment.

Three 27G trocars with a lumen of 0.4 mm were inserted 1 mm behind the limbus. The insertion was performed perpendicularly (not lamellar). A central and peripheral vitrectomy was performed. The vitrectomy was performed with an EVA vitrectomy machine (DORC), a cutting speed of 7000 cuts/min and a vacuum of 500 mmHg. At the end, 0.65 mg bevacizumab was injected into the vitreous cavity. No PVD, no peeling and no tamponade were performed. The trocars were removed and the sclerotomies were not sutured. The surgical time of each eye was less than 20 min.

On the first postoperative day, the conjunctiva was white, the globe normotensive. The retina was completely attached on the LE and partially reattached on the RE. After 14 days follow-up, the retina was peripherally and centrally attached in both eyes (Figs. 21.5 and 21.7).

Further Reading

1. Capone A Jr, Trese MT. Lens-sparing vitreous surgery for tractional stage 4A retinopathy of prematurity retinal detachments. Ophthalmology. 2001;108(11):2068–70.
2. Hubbard GB 3rd, Cherwick DH, Burian G. Lens-sparing vitrectomy for stage 4 retinopathy of prematurity. Ophthalmology. 2004;111(12):2274–7.
3. Hartnett ME. Features associated with surgical outcome in patients with stages 4 and 5 retinopathy of prematurity. Retina. 2003;23(3):322–9.
4. Joshi MM, Trese MT, Capone A Jr. Optical coherence tomography findings in stage 4A retinopathy of prematurity: a theory for visual variability. Ophthalmology. 2006;113(4):657–60.
5. Kono T, Oshima K, Fuchino Y. Surgical results and visual outcomes of vitreous surgery for advanced stages of retinopathy of prematurity. Jpn J Ophthalmol. 2000;44(6):661–7.
6. Lakhanpal RR, Sun RL, Albini TA, Holz ER. Anatomic success rate after 3-port lens-sparing vitrectomy in stage 4A or 4B retinopathy of prematurity. Ophthalmology. 2005;112(9):1569–73.
7. Lakhanpal RR, Sun RL, Albini TA, Coffee R, Coats DK, Holz ER. Visual outcomes after 3-port lens-sparing vitrectomy in stage 4 retinopathy of prematurity. Arch Ophthalmol. 2006;124(5):675–9.
8. Moshfeghi AA, Banach MJ, Salam GA, Ferrone PJ. Lens-sparing vitrectomy for progressive tractional retinal detachments associated with stage 4A retinopathy of prematurity. Arch Ophthalmol. 2004;122(12):1816–8.
9. Moshfeghi AA, Awner S, Salam GA, Ferrone PJ. Excellent visual outcome and reversal of dragging after lens sparing vitrectomy for progressive tractional stage 4a retinopathy of prematurity retinal detachment. Retina. 2004;24(4):615–6.
10. Prenner JL, Capone A Jr, Trese MT. Visual outcomes after lens-sparing vitrectomy for stage 4A retinopathy of prematurity. Ophthalmology. 2004;111(12):2271–3.
11. Repka MX, Tung B, Good WV, Shapiro M, Capone A Jr, Baker JD, Barr CC, Phelps DL, van Heuven WA. Outcome of eyes developing retinal detachment during the Early Treatment for Retinopathy of Prematurity Study (ETROP). Arch Ophthalmol. 2006;124(1):24–30.
12. Repka MX, Tung B, Good WV, Capone A Jr, Shapiro MJ. Outcome of eyes developing retinal detachment during the Early Treatment for Retinopathy of Prematurity study. Arch Ophthalmol. 2011;129(9):1175–9.
13. Trese MT, Droste PJ. Long-term postoperative results of a consecutive series of stages 4 and 5 retinopathy of prematurity. Ophthalmology. 1998;105(6):992–7.

Chapter 22
Scleral Buckling for ROP Stage 4A and 4B

A scleral buckling is not a logical therapy in a non-rhegmatogenous retinal detachment because there is no retinal hole to seal. The band impresses the sclera and presses the retinal pigment epithelium against the retina. The reattachment after a buckling procedure is therefore a slow process and may take several weeks. A vitrectomy, in contrast, is a logical therapy in a retinal detachment secondary to ROP because the contracted vitreous is removed allowing the retina to reattach. The healing process after a vitrectomy is fast and reattachment needs only a few days.

If a stage 4A detachment with a temporal detachment is present, then a segmental buckle is sufficient. If a stage 4A detachment involves the nasal and temporal periphery then an encircling band is necessary.

Segmental buckle: Perform a peritomy from 12 to 6 o'clock. Place three holding sutures under the superior, temporal and inferior straight muscles. Place the segmental buckle on the equator from 2 o'clock to 4 o'clock in a left eye and from 8 to 10 o'clock in a right eye.

Encircling band: Perform a 360 deg peritomy and place four holding sutures. Fasten a 2.5 mm band on the equator with non-resorbable sutures. Aspirate aqueous from the anterior chamber with a 30G needle to achieve hypotony and then tighten the band.

The anatomic success of encircling bands takes several weeks and is fairly good. The functional outcome, however, is poor. The encircling band induces a high myopia of approximately 10 diopters and diminishes the ocular blood flow [1]. The encircling band must be removed or cut after 6 months because it inhibits the growth of the neonate's globe. If the cerclage is removed or relaxed after 6 months, then the myopia reduces to −5 diopters.

Electronic Supplementary Material The online version of this chapter (https://doi.org/10.1007/978-3-030-13701-4_22) contains supplementary material, which is available to authorized users.
The videos can be accessed under http://extras.springer.com/Search. Enter the ISBN number of your book and download the videos.

U. Spandau, S. J. Kim, *Pediatric Retinal Vascular Diseases*,
https://doi.org/10.1007/978-3-030-13701-4_22

Case report
A neonate with ROP stage 4 in the left eye was operated with an encircling band only on the left eye. His postoperative refraction was +1.5 diopters in the right eye and −12 diopters in the left eye. The left eye had an esotropia and amblyopia. Ten months later, the encircling band was removed and the myopia reduced to −11 diopters. Conclusion: A (too) late encircling band removal results in grave myopia.

Reference

1. Lincoff H, Stopa M, Kreissig I, Madjarov B, Sarup V, Saxena S, Brodie S. Cutting the encircling band. Retina. 2006;26(6):650–4.

Chapter 23
Posterior Hyaloid Contraction Syndrome

Retinal detachments in pediatric vasoproliferative disorders such as retinopathy of prematurity (ROP) and familial exudative vitreoretinopathy (FEVR) have an exudative and tractional component. Young eyes have a very adherent posterior hyaloid. Contraction of the posterior hyaloid interface may lead to a tractional retinal detachment [1].

The posterior hyaloid contraction syndrome may occur after a primary vitrectomy. In the initial surgery a core vitrectomy without posterior vitreous detachment (PVD) was performed (Fig. 23.1a). A few weeks after the primary vitrectomy a posterior vitreous detachment may occur (Fig. 23.1b). The detached posterior vitreous contracts resulting in a retinal traction with a retinal detachment. In case of strong tractions subretinal hemorrhages may develop (Figs. 23.1b and 23.2).

Surgical treatment
Schedule immediately a second vitrectomy. A 25G or 27G setup is advisable. Remove the posterior vitreous and hyaloid and repeat an anti-VEGF injection. A complete induction of posterior vitreous is not recommended because it may induce retinal tears. A lensectomy is not necessary. An air tamponade is not required.

Electronic Supplementary Material The online version of this chapter (https://doi.org/10.1007/978-3-030-13701-4_23) contains supplementary material, which is available to authorized users.
The videos can be accessed under http://extras.springer.com/Search. Enter the ISBN number of your book and download the videos.

U. Spandau, S. J. Kim, *Pediatric Retinal Vascular Diseases*,
https://doi.org/10.1007/978-3-030-13701-4_23

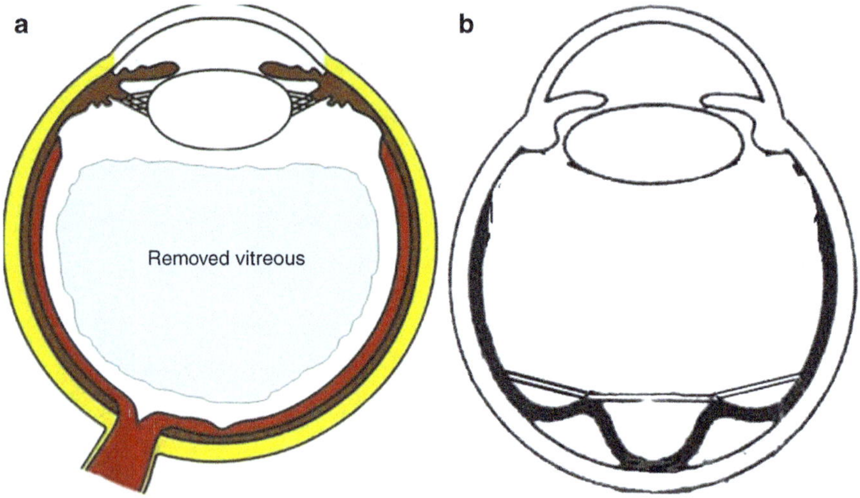

Fig. 23.1 Status after core vitrectomy (**a**). A few weeks later a PVD may occur resulting in retinal traction (**b**)

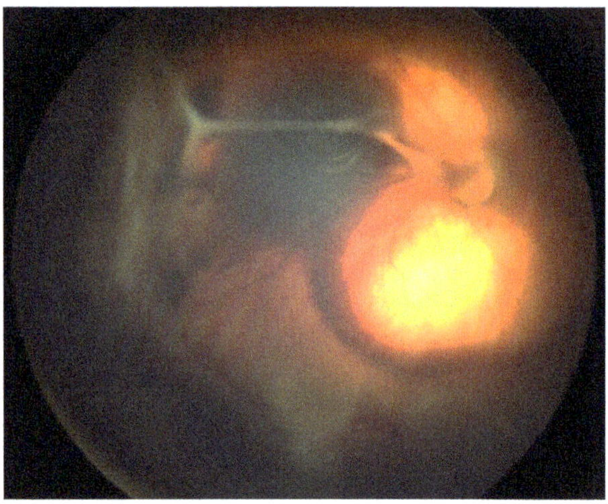

Fig. 23.2 A posterior hyaloidal contraction syndrome. The posterior hyaloid detached and contracted. In this case a recurrent retinal detachment stage 4B with subretinal bleeding occurred

Reference

1. Joshi MM, Ciaccia S, Trese MT, Capone A Jr. Posterior hyaloid contracture in pediatric vitreoretinopathies. Retina. 2006;26(7 Supplement):S38–41.

Chapter 24
Retinal Detachment Stage 4A and 4B with Fibrovascular Membranes

In a small group of newborns with ROP a tractional retinal detachment caused by fibrovascular membranes may develop (Figs. 24.1, 24.2, and 24.3). These fibrovascular membranes extend from the peripheral retina to the lens and pull the retina forwards towards the lens and ciliary body. Even more fibrovascular membranes can develop within the vitreous cavity (Fig. 24.1).

All these fibrovascular membranes can extend for many clock hours narrowing the available space for surgical approach. The surgical entry space may be too narrow or closed for insertion of trocars. The surgical aim is to remove the vectors of traction to relax the retina while preserving the lens and avoiding retinal breaks. In these difficult cases, however, a lensectomy is often required. The surgical repair is difficult, and the outcome of these eyes is poor.

Two surgical techniques are possible:

1. Removal of the membranes with a vitreous cutter.
2. Removal of membranes with a knife.

1. **Removal of the membranes with a vitreous cutter** (Figs. 24.4, 24.5, and 24.6): A vitrectomy becomes very difficult if fibrovascular membranes from the retina to the lens are present. A prominent retinal fold develops from the ridge and adheres to the posterior lens capsule. These membranes prevent an insertion of trocars. Determine first the location of the membranes with binocular ophthalmoscopy and then insert the trocars in a membrane-free space. This is often the nasal side of the eye. If you don't find an entry for the trocars, then a lensectomy has to be performed. Perform a core vitrectomy and then cut and remove the fibrous vascular membranes.

Electronic Supplementary Material The online version of this chapter (https://doi.org/10.1007/978-3-030-13701-4_24) contains supplementary material, which is available to authorized users.
The videos can be accessed under http://extras.springer.com/Search. Enter the ISBN number of your book and download the videos.

U. Spandau, S. J. Kim, *Pediatric Retinal Vascular Diseases*,
https://doi.org/10.1007/978-3-030-13701-4_24

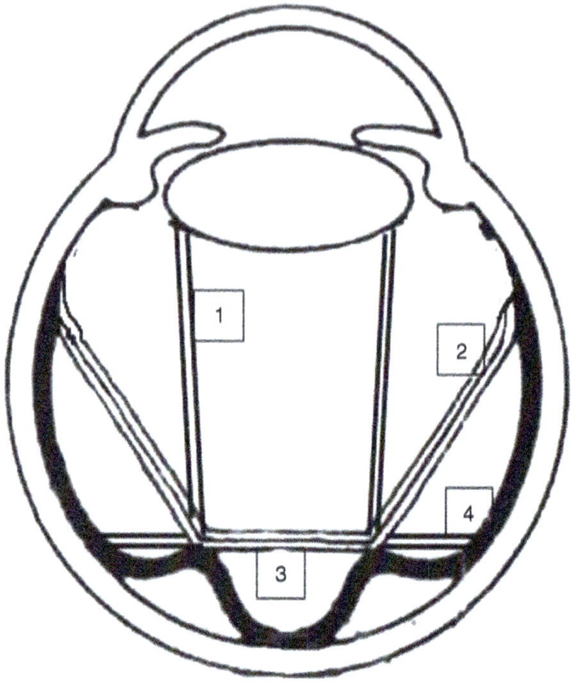

Fig. 24.1 Drawing demonstrating the tractional vectors in advanced retinopathy of prematurity from ridge to lens (1), from retina to the ciliary body (2) from the ridge to ridge (3) and from the ridge to the retina (4)

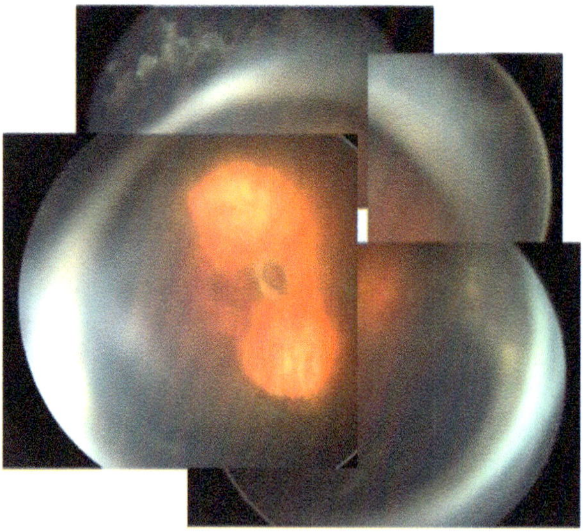

Fig. 24.2 Fibrovascular membranes growing from the ridge to the posterior part of the lens. The membranes grow at the temporal, superior side and nasal pole. Trocars can only be inserted inferior. A lensectomy may be the best choice in this case

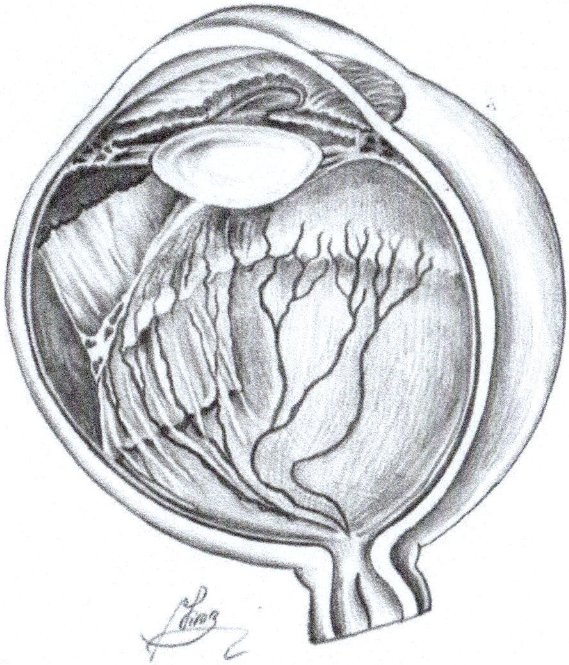

Fig. 24.3 Fibrovascular membrane stretching from the ischemic retina up to the lens. Drawing from Dr. Antoni Firoz

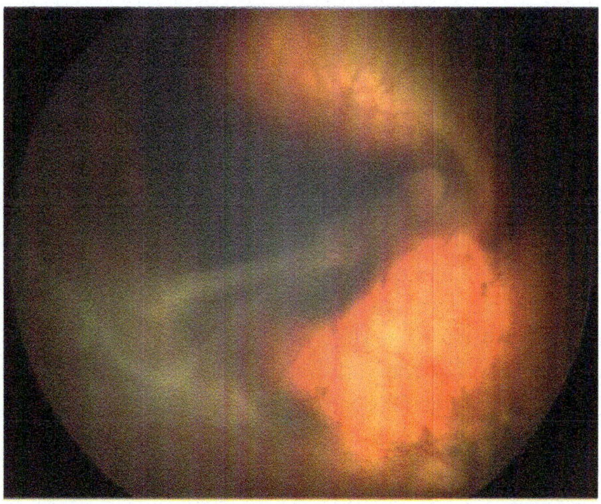

Fig. 24.4 Primary retinal detachment stage 4B with subretinal bleeding and a fibrovascular membrane from the ridge to the posterior part of the lens

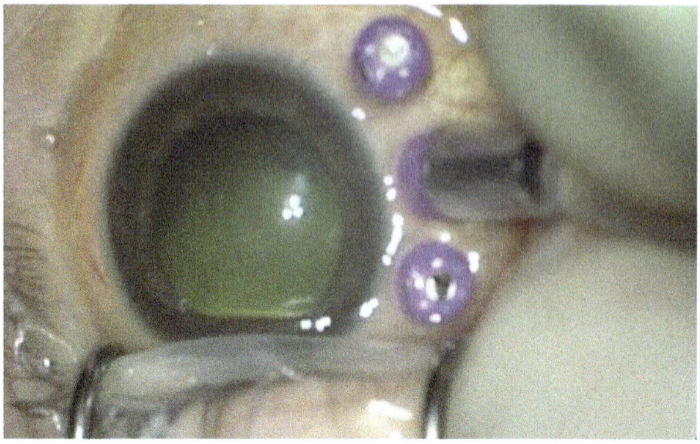

Fig. 24.5 The same eye as Fig. 24.3. An insertion of trocars on the temporal side is not possible. All trocars are inserted on the nasal side

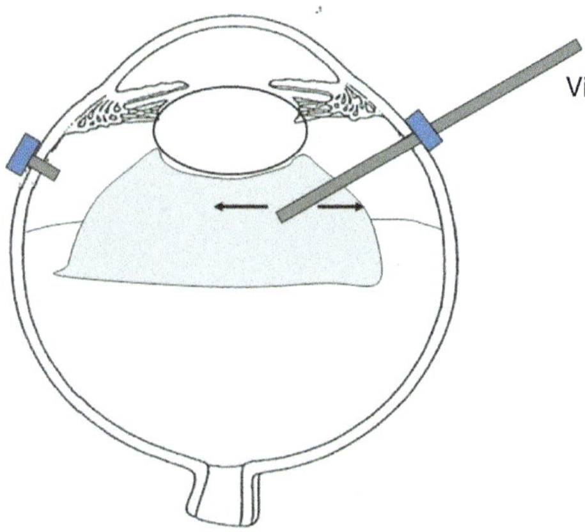

Fig. 24.6 Insert the trocars in a membrane-free area. Then remove the membrane with a vitreous cutter

2. **Removal of membranes with a knife** (Fig. 24.7): These complications can be avoided by using a vitreoretinal microblade for membrane incisions. Once the sclera is entered, the microblade is first directed carefully into the space between the retina and posterior lens capsule. The membrane extending anteriorly from the ridge is cut using the blade for sharp dissection. This relieves anterior retinal traction, and posterior relaxation of the retina is immediately apparent. This incision can be extended for many clock hours by sweeping in the surgical space parallel to the lens capsule using the sclerotomy as a pivot point or by sliding the blade like a saw to release any tractional vectors. Now adequate space has been created for the ensuing vitrectomy. Dissect the proliferation along the retinal surface. Care must be taken to avoid injuring the crystalline lens or causing an unintentional retinal break [1].

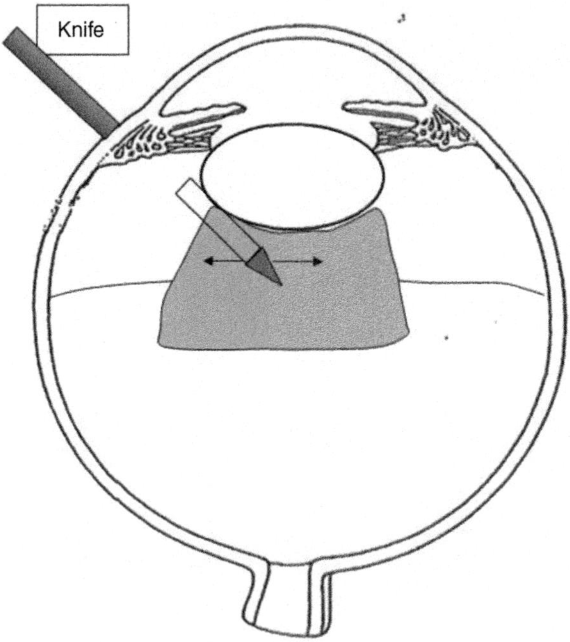

Fig. 24.7 Ab interno transection of retrolental membrane. A microblade is inserted through the pars plicata into the surgical space between the lens and the retinal fold. The membrane is first punctured and then swept laterally. This allows a safer entry site for the vitreous cutter

Reference

1. Repka MX, Tung B, Good WV, Shapiro M, Capone A Jr, Baker JD, Barr CC, Phelps DL, van Thomas BJ, Yonekawa Y, Trese MT. Complete resolution of large retinal fold after transection of retrolental membrane during lens-sparing vitrectomy for retinopathy of prematurity: a 15-year follow-up. Retin Cases Brief Rep. 2016;10:93–5.

Chapter 25
Stage 5 ROP

Vitreoretinal surgery of stage 5 ROP is very controversial among vitreoretinal surgeons due to limited anatomical and functional results. Some surgeons such as Dr. Zivojnovic claim that stage 5 ROP is not operable (oral communication). Other surgeons claim that even a minimal functional outcome is positive for the newborn meaning that surgery is worth trying. The ETROP study found that surgery for stage 5 ROP was associated with some anatomical success but poor functional outcome. Surgery resulted in anatomical success in none of newborns and none achieved a visual acuity of >0.1 (Table 25.1) [1]. Cusick M shows better results. His surgery resulted in anatomical success in about one third of newborns and 4% achieved a visual acuity of >0.05 [2].

The retina of eyes at stage 5 ROP is more vulnerable to a recurrence of the RD than in eyes at stage 4B after being attached by vitrectomy. A recurrent RD occurred in 5% at stage 4B ROP and 22% of eyes with stage 5 ROP. The recurrence developed at 2–10 years of age (median, 4 years) [3].

Table 25.1 Outcome of vitreoretinal surgery in stage 4A, stage 4B and stage 5 according to the ETROP study with 401 patients [1]

ETROP study (n = 401)	All RD's	Stage 4A	Stage 4B	Stage 5
Rate of RD's	n = 89 (11%)	n = 28 (40%)	n = 14 (20%)	n = 13 (19%)
Overall attachment After vitreoretinal surgery	33%	31%	60%	0%
Vitrectomy with encircling band	71% (34% with attached macula)			
Encircling band	12% (67% with attached macula)			
Favorable VA	10%	10%	0%	0%

U. Spandau, S. J. Kim, *Pediatric Retinal Vascular Diseases*,
https://doi.org/10.1007/978-3-030-13701-4_25

Stage 5 ROP may present in different anatomic shapes of the funnel. The funnel may be anterior open and posterior open (Fig. 25.1a). The funnel may be anterior open and closed in the posterior part (Fig. 25.1b). Surgery becomes very difficult if the anterior part of the funnel is closed (Fig. 25.1c, d). Some surgeons perform in these cases an open sky vitrectomy. They open the cornea, remove the lens, perform a vitrectomy and suture the cornea back to place [4].

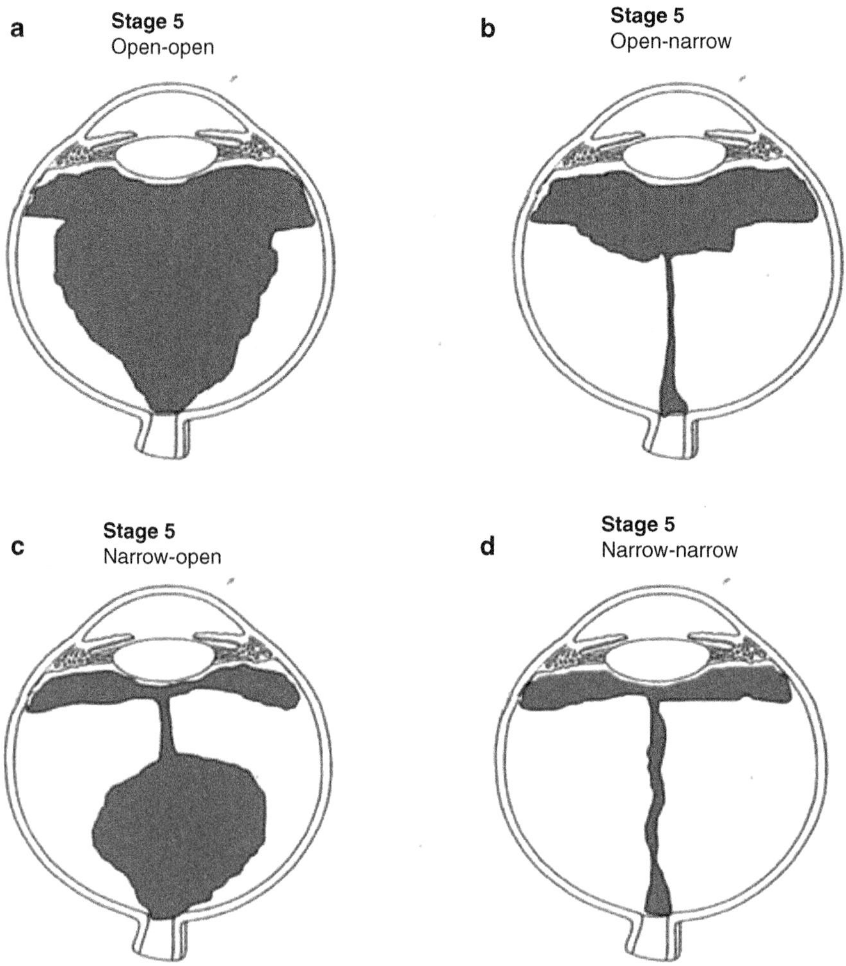

Fig. 25.1 (**a–d**) The different stages of ROP stage 5 are depicted

Further Reading

1. Repka MX, Tung B, Good WV, Capone A Jr, Shapiro MJ. Outcome of eyes developing retinal detachment during the Early Treatment for Retinopathy of Prematurity study. Arch Ophthalmol. 2011;129(9):1175–9.
2. Cusick M, Charles MK, Agrón E, Sangiovanni JP, Ferris FL 3rd, Charles S. Anatomical and visual results of vitreoretinal surgery for stage 5 retinopathy of prematurity. Retina. 2006;26(7):729–35.
3. Kondo H, Arita N, Osato M, Hayashi H, Oshima K, Uchio E. Late recurrence of retinal detachment following successful vitreous surgery for stages 4B and 5 retinopathy of prematurity. Am J Ophthalmol. 2009;147(4):661–666.e1.
4. Hirose T, Katsumi O, Mehta MC, Schepens CL. Vision in stage 5 retinopathy of prematurity after retinal reattachment by open-sky vitrectomy. Arch Ophthalmol. 1993;111(3):345–9.
5. Fuchino Y, Hayashi H, Kono T, Ohshima K. Long-term follow up of visual acuity in eyes with stage 5 retinopathy of prematurity after closed vitrectomy. Am J Ophthalmol. 1995;120(3):308–16.
6. Hartnett ME. Features associated with surgical outcome in patients with stages 4 and 5 retinopathy of prematurity. Retina. 2003;23(3):322–9.
7. Kono T, Oshima K, Fuchino Y. Surgical results and visual outcomes of vitreous surgery for advanced stages of retinopathy of prematurity. Jpn J Ophthalmol. 2000;44(6):661–7.
8. Mintz-Hittner HA, O'Malley RE, Kretzer FL. Long-term form identification vision after early, closed, lensectomy-vitrectomy for stage 5 retinopathy of prematurity. Ophthalmology. 1997;104(3):454–9.
9. Repka MX, Tung B, Good WV, Shapiro M, Capone A Jr, Baker JD, Barr CC, Phelps DL, van Heuven WA. Outcome of eyes developing retinal detachment during the Early Treatment for Retinopathy of Prematurity Study (ETROP). Arch Ophthalmol. 2006;124(1):24–30.
10. Trese MT, Droste PJ. Long-term postoperative results of a consecutive series of stages 4 and 5 retinopathy of prematurity. Ophthalmology. 1998;105(6):992–7.
11. Trese MT. Visual results and prognostic factors for vision following surgery for stage V retinopathy of prematurity. Ophthalmology. 1986;93(5):574–9.
12. Seaber JH, Machemer R, Eliott D, Buckley EG, deJuan E, Martin DF. Long-term visual results of children after initially successful vitrectomy for stage V retinopathy of prematurity. Ophthalmology. 1995;102(2):199–204.
13. Trese MT. Surgical results of stage V retrolental fibroplasia and timing of surgical repair. Ophthalmology. 1984;91(5):461–6.

Chapter 26
Visual Outcome of Very Preterm Neonates at 6.5 Years of Age

We, who work with ROP neonates, wonder about the outcome of our small patients. How is their vision, how is their mental status, how will they do in life? Well, the answer is not easy, and the outcome is very different from neonate to neonate. Regarding the visual outcome a big Swedish study has recently been published examining ROP children at 6.5 years of age [1].

This Swedish study compares the visual outcome of very preterm neonates (<27 weeks GA) with a control group of term born neonates (40 weeks GA). All extremely premature born neonates within the time period of 2004 to 2007 were included in the study. The study included 486 participants with ROP and was compared with 300 control group children. The percentage of blind children with ROP was 2.5% compared to 0% in the control group. The percentage of visually impairment (VA from 0.1 to 0.5) occurred in 5.6% of ROP neonates compared to 1% in the control group. The overall visual impairment in very preterm neonates with ROP is 9% compared to the control group with 1%.

The percentage of very preterm neonates with strabism was 17.4% compared to 0% in the control group. And the percentage of refractive errors in the ROP group was 29.7% compared to 6% in the control group. The spherical range of refractive errors in the very preterm group varied from −13.50 to +10.25 D compared to −1.13 to +6.81 D in the control group.

Another study investigated the rate of non-visual impairment of children with severe ROP at 5.5 years of age [2]. Nonvisual impairments included severe hearing loss, motor and cognitive. Of the children with severe retinopathy, 39.5% had at least 1 nonvisual disability at 5 years compared with 15.8% of children without it ($P < .001$).

In order to illustrate the different outcome, we will show the visual outcome of three neonates who were born in week 23 and 24 and treated for ROP in zone I. Two neonates were twins and treated with Avastin only and one neonate was treated with laser and Avastin.

U. Spandau, S. J. Kim, *Pediatric Retinal Vascular Diseases*,
https://doi.org/10.1007/978-3-030-13701-4_26

Case 1 (Fig. 26.1) This neonate was born in week 24 with a birth weight of 716 g. A difficult necrotizing enterocolitis occurred with short-bowel syndrome after bowel resections. The neonate was treated with laser photocoagulation for ROP in zone I. Two weeks later a recurrence occurred, and he was treated with a completing laser. Again, 2 weeks later a plus disease occurred. We injected in both eyes anti-VEGF and the plus disease disappeared.

The *8-year follow-up* showed a fine anatomical outcome in the right eye (Fig. 26.1). The visual acuity is 0.25 with own glasses. The left eye has a macular dragging and amblyopia. The refractive error is −5.25/− 2.5 cylinder 40° in the right eye and −4.25/−2 cylinder 150° in the left eye.

Case 2 A premature born triplet, born after 23 weeks with a weight of 495 g. Operated with acute laparotomy due to NEC. He developed sepsis a couple of times as well as liver affection due to CMV infection. He was diagnosed with ROP 3+ in zone I and received an intravitreal injection of Avastin 0.65 mg bilaterally. The ROP disease disappeared and no further treatment was required.The *7-year follow-up* showed a refractive error and visual acuity of +5.25/−1.25/152 = 0.3 (right eye) and + 6.25/−1.75/41 = 0.3 (left eye). The binocular visual acuity was 0.4. An esotropia and nystagmus was present in the left eye. According to the mother he was not doing as well as his brother.

Case 3 The twin brother of case 2 had a much better visual acuity outcome. This male triplet was born in week 23 and a birth weight of 585 g. He had a laparotomy for NEC. In addition, hypothyroidism and pulmonary hypertension were diagnosed. A ROP 3+ occurred in zone I and was treated with a bilateral injection of 0.5 mg Avastin. The plus disease disappeared and did not recur again.At the *7 years follow-up* a visual acuity of +2.75sph = 0.8 (right eye) and + 2.75sph = 0.9 (left eye) was recorded. According to the mother he is well functioning. He has a normal viewing status, even if a stereo function could not be detected with certainty. The retina looked normal, but some tortuous vessels are present (Fig. 26.2).

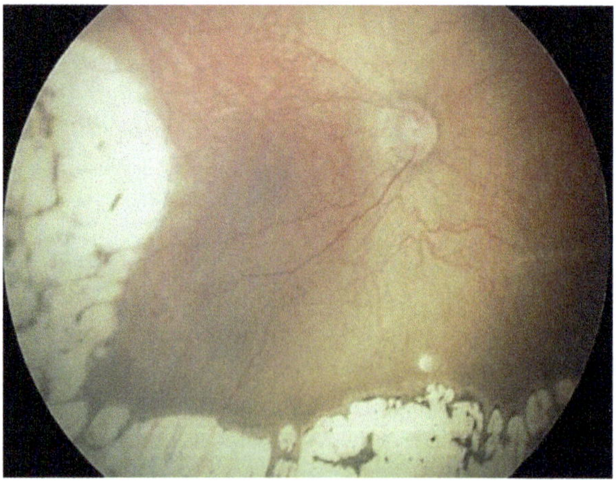

Fig. 26.1 RE: The retina after two laser treatments and one Avastin injection. VA is 0.25

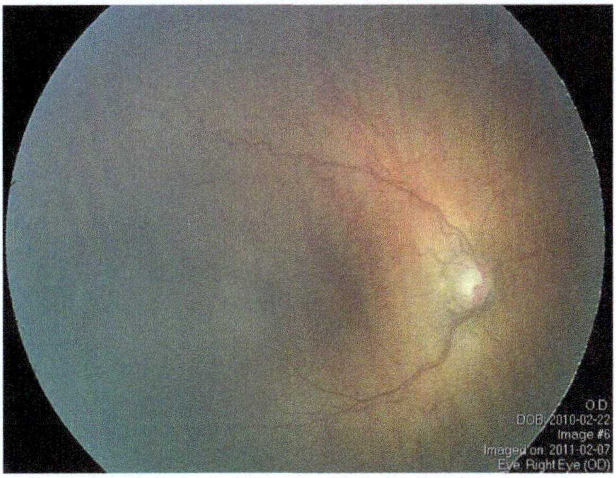

Fig. 26.2 RE: 1 year after treatment with 1× Avastin. The retina is fully vascularized. VA at 7 years follow-up is 0.8

References

1. Hellgren KM, Tornqvist K, Jakobsson PG, Lundgren P, Carlsson B, Källén K, Serenius F, Hellström A, Holmström G. Ophthalmologic outcome of extremely preterm infants at 6.5 years of age: extremely preterm infants in Sweden Study (EXPRESS). JAMA Ophthalmol. 2016; https://doi.org/10.1001/jamaophthalmol.2016.0391.
2. Schmidt B, Davis PG, Asztalos EV, Solimano A, Roberts RS. Association between severe retinopathy of prematurity and nonvisual disabilities at age 5 years. JAMA. 2014;311(5):523–5. https://doi.org/10.1001/jama.2013.282153.

Part VIII

Case Series Reports

The case series report is divided up in *three* chapters. The *first chapter* (1) shows pediatric retinal diseases such as FEVR, Incontinentia pigmenti and successful ROP cases. The *second chapter* (2) shows treatment failures of ROP disease from the authors' clinics. The *third chapter* (3) documents ROP treatment failures from the literature.

Chapter 27
Pediatric Retinal Diseases

27.1 Case Report No. 1: Neurofibromatosis Type 2 (Figs. 27.1 and 27.2)

A 5 y/o boy was referred to our hospital for surgery of an epiretinal membrane in the right eye. He was diagnosed with neurofibromatosis type 2. In December 2012 a large tumor in his brain was surgically removed. He has a remaining tumor affecting balance and hearing; furthermore, an intraspinal tumor. He is treated for epilepsy.

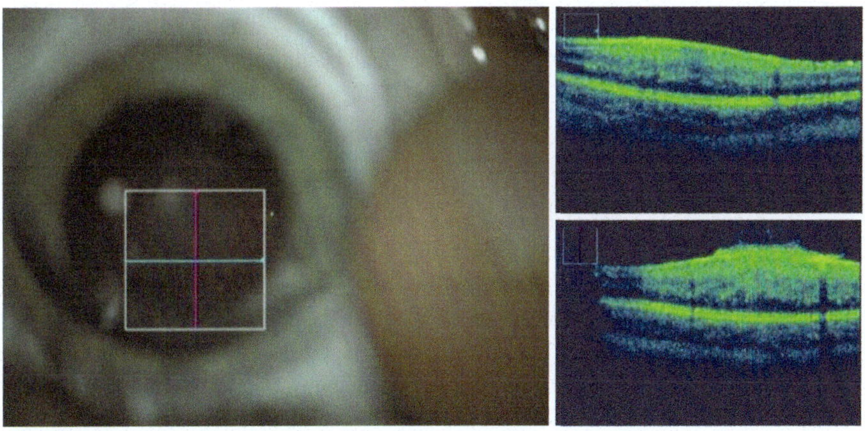

Fig. 27.1 Intraoperative OCT (Zeiss, Rescab 700) of a boy with an epiretinal membrane secondary to neurofibromatosis type 2

Electronic Supplementary Material The online version of this chapter (https://doi.org/10.1007/978-3-030-13701-4_27) contains supplementary material, which is available to authorized users.
The videos can be accessed under http://extras.springer.com/Search. Enter the ISBN number of your book and download the videos.

U. Spandau, S. J. Kim, *Pediatric Retinal Vascular Diseases*,
https://doi.org/10.1007/978-3-030-13701-4_27

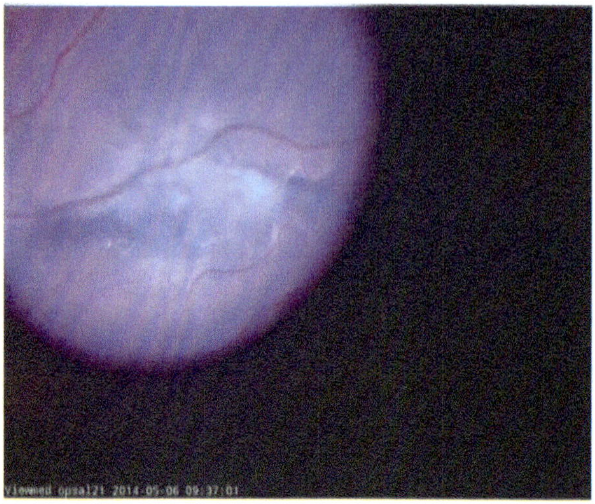

Fig. 27.2 Photograph of the epiretinal membrane

Visual acuity was measured with 0.8 on both eyes; it was not possible to measure the visual acuity of each eye. A fundus examination showed a whitish epiretinal membrane on the macula (Fig. 27.1).

Three months later a 27G lens sparing vitrectomy was performed (Fig. 27.2). The membrane was delaminated with the 27G Atkinson cannula and removed with the 27G endgripping forceps (DORC).

An examination 9 months later showed a visual acuity of 0.2 on the right eye, 1.0 on the left eye and OCT revealed a thickening of the macula very similar to the preoperative OCT. The surgery achieved no functional improvement.

27.2 Case Report No. 2: Persistent Hyperplastic Primary Vitreous (PHPV) (Figs. 27.3, 27.4, and 27.5)

A 23 days old newborn was admitted to us for surgery of a retinal detachment of the right eye (Fig. 27.4). At birth the right eye had a big pupil which did not react to light. There was no red reflex. The fellow eye was normal. An examination in general anaesthesia was performed. The axial length on the right eye was measured with 14.60 mm and white-to-white with 10 mm. An anterior segment examination showed a strong iris hyperemia, posterior synechiae at 6 o'clock and a zonular lysis from to 11 to 1 o'clock. A white vascularized tissue behind the lens was present (Fig. 27.5). B-scan revealed a funnel shaped hyperreflectivity from the optic nerve to the lens. The retina seemed to be attached. The examination of the left eye

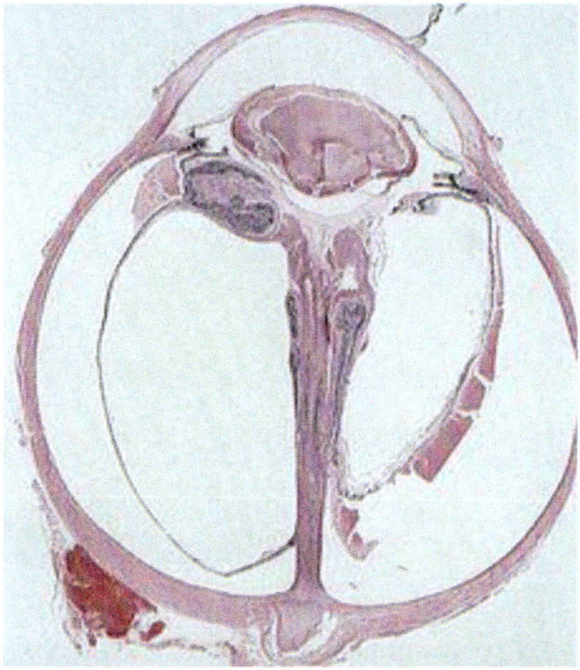

Fig. 27.3 Persistent-hyperplastic-primary-vitreous (PHPV). A closed funnel from the optic head to the lens. (Photocourtesy Wikipedia)

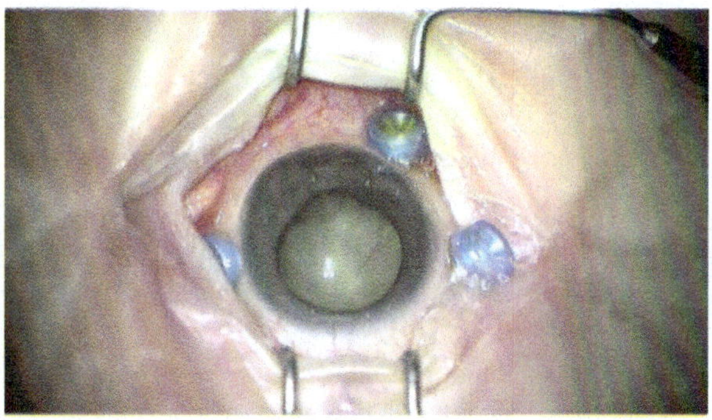

Fig. 27.4 A newborn with unlitateral PHPV. Note the retolental mass

revealed an axial length of 16.81 mm and a W-t-W of 11 mm. Anterior segment and posterior segments were regular.

The parents were informed about the findings and consented into an operation. A 27G lens sparing vitrectomy was performed and the retrolental tissue was removed (Figs. 27.4 and 27.5). The view to fundus was poor and it seemed that retinal vessels were visible.

An ERG is scheduled in 6 months.

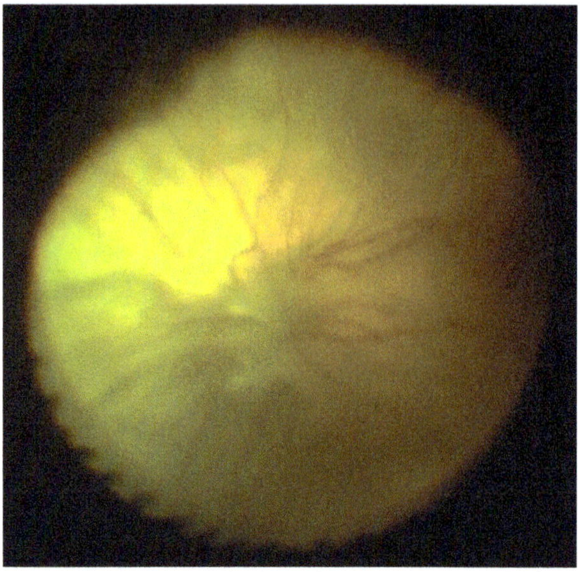

Fig. 27.5 The retrolental tissue

27.3 Case Report No. 3: FEVR (Figs. 27.6, 27.7, 27.8, 27.9, 27.10, 27.11, 27.12, 27.13, 27.14, 27.15, 27.16, 27.17, 27.18, 27.19, and 27.20)

General history: A 9-year-old girl was referred for unclear retinal pathology in the right eye and visual acuity decrease in the left eye in the last 6 months. A squint was observed in the left eye. Positive trauma history for 1 year ago.

Ocular examination:

- Visual acuity: RE: 0.7 and LE:0.05.
- The right eye had clear optical media. The retina showed fibrovascular proliferations at the temporal pole (Fig. 27.6) and reduced retinal vascularization in the periphery. The left eye had no view to retina due to a dense vitreous hemorrhage (Fig. 27.7). A bilateral intravitreal Lucentis injection in general anaesthesia was performed. Three weeks later an Optos photo revealed an almost unchanged fundus on the right eye (Fig. 27.8) and a diminished and dense vitreous hemorrhage in the left eye (Fig. 27.9).

One month later an examination of the right eye and a surgery of the left eye was performed. In the RE a Retcam angiography showed a peripheral retinal ischemia with proliferations (Fig. 27.10). A laser photocoagulation with indirect ophthalmoscopy (LIO) was performed (Fig. 27.11). In the LE a lens sparing vitrectomy was performed (see video 27.4).

One month after surgery an Optos photo and angiography was performed. The Optos photography showed pigmented laser scars in the temporal periphery

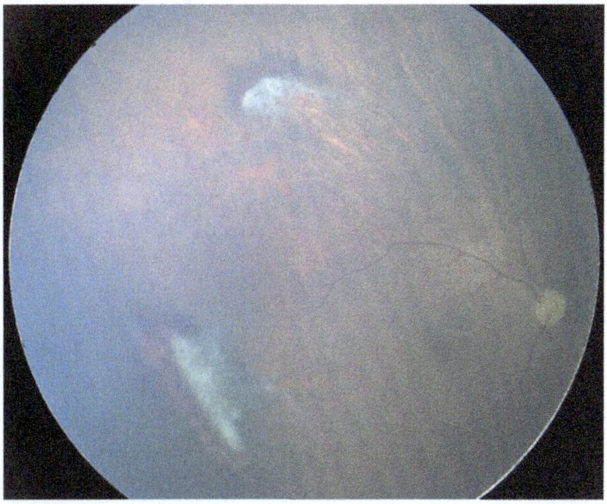

Fig. 27.6 RE: Initial examination with Retcam

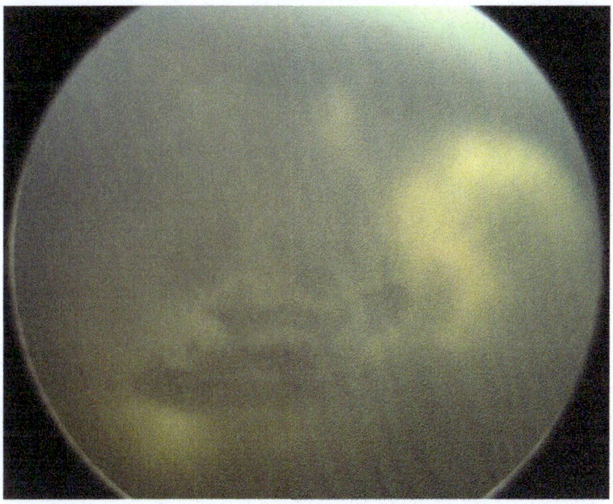

Fig. 27.7 LE: Vitreous hemorrhage

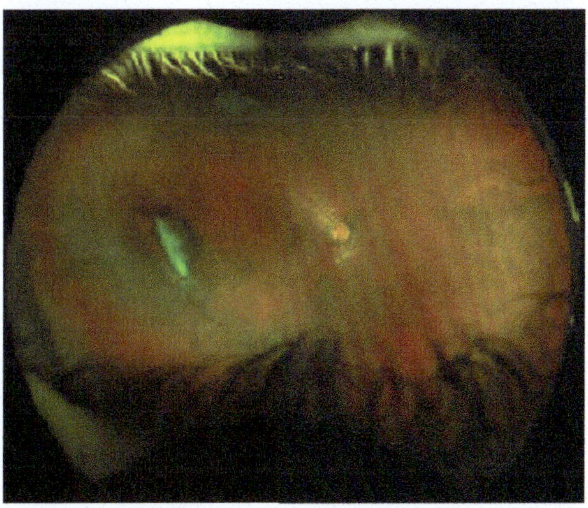

Fig. 27.8 **RE:** One month after Lucentis treatment

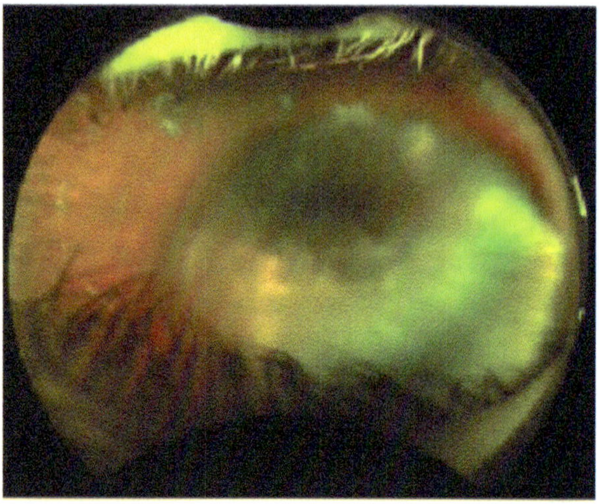

Fig. 27.9 LE: One month after Lucentis treatment

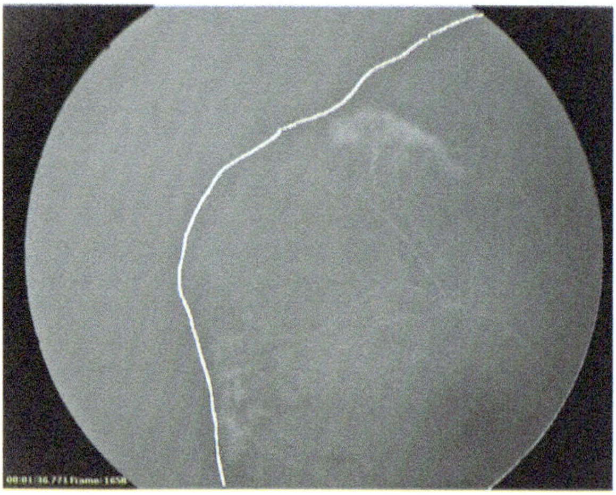

Fig. 27.10 RE: Retcam angiography. The white line demarcates the physiologic from the ischemic retina

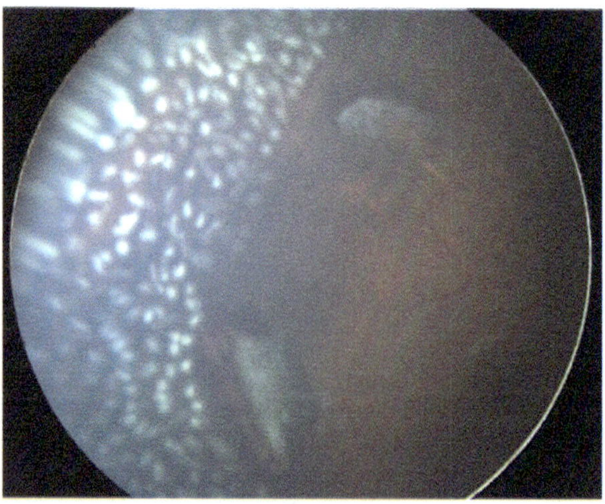

Fig. 27.11 RE: Retcam photography. The ischemic retina was treated with peripheral LIO laser. The picture was taken directly after laser treatment

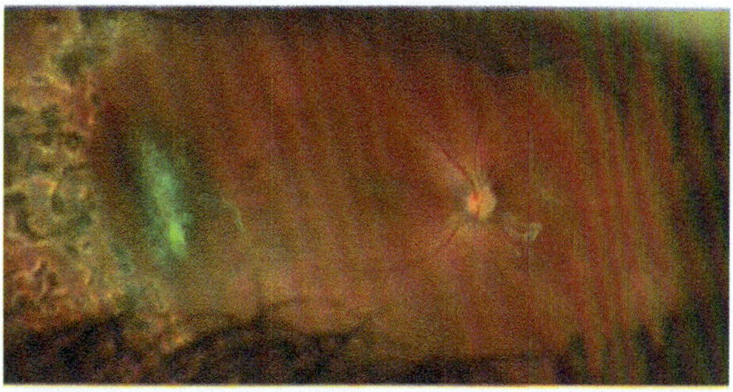

Fig. 27.12 RE: Optos photography. One month after laser (LIO) treatment

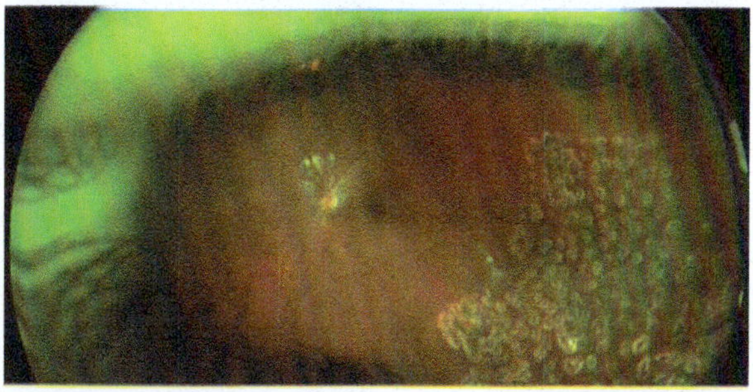

Fig. 27.13 LE: Optos photography. One month after lens sparing vitrectomy

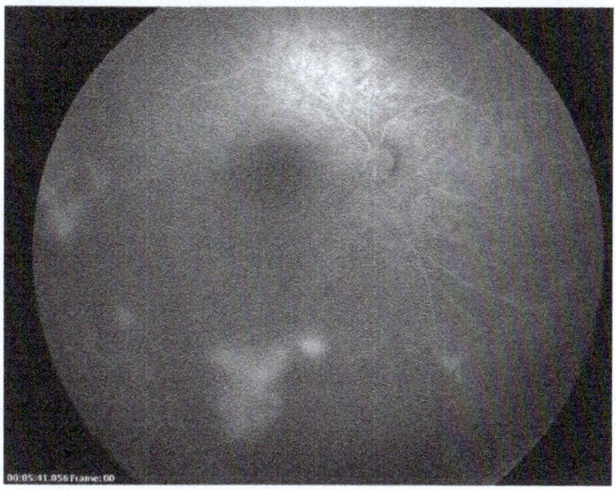

Fig. 27.14 RE: Retcam angiography reveals a residual retinal ischemia inferior and temporal

(Fig. 27.12). In the left eye a temporal and quite central laser coagulation is visible (Fig. 27.13). The fibrovascular proliferations were removed during vitrectomy.

We scheduled an examination with Retcam in general anaesthesia. The Retcam angiography (and not photography) revealed avascular areas, which were not yet laser treated (Fig. 27.14). We performed therefore an angiography assisted laser photocoagulation (see Chap. 12) (Fig. 27.15).

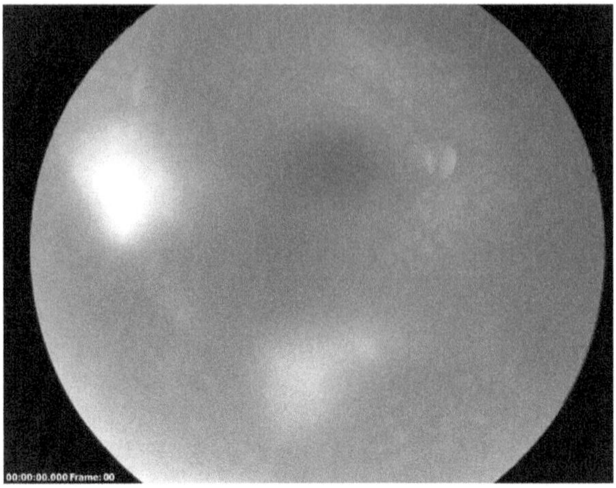

Fig. 27.15 RE: Retcam angiography. An angiography assisted Retcam angiography was performed. The skip lesion at 6 o'clock is treated with laser. Note the small visual field of the Retcam angiography and compare with Fig. 27.16

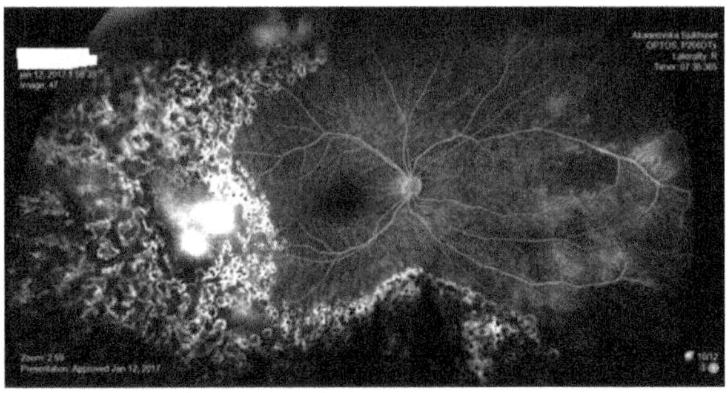

Fig. 27.16 RE: Optos angiography. Two laser coagulations with help of Retcam angiography had been performed. Today an Optos angiography is performed and reveals extensive ischemia in the nasal periphery

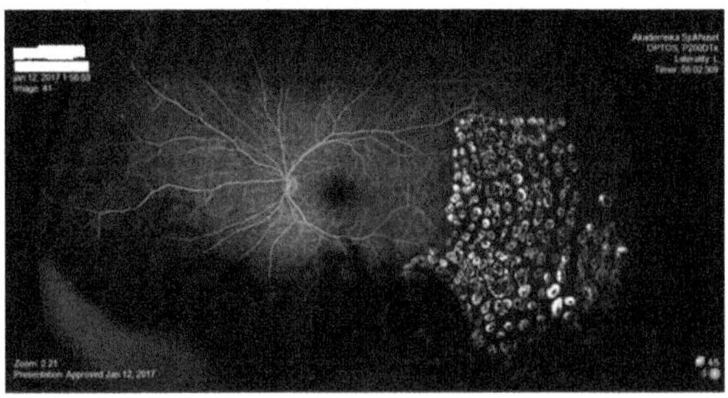

Fig. 27.17 LE: Optos angiography. This eye has been vitrectomized due to a vitreous hemorrhage. Note the retinal ischemia in the nasal periphery and even in the temporal periphery

In the meantime, our department received the Optos California and we scheduled immediately an Optos angiography. The Optos angiography (and not Optos photography) revealed extensive ischemic areas in the periphery of both eyes which were NOT detected with the Retcam angiography (Figs. 27.16 and 27.17). An additional laser photocoagulation was performed with LIO (Laser indirect ophthalmoscopy).

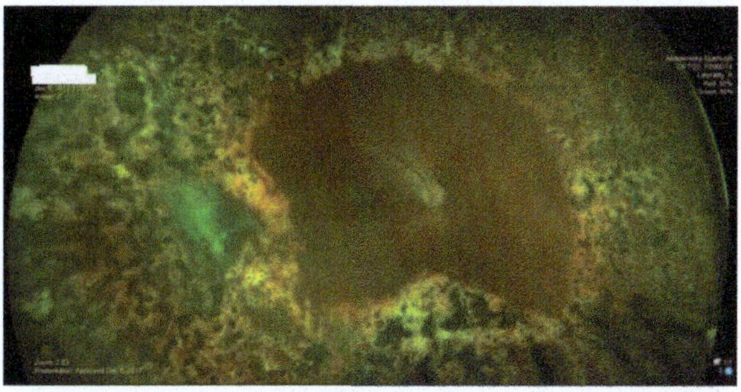

Fig. 27.18 RE: Optos photography. Final follow-up

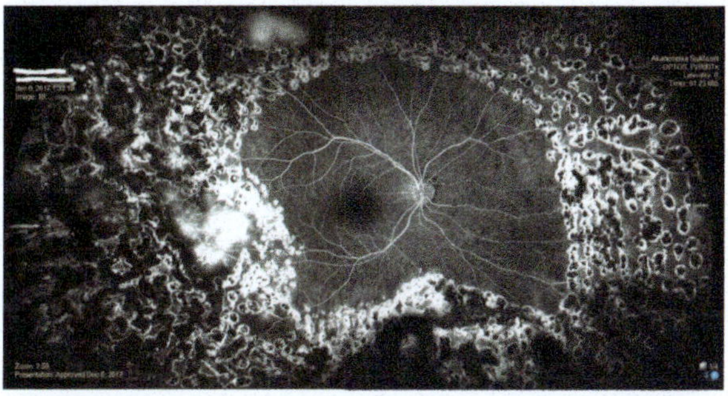

Fig. 27.19 RE: Optos angiography. Final follow-up

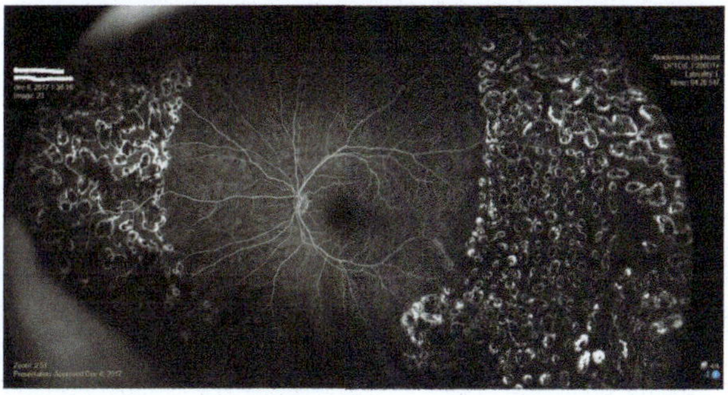

Fig. 27.20 LE: Optos angiography. Final follow-up 6 months after the laser photocoagulation

The 6-month follow-up after the last laser treatment shows an extensive laser photocoagulation of both eyes. The proliferations in the right eye are still leaking (Figs. 27.18, 27.19, and 27.20). The visual acuity was 1.0 in both eyes.

27.4 Case Report No. 4: Congenital Familial Exudative Vitreoretinopathy (FEVR) (Figs. 27.21, 27.22, 27.23, and 27.24)

General history: Full-term born and healthy child.

Ocular history: A six-month-old girl with pathological visual behaviour and nystagmus. Pronounced retinal changes were observed. The patient was referred for further investigation including angiography.

Examination in general anaesthesia:

- *Retinoscopy in cycloplegia:*
  - RE: −1.0/ −1.0 cyl 70°.
  - LE: −6.0/ −2.5 cyl 160°.
- *Axial length:*
  - RE: 19.0 mm
  - LE: 18.9 mm

Retcam photography and angiography (Figs. 27.21, 27.22, 27.23, and 27.24):

- RE: Clear optical media. Good view to fundus. A retinal fold from the optic disc to the temporal periphery. Engagement of macula. Angiography shows a retinal ischemia in the periphery of the eye with slight leakage from the vessels (Fig. 27.21).
- LE: Clear optical media. A retinal fold from the optic disc to the temporal periphery (Fig. 27.22). The retinal fold is very thick in the periphery and touches the lens. Avascular retina is visible in the periphery. A mild leakage is present (Figs. 27.23 and 27.24).

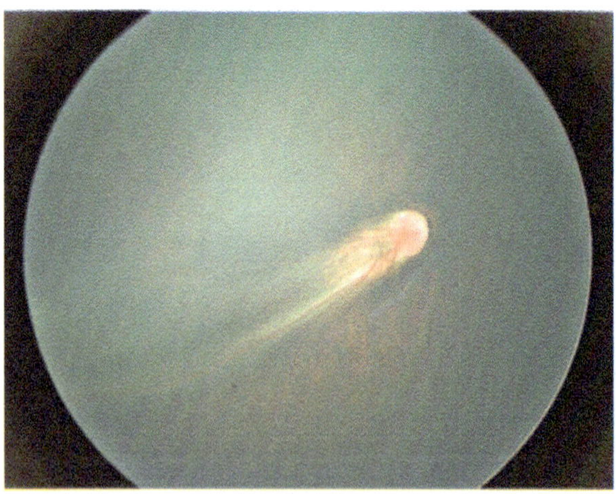

Fig. 27.21 RE: A retinal fold from the optic disc to the temporal periphery

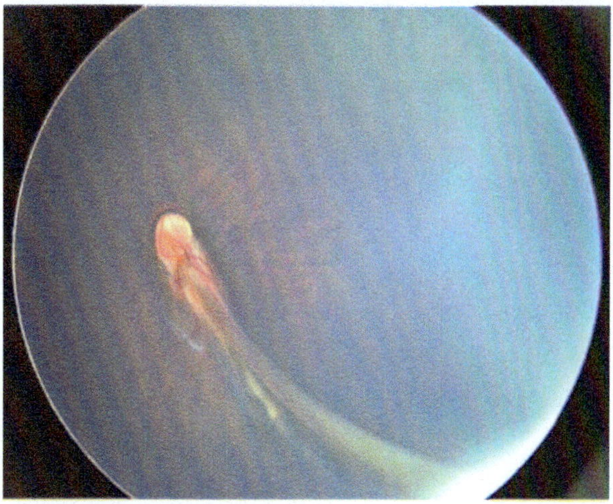

Fig. 27.22 LE: A retinal fold from the optic disc to the temporal periphery touching the lens

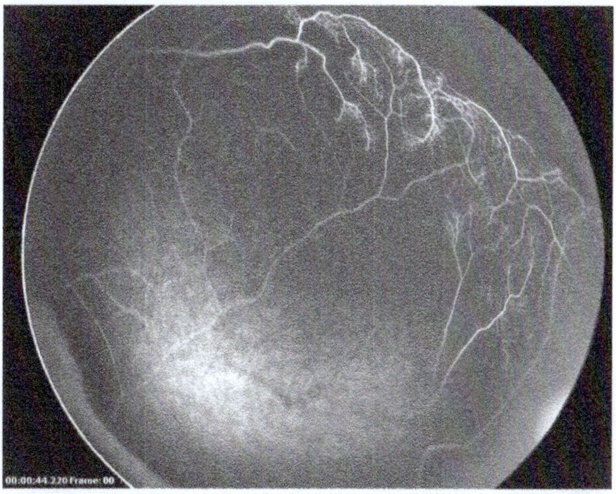

Fig. 27.23 LE: Angiography reveals peripheral ischemia and curved vessels

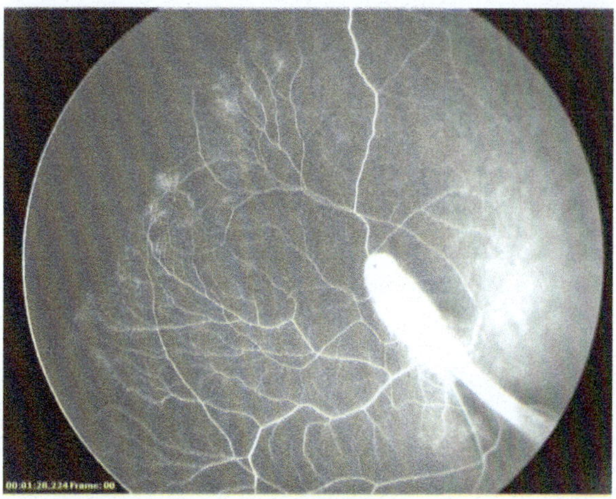

Fig. 27.24 LE: Angiography reveals a strong hyperfluorescence from the retinal fold. Note the ischemia and leakage in the periphery (left)

Conclusion:

The diagnosis is most likely FEVR because the neonate is not preterm born and because the retinal fold is located temporal which is typical for FEVR. There is no indication to laser treatment. A new examination is planned in 3–6 months. The risk for secondary complication such as retinal detachment (tractive, exudative and rhegmatogenous) is 30% [1].

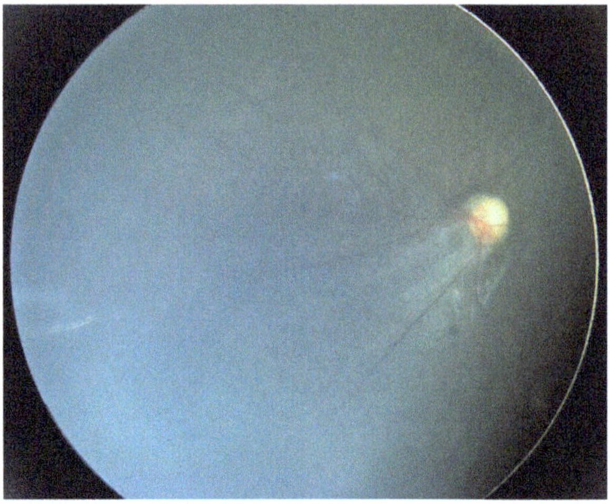

Fig. 27.25 RE: A macular dragging

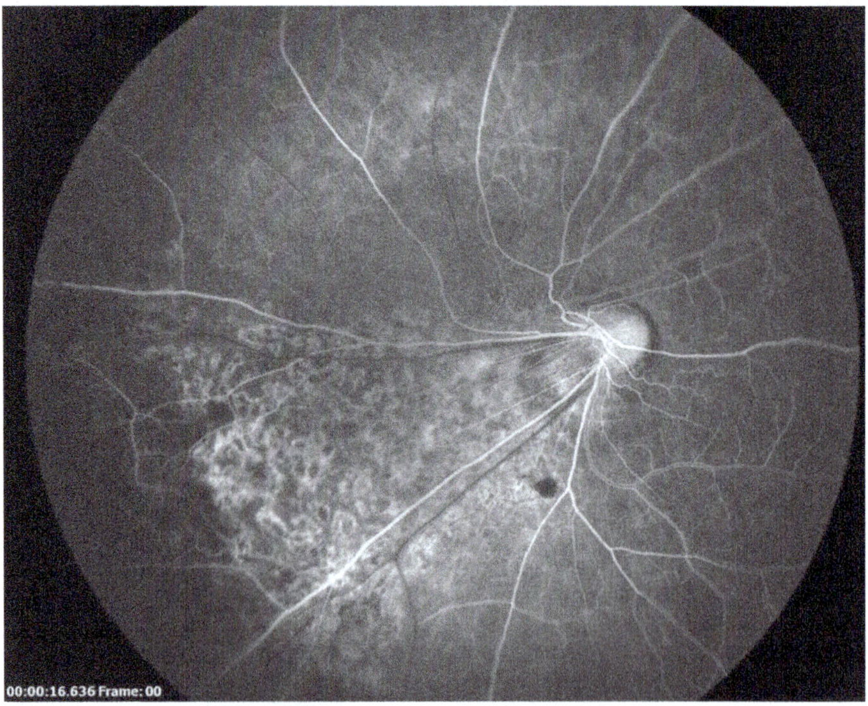

Fig. 27.26 RE: Severe RPE changes presumably secondary to the macular dragging

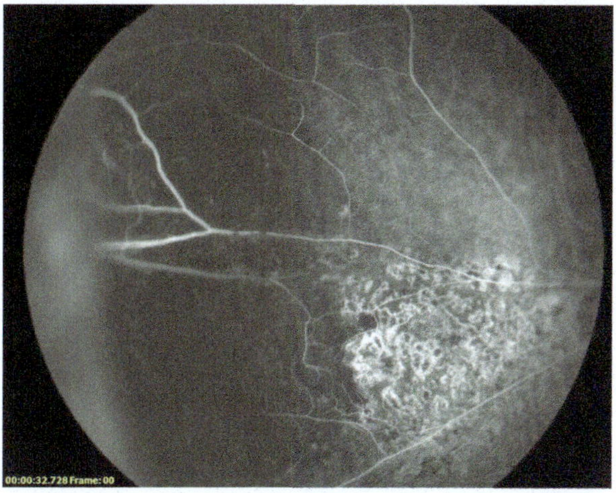

Fig. 27.27 RE: Vessel malformation in the periphery

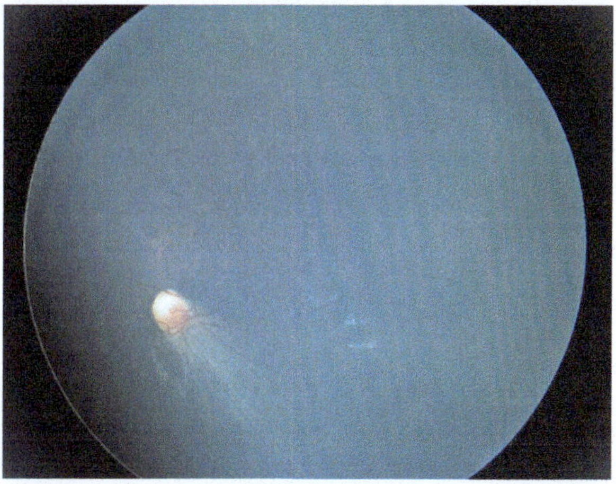

Fig. 27.28 LE: Macular dragging on the temporal side

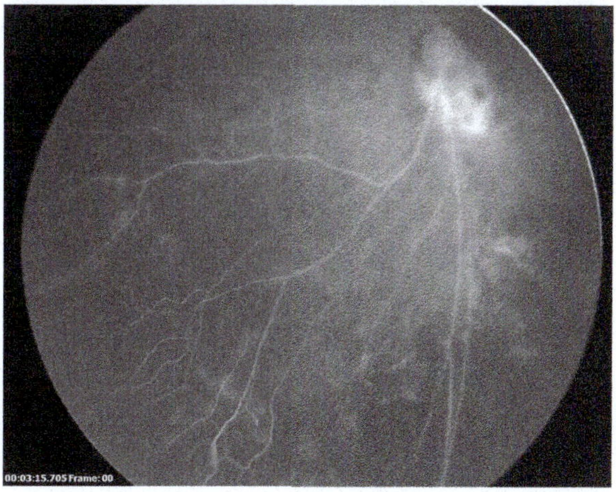

Fig. 27.29 LE: Pronounced vessel malformations with leakage

27.5 Case Report No. 5: Is this FEVR and ROP = ROPER? (Figs. 27.25, 27.26, 27.27, 27.28, 27.29, and 27.30)

General history: A 3y/o boy from South-East Asia, where he was born prematurely.

Ocular history: Parents judge his vision as seriously impaired. An examination in general anaesthesia was scheduled.

Examination in general anaesthesia:

- Retinoscopy in cycloplegia:
  - Right eye:−7.5/ −5.0 cyl 30°.
  - Left eye: −9.5 / −2.0 cyl 160°.

An examination with Retcam and Retcam angiography was performed. Retcam showed a temporal macular fold in both eyes (Figs. 27.25, 27.26, 27.27, 27.28, 27.29, and 27.30). The macula had a "pepper-salt" appearance. The retina was attached. Retcam angiography revealed RPE changes in the macula. In the periphery, vessel malformations with leakage and an avascular retina were detected.

Conclusion:

A macular dragging on the temporal side and a normal retina on the nasal side is present. The diagnosis may be ROP because the boy was premature born or FEVR. In a recent study a new entity called "ROPER" was proposed for neonates with are premature born and have a retina with signs of ROP and FEVR [2]. In addition, a grave myopia was detected.

27.6 Case Report No. 6: Incontinentia Pigmenti (Figs. 27.31, 27.32, 27.33, 27.34, 27.35, 27.36, 27.37, 27.38, 27.39, 27.40, and 27.41)

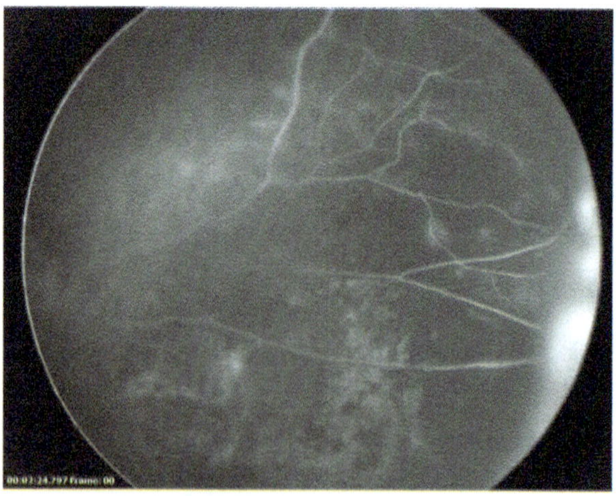

Fig. 27.30 LE: Stretched vessels with a strong leakage in the periphery

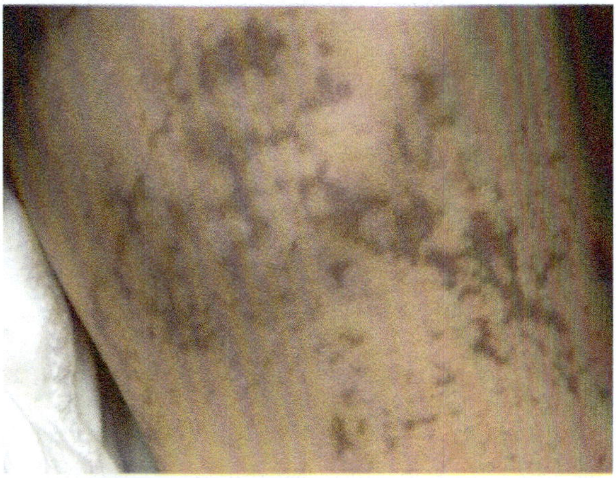

Fig. 27.31 Hyperpigmented skin of the leg

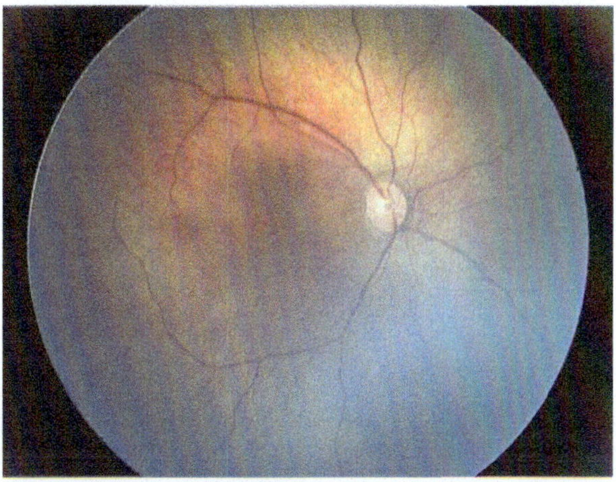

Fig. 27.32 RE: The colour picture shows no pathology

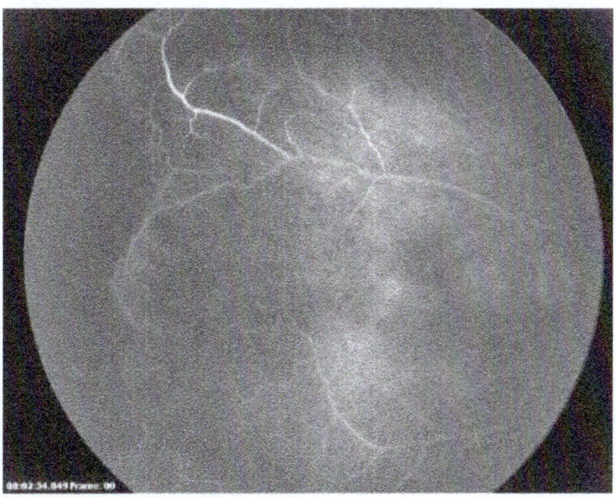

Fig. 27.33 RE: Fluorescein angiography shows an ischemic retina without leakage from the vessels

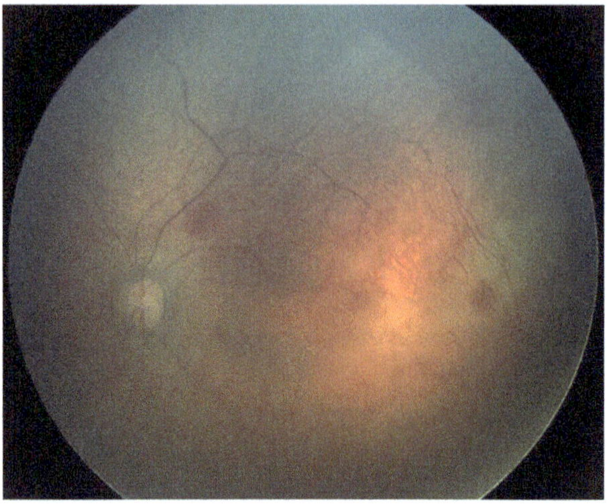

Fig. 27.34 LE: Colour photography shows two retinal hemorrhages

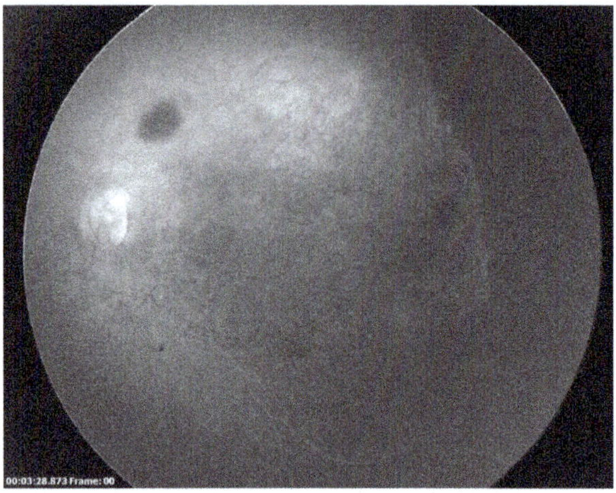

Fig. 27.35 LE: The ischemic retina can only be visualized with fluorescein angiography

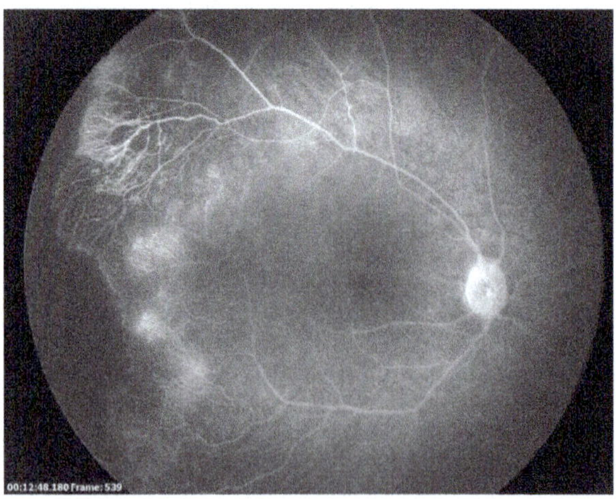

Fig. 27.36 RE: 1 month later the picture has changed very much. Leakage and proliferations have occurred. A laser coagulation is initiated

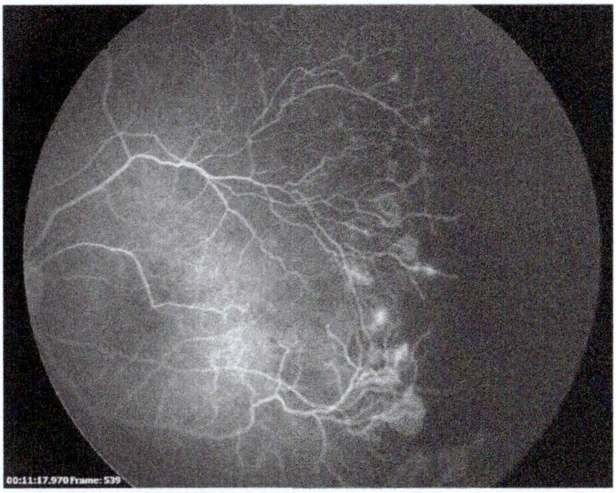

Fig. 27.37 LE: 1 month later, Retcam angiography reveals an ischemic retina in the periphery and leakage from the retinal vessels. A laser coagulation is initiated. But the border between physiologic and pathologic retina is difficult to discern

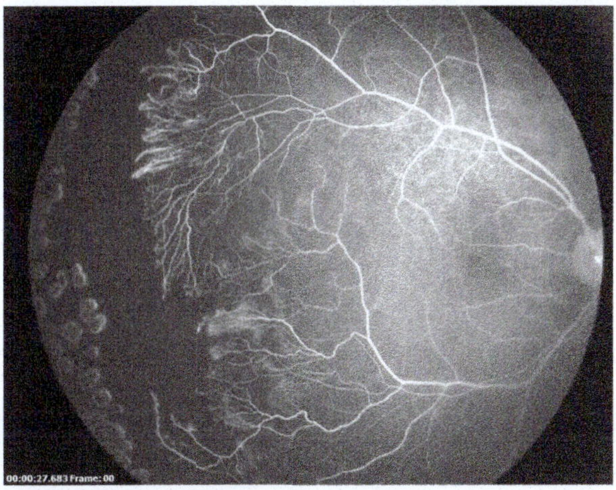

Fig. 27.38 RE: 1 month after laser coagulation: Angiography reveals a residual ischemia in the right eye

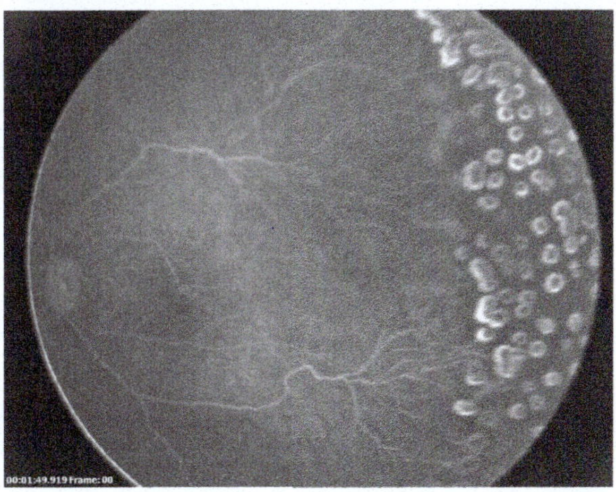

Fig. 27.39 LE: 1 month after laser coagulation: Angiography reveals no residual ischemia in the left eye

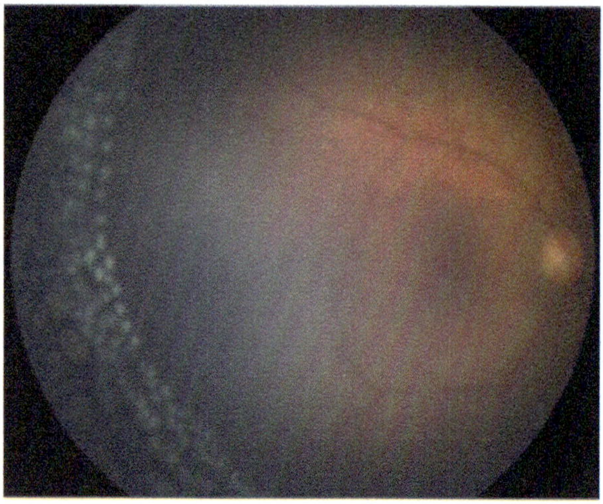

Fig. 27.40 RE: In the same sitting, a completing laser coagulation is performed. This picture is taken immediately after laser treatment. Old and new laser effects can be discerned

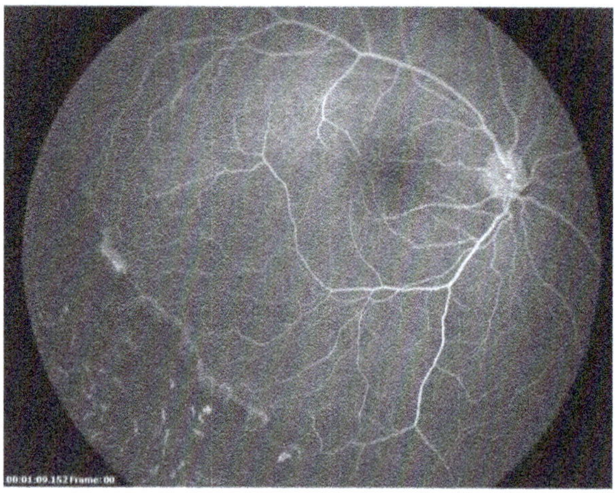

Fig. 27.41 RE: One year later fluorescein angiography shows a quiet retina and no retinal ischemia

Incontinentia pigmenti is a rare congenital skin disease with an eye affection. A retinal ischemia may be present resulting in a retinal detachment [3, 4].

General history:

An in term born neonate was diagnosed with Incontinentia pigmenti (Fig. 27.31) and referred to us for ocular examination.

Examination in general anaesthesia:

In the first examination two retinal hemorrhages were present in the left eye (Fig. 27.34). The RE looked normal (Fig. 27.32). But fluorescein angiography showed a peripheral ischemia without leakage (Figs. 27.33 and 27.35). We decided to repeat an examination in 1 month.

One month later the retinal pathology had become worse (Figs. 27.36 and 27.37). Fluorescein angiography revealed proliferations and leakage. A laser coagulation is performed in the same sitting. The right eye is treated with 1227 effects and the left eye with 1066 effects. But during laser coagulation the border between physiologic and pathologic retina is difficult to see.

Surgery:

Therefore, an angiography assisted laser coagulation is scheduled 1 month later (for details see chapter "Angiography assisted laser coagulation"). Fluorescein angiography reveals a complete laser in the left eye but residual ischemia in the right eye (Figs. 27.38 and 27.39). A complete laser coagulation is performed in the same session (Fig. 27.40).

1-year follow up:

Retinoscopy showed emmetropia in both eyes and no pathologic changes of the retina (Fig. 27.41).

27.7 Case Report No. 7: Morning Glory Syndrome (Figs. 27.42, 27.43, 27.44, and 27.45)

A 1.5 y/o girl presented in OPD for visual acuity decrease. The visual acuity of the right eye is 0.2 and of the left eye 0.02. Refraction is +1.5/−1.5 cylinder at 0° in the right eye and +1.5/−0.5 cylinder at 0° in the left eye.

An examination in general anaesthesia with Retcam and Retcam angiography revealed the following:

- The right eye had normal findings. The left eye showed a typical morning glory optic disc dysplasia (Fig. 27.42). Temporal to the macula an arc formed light brown pigmentation was found (Fig. 27.43). Angiography revealed a very immature retina; a macula cannot be found. A large non-vascularized zone is present 360 deg in the periphery (Figs. 27.44 and 27.45).

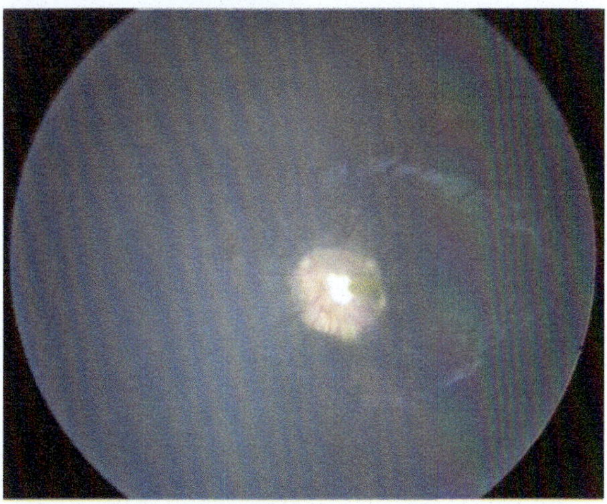

Fig. 27.42 LE: Morning glory syndrome

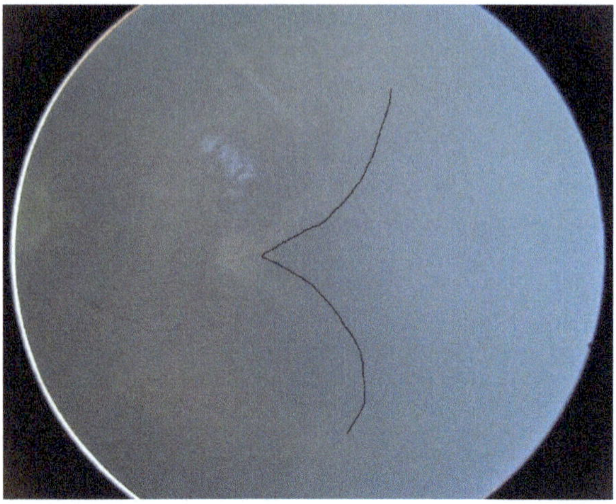

Fig. 27.43 LE: Morning glory syndrome. An arc formed light-brown retinal pigmentation is present temporal to the macula

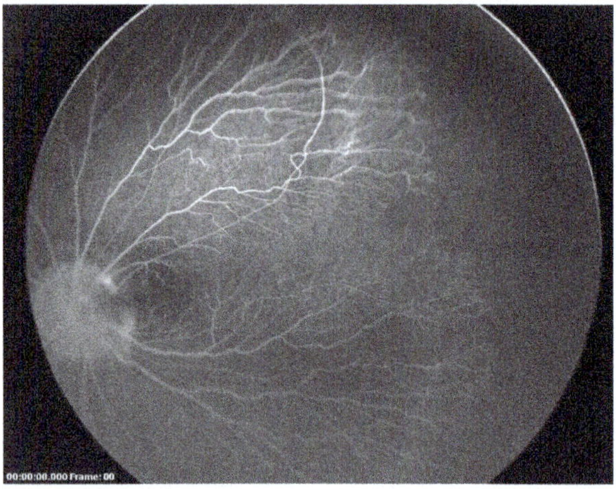

Fig. 27.44 LE: Angiography reveals an immature retina. A macula cannot be discerned

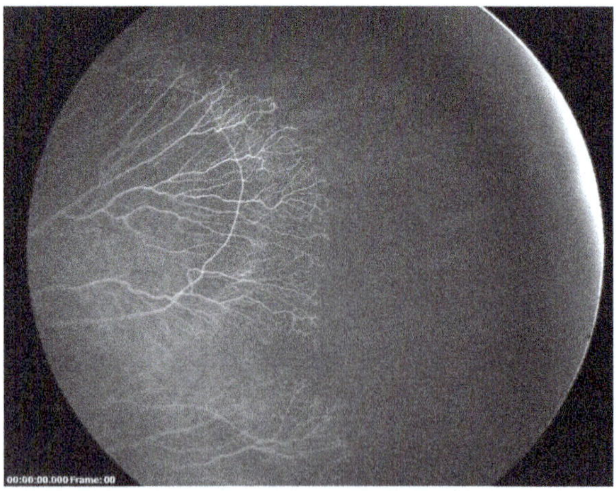

Fig. 27.45 LE: A peripheral 360 deg ischemia is present. Leakage or proliferations were not found

Conclusion:

Morning glory syndrome is an optic disc anomaly. Symptoms include low visual acuity and amblyopia. The most severe complication is retinal detachment, and can occur in about 26–38% of people with Morning glory syndrome [5]. The retina is very immature and resembles the next case report of a neonate very much with microcephalus.

27.8 Case Report No. 8: Microcephalus (Figs. 27.46, 27.47, and 27.48)

Microcephalus is a rare disease which may be caused by an infection (Zika), Crystal Meth or alcohol abuse during pregnancy. Chromosome abnormalities may also be causative [6]. In this case no infection or drug abuse was reported. The baby was

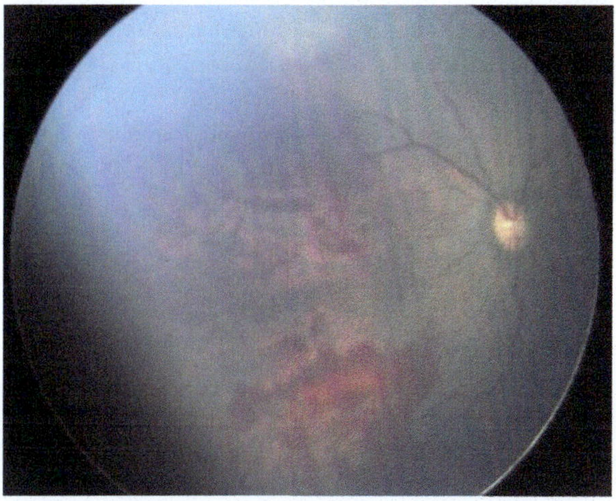

Fig. 27.46 A full term born baby with micro-cephalus. Extensive preretinal hemorrhage is present

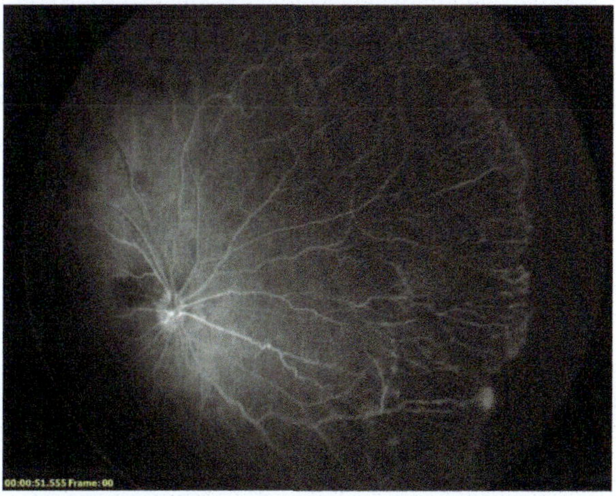

Fig. 27.47 Fluorescein angiography shows peripheral ischemia with leakage from vessels

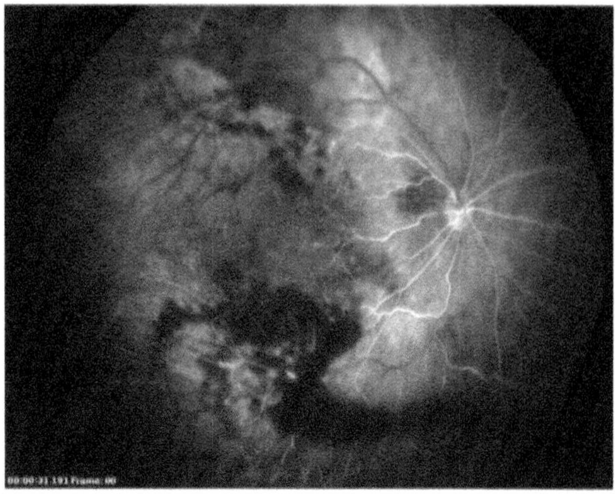

Fig. 27.48 The FA picture shows a very immature retina. A macula cannot be visualized

born full term. The parents were cousins. Indirect ophthalmoscopy revealed a preretinal hemorrhage (Fig. 27.46). Angiography shows a very immature retina with ischemia in the periphery (Figs. 27.47 and 27.48).

Conclusion:

The retina of this infant with microcephalus is very immature and peripheral ischemia is present. This case resembles the previous case with morning glory syndrome.

27.9 Case Report No. 9: Coats Disease (Figs. 27.49, 27.50, 27.51, 27.52, and 27.53)

General history:

Term born, no diseases

Ocular history:

A 3y/o boy presented at OPD for pain in the left eye. Visual acuity was RE = 0.63 and LE = 0.8. Funduscopy was normal. At 13 years of age the boy presents again in OPD due to visual field loss for 2 weeks. Visual acuity in the RE = 1.0 and in the LE = 0.2. Funduscopy of the RE is normal (Fig. 27.49) and in the LE an exudative retinopathy is present (Fig. 27.50). The diagnosis of Coats disease stage 2B was made. For details see chapter "Coats disease".

Therapy:

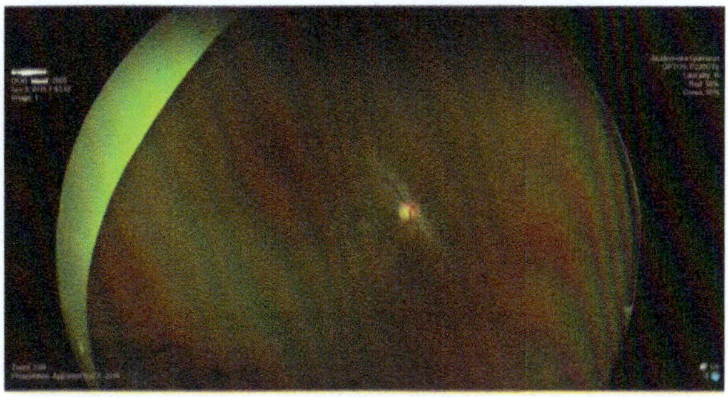

Fig. 27.49 Normal fellow eye

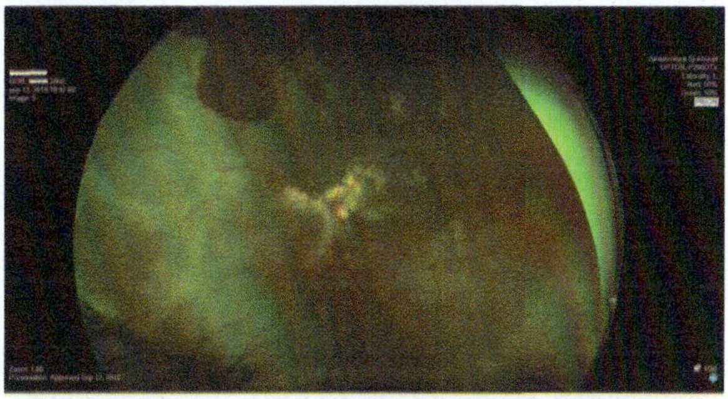

Fig. 27.50 An exudative retinopathy with peripheral hemorrhage

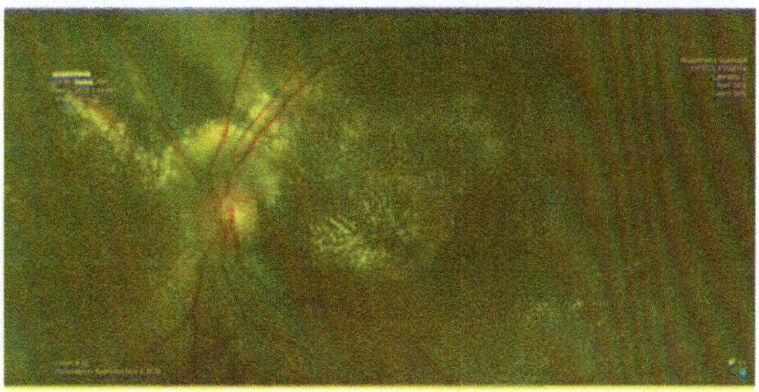

Fig. 27.51 Foveal exudation, VA = 0.2

Fig. 27.52 Extensive leakage from the vessels

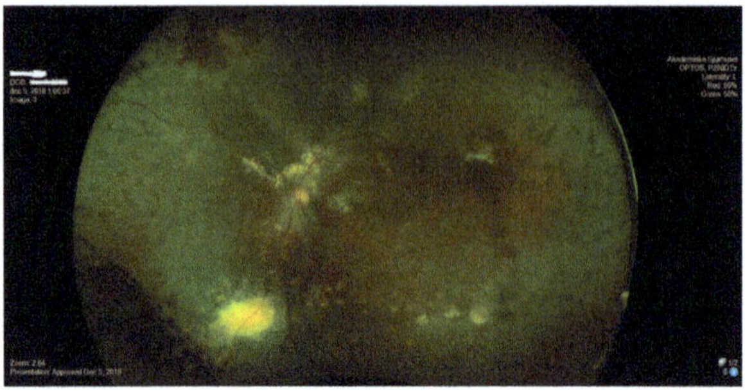

Fig. 27.53 One month follow-up after LIO (laser) and Eylea injection. VA = 0.7. Observe the pigmented laser effects in the periphery

An intravitreal injection of Eylea was performed and a laser coagulation in general anaesthesia was scheduled. Then a laser indirect ophthalmoscopy with 1487 effects was performed. In addition, a second Eylea injection was performed.

Follow-up:

One month later visual acuity was 0.7 (Figs. 27.51, 27.52, and 27.53).

27.10 Case Report No. 10: Avastin and Laser Treatment for ROP Zone I (Figs. 27.54, 27.55, 27.56, 27.57, and 27.58)

General history: A 23 weeks gestational age born girl. The child is sick.

Ocular history:

- October13th: **Aggressive posterior ROP in zone I** was diagnosed. Note that the temporal ischemia is located in zone I (Figs. 27.54 and 27.55)
- October13th**: In**jection of 0.6 mg **Avastin.**
- October 18th**: Follow**-up: Improvement, less plus disease
- October 21s**t: Improveme**nt
- October 26th: **Recurrence**: No iris rubeosis. Relatively clear media. Optic disc normal. Pre plus. Preretinal hemorrhages of an optic disc diameter around the entire circular vascular zone. No traction. The avascular zone is relatively central and lies in zone I.
- October, 27nd: Second intravitreal injection of 0.6 mg **Avastin**.
- November 1st: Improvement
- November, 08th: **Recurrence in zone II**. In the meantime, the retina had vascularized to zone II resulting in an increased visual field (Fig. 27.56). In zone II we perform laser photocoagulation.
- November 10th: **Laser**; Right eye: 1859 effects, Left eye: 1730 effects (Figs. 27.57 and 27.58)

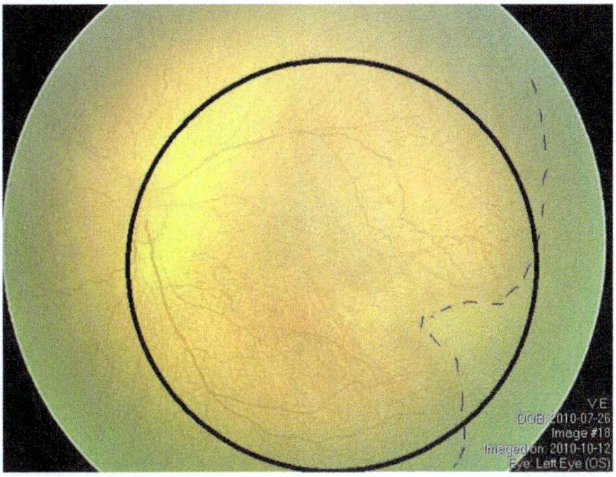

Fig. 27.54 LE: Before Avastin treatment. Note that this is zone I

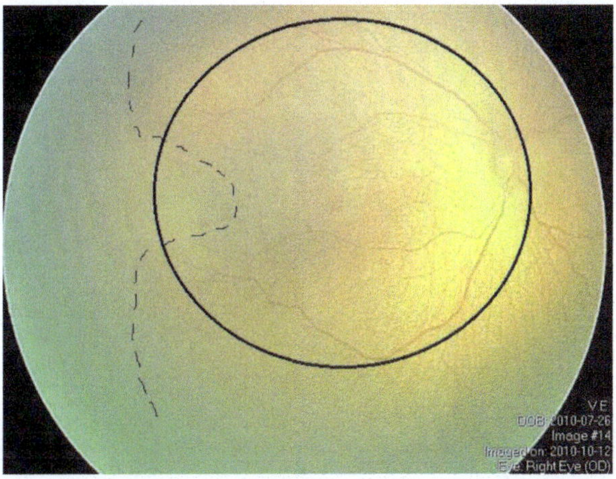

Fig. 27.55 RE: Before Avastin treatment. Also zone I

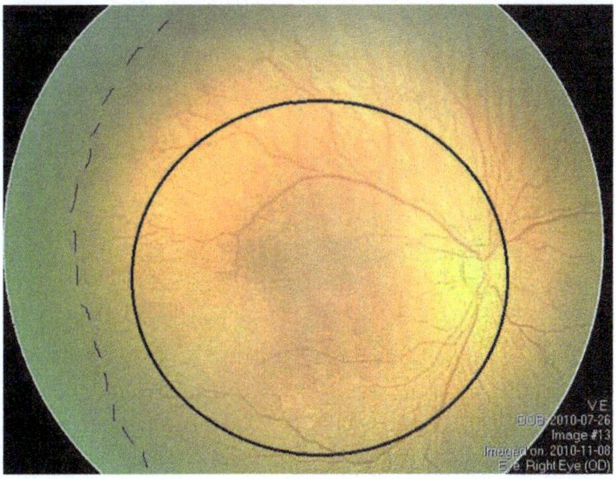

Fig. 27.56 RE: After Avastin treatment. Note that the retina has vascularized until zone II (dashed line)

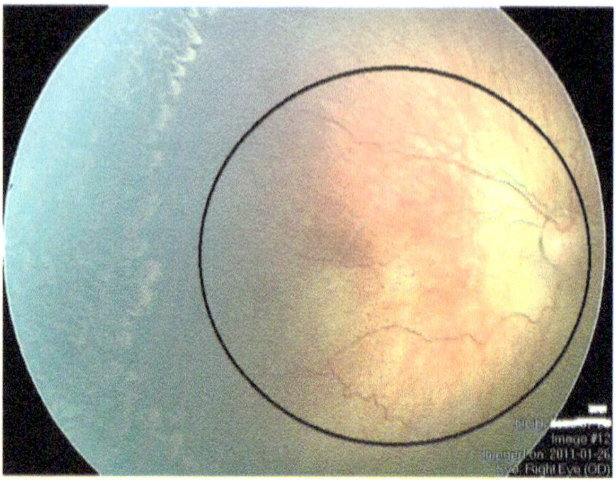

Fig. 27.57 RE: After laser treatment. Note that a zone II is present

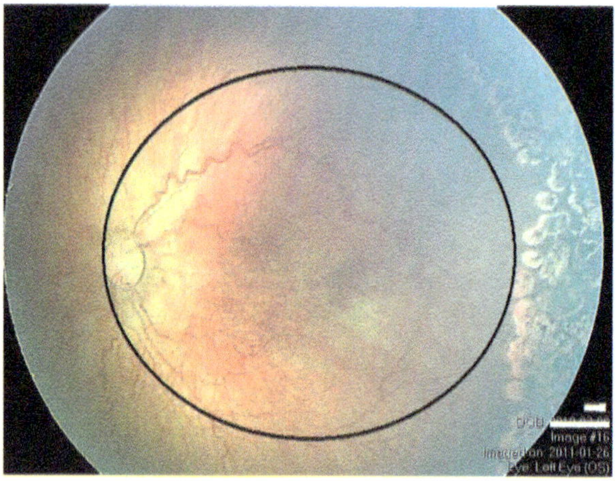

Fig. 27.58 LE: After laser treatment. Note that this is zone II

<u>1-year follow-up:</u> Esotropy was noted on the left eye. Glasses and patching were prescribed.
<u>3-years follow-up:</u>

- RE: +2.5/−1.25/13 = 0.25
- LE: +2.25/ -1.0/11 = 0.25

<u>Conclusion:</u>

Two intravitreal anti-VEGF injections for zone I and one laser coagulation for zone II were required to treat the ROP. This case is unusual because within a time period of 4 weeks two recurrences occurred. The neonate was very sick. The first recurrence is treated again with anti-VEGF because the retinopathy is still present in zone I, whereas the second recurrence is treated with laser coagulation because a zone II disease is present. Remember: In case of ROP plus in zone I an anti-VEGF injection is the therapy of choice and in case of zone II an injection or laser treatment are equally good.

Remark: Zone II = Distance of 2× (nasal part of optic disc to macula).

27.11 Case Report No. 11: Lucentis Treatment for ROP Zone I (Figs. 27.59, 27.60, 27.61, 27.62, 27.63, and 27.64)

General history. A premature born boy in week 22 + 5 and a weight of 435 g.
Sick boy. Underwent a ductus surgery in week 31 without complications.

Ocular history:

- Week 30: no ROP detected. Bad view to fundus.
- Week 31: no ROP. Bad view to fundus.
- Week 32: no ROP. Bad view to fundus.

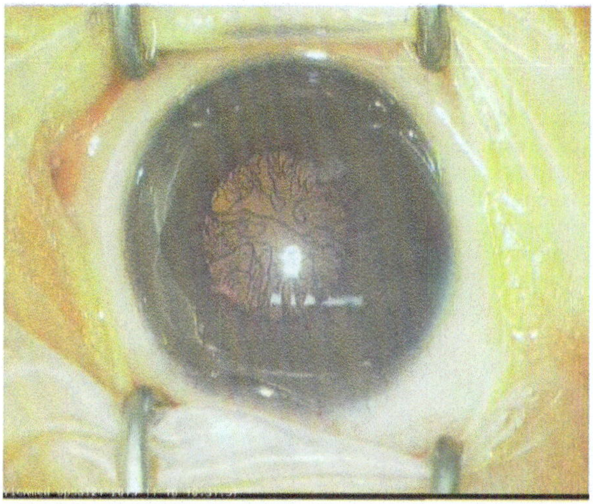

Fig. 27.59 Tunica vasculosa lentis and a rubeotic iris are present

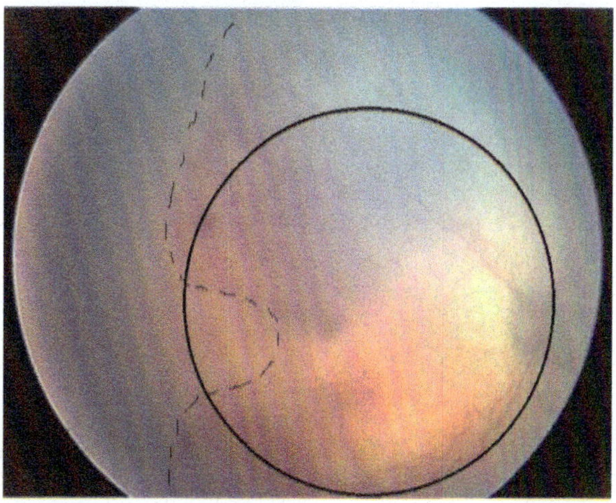

Fig. 27.60 RE: The left eye before treatment. ROP 3+ in zone I is present

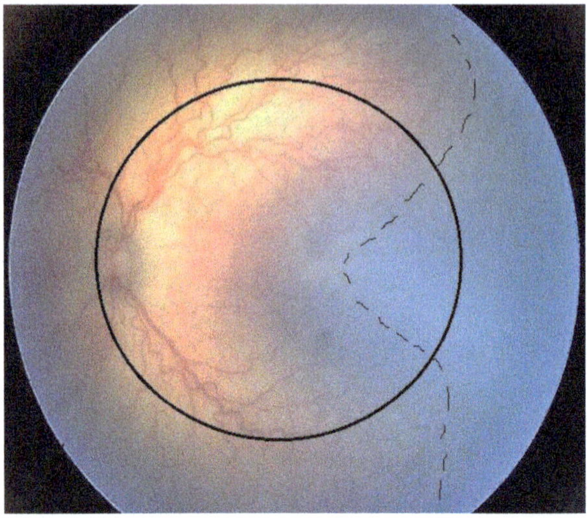

Fig. 27.61 LE: The central vessels are tortuous and a zone I is present

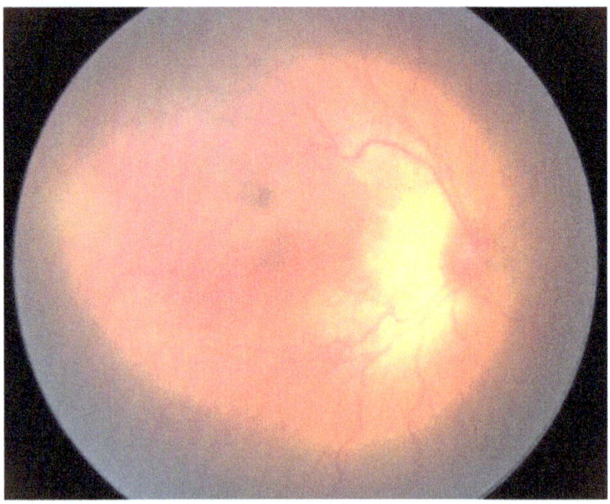

Fig. 27.62 RE: Retcam colour picture. Two months after first Lucentis treatment. Note the tortuous vessels at the posterior pole. A recurrence of ROP 3+ is present

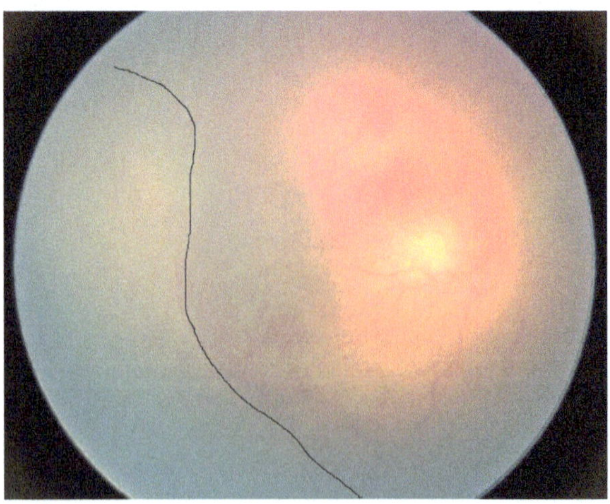

Fig. 27.63 RE: Retcam colour picture. Two months after first Lucentis treatment. Many new proliferations at the ridge (black line). A second Lucentis injection is scheduled

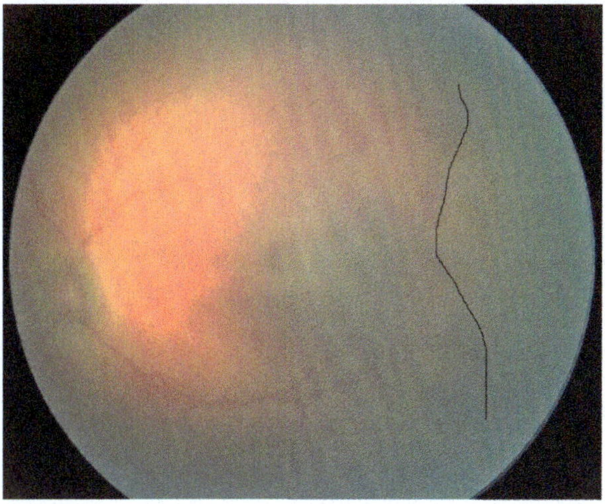

Fig. 27.64 LE: Retcam picture. Two months after Lucentis treatment. The black line indicates the ridge. A second Lucentis injection is scheduled

- Week 33: ROP 3.
- Week 34: ROP 3+. Tunica vasculosa lentis and iris rubeosis are present (Fig. 27.59). A Retcam photography show that the ridge is located in zone I (Figs. 27.60 and 27.61). Therefore, a treatment with **intravitreal Lucentis** (50% adult's dose) was performed
- Week 42: Recurrence of ROP 3+ in the right eye and less pronounced in the LE (Figs. 27.62, 27.63, and 27.64). Difficult to assess if zone I or zone is affected.

- Week 42: Treatment with **intravitreal Lucentis** (50% adult's dose)
- No recurrence occurred during the follow-up.

Conclusion:

This is a typical case in so far that the recurrence occurred 8 weeks after the Lucentis injection. This case is also unusual because we usually perform a laser coagulation as second treatment. But in this case a zone I was still present.

27.12 Case Report No. 12: Three-Year Follow-Up After ROP in Zone I and Treatment with 1× Lucentis (Figs. 27.65, 27.66, 27.67, 27.68, 27.69, and 27.70)

General history. A premature born boy in week 24. Developed a necrotizing enterocolitis and was operated two times for this with very critical postoperative status.
Ocular history:

- Week 32: Diagnosed with ROP 3+ in zone I (Figs. 27.65 and 27.66)
- Week 32: Treated bilateral with intravitreal Lucentis (50% adults dose)

One-year follow-up:

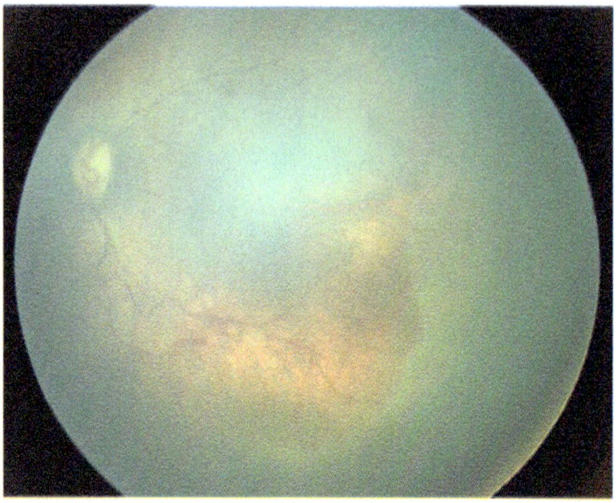

Fig. 27.65 LE: Temporal side. Very central pathology. ROP 3+ in zone I

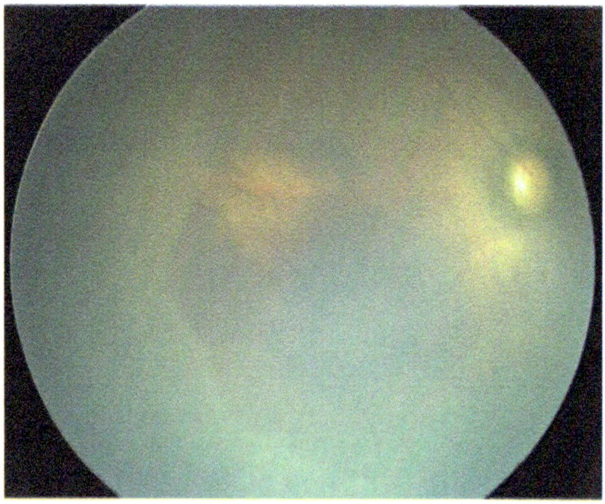

Fig. 27.66 LE: Nasal side. Very big ischemic area

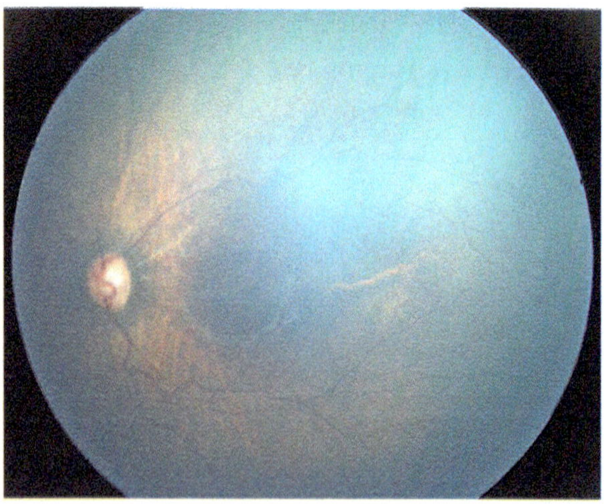

Fig. 27.67 LE: 1-year follow up. Note the vascularized retina in the temporal periphery

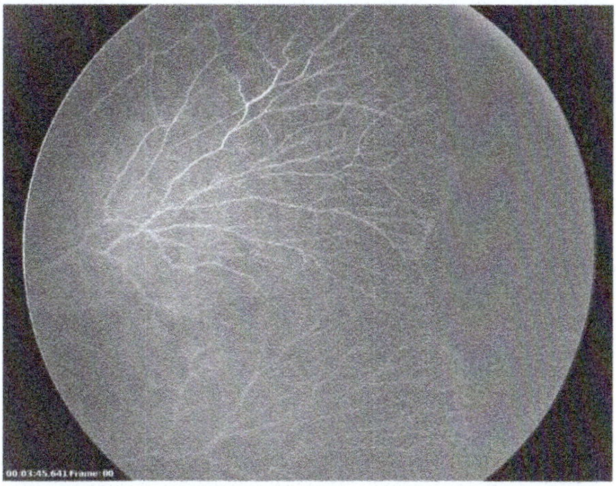

Fig. 27.68 LE: 1-year follow up. A big non-vascularized area is present

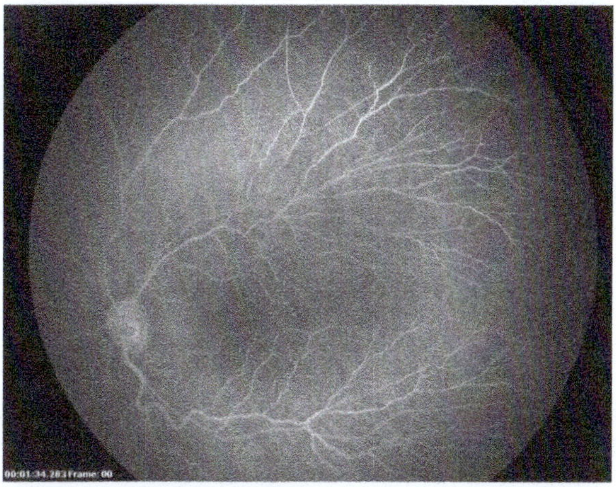

Fig. 27.69 LE: 3-years follow up. Myopia of −10.0D

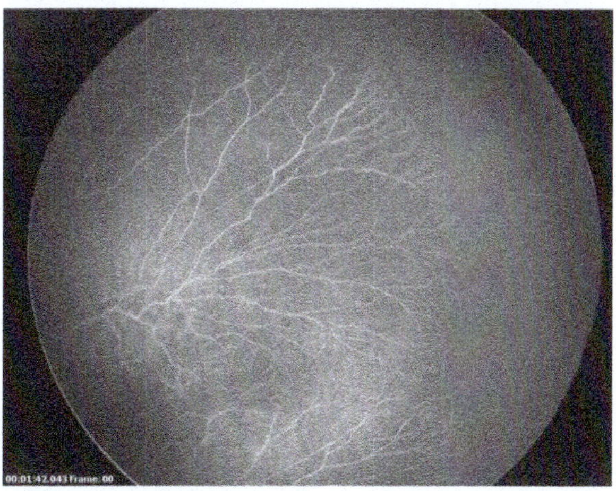

Fig. 27.70 LE: 3-years follow up. The non-vascularized area is almost unchanged

Bilateral high myopia. Peripheral non-vascularized retina. No leakage and no proliferations. No indication for laser treatment. (Figs. 27.67 and 27.68)

Three-year follow-up:

Bilateral grave myopia. Peripheral ischemia but no leakage and no proliferation. No indication for laser treatment. (Figs. 27.69 and 27.70)

- RE: −8.5/ −3.0 cyl i cirka 150°.
- LE: −12/ −3.0 cyl i cirka 45°.

Conclusion:

One bilateral Lucentis injection treated successfully a ROP 3 plus disease in zone I. After 3 years an angiography demonstrates that the eye is not yet fully vascularized. There is no consensus yet if these eyes should be laser treated or not.

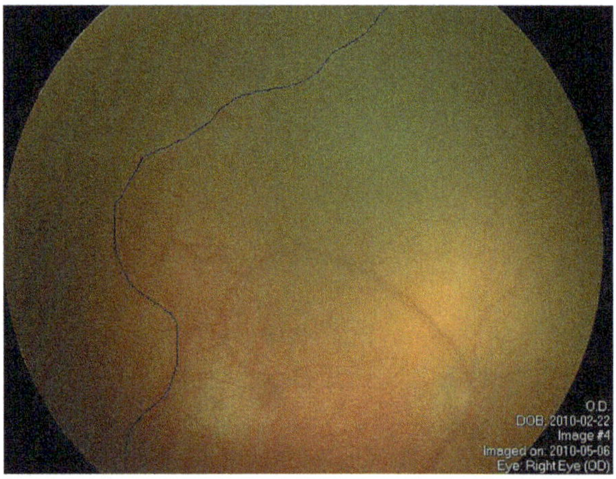

Fig. 27.71 RE: Before treatment. ROP 3 in zone I. Note that the temporal ridge is located in zone I

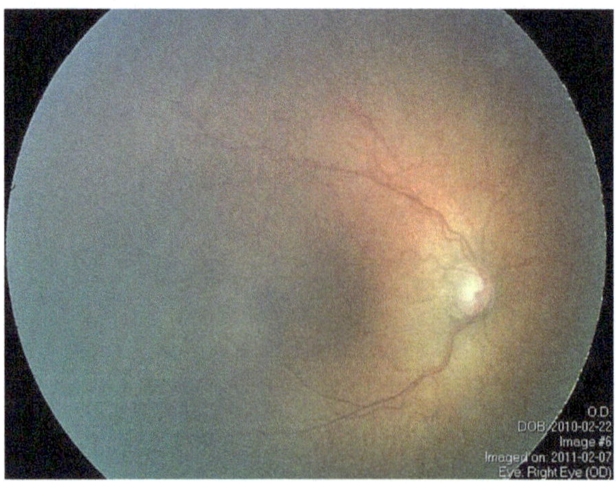

Fig. 27.72 RE: 1 year after treatment. The retina is fully vascularized

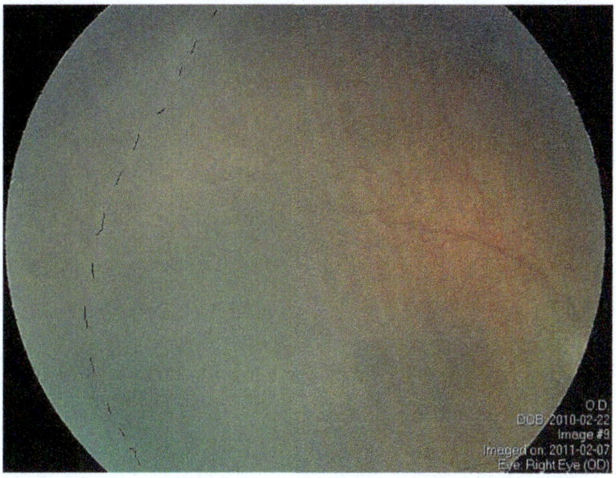

Fig. 27.73 RE: 1 year after treatment. A slight ridge is still present

27.13 Case Report No. 13: Seven-Year Follow-Up After ROP in Zone I and Treatment with 1× Avastin (Figs. 27.71, 27.72, and 27.73)

General history: In summary, a premature born triplet, born after 23 + 1 weeks with a weight of 495 g. Operated with acute laparotomy due to NEC. He developed sepsis a couple of times as well as liver affection due to CMV infection.

Ocular history: (Fig. 27.71)

05/2010: Diagnosis of ROP 3+ in zone I: Injection of Avastin 0.65 mg bilaterally

1-year follow-up: Investigation with Retcam in anesthesia (Figs. 27.72 and 27.73)

Visual acuity

- RE: +3.5/ −1.0150 deg = 0.13
- LE: +3.5/−1.0 60 deg = 0.2

7-year follow-up:

- RE: +5.25/−1.25/152 = 0.3
- LE: +6.25/−1.75/41 = 0.3
- Binocular:0.4
- Esotropia and nystagmus in the left eye.

Conclusion:

A single treatment of an advanced retinopathy with Avastin of a sick neonate resulted in a satisfactory outcome. The 2-year follow-up reveals that the child is visually handicapped. See also chapter "Visual outcome of very preterm neonates at 6.5 years of age".

27.14 Case Report No. 14: Seven-Year Follow-Up After ROP in Zone I and Treatment with 1× Avastin

General history: A male triplet, pregnant premature born v 23 + 3 with birth weight 585 g. Laparotomy for NEC. In addition, hypothyroidism and pulmonary hypertension ROP grade III.

Ocular history:

05/2010: Diagnosed with ROP 3+ in zone I: Both Eyes: Injection of 0.5 mg Avastin intravitreal

Follow-up 3 years:

He is just over 3 years of age. Going to kindergarten and, according to the mother, is well functioning. Had a normal viewing status, even if a stereo function could not be detected with certainty. The retina looked normal, but some tortuous vessels and some thin vessels with a rather divergent course in the periphery are present. No proliferation or bleeding can be detected.

Visual acuity:

- RE: 0.63 LH 3 meter.
- LE: 0.63 LH 3 meter.

Follow-up 7 years:

- RE: +2.75sph = 0.8
- LE: +2.75sph = 0.9
- He wears glasses

No pictures available. The fundus pictures are similar to his brother (case 12).

Conclusion:

The comparison of the twins of case 12 and case 13 shows how different the visual outcome can be. This child has an excellent visual outcome compared to his brother.

27.15 Case Report No. 15: Two-Years Follow-Up After ROP in Zone I and Treatment with 1× Lucentis (Figs. 27.74, and 27.75)

This neonate was treated with 1× Lucentis (50% adult's dose) for posterior aggressive ROP in zone I. No laser coagulation was performed. A follow-up after 2 years shows refraction of +0.5D (RE) and – 7.0D (LE). The retina of the left eye looks normal (Fig. 27.74) and Retcam angiography reveals a persistent non-vascularized retina in zone III (Fig. 27.75).

Conclusion: There is no consensus whether eyes with an incomplete vascularization should be laser treated or not (Fig. 27.75).

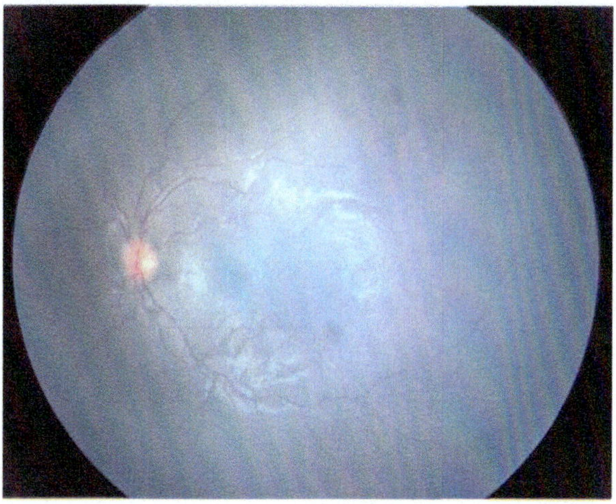

Fig. 27.74 Normal fundus picture 2 years after treatment with Lucentis for ROP in zone I

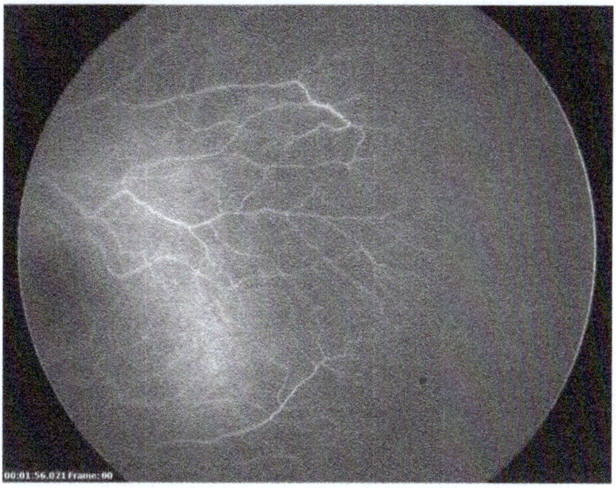

Fig. 27.75 Angiography reveals a non-vascularized retina in the temporal periphery corresponding to zone III. No leakage and no proliferations are present

27.16 Case Report No. 16: Retinal Bleedings 8 Years After Surgical Treatment for ROP (Figs. 27.76, 27.77, 27.78, 27.79, and 27.80)

General history: A premature born boy in week 24. Necrotizing enterocolitis and intestinal perforation neonatally. Got stoma.
Ocular history:

- January 7th: Diagnosis as **posterior aggressive ROP** with ROP 3+ in zone I.
- January 7th: Bilateral **Avastin** 0.6 mg injection
- February 1st: Bilateral **Avastin** 0.6 mg injection
- March 25th: **Recurrence in zone II**

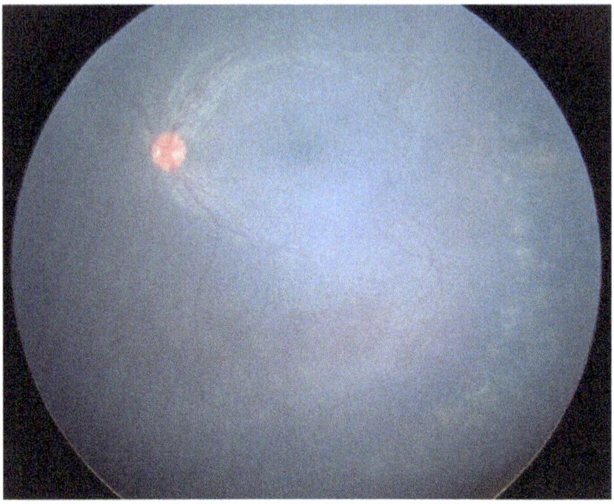

Fig. 27.76 Seven years after 2× Avastin and 1× laser photocoagulation. Note the preretinal bleeding at the inferior pole

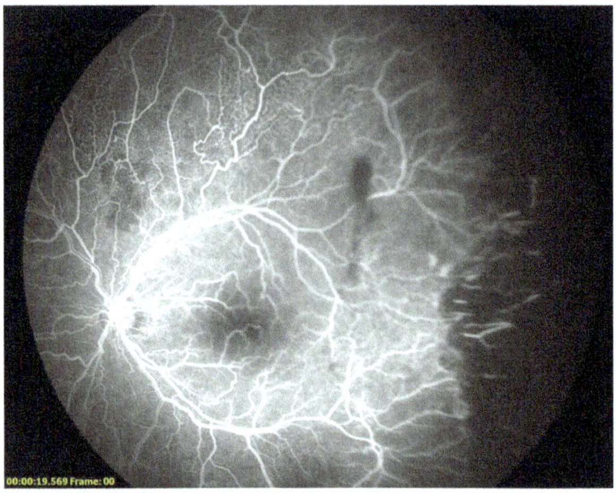

Fig. 27.77 Angiography reveals pathologic retinal vessels at the superior pole and a bleeding superotemporal to the macula

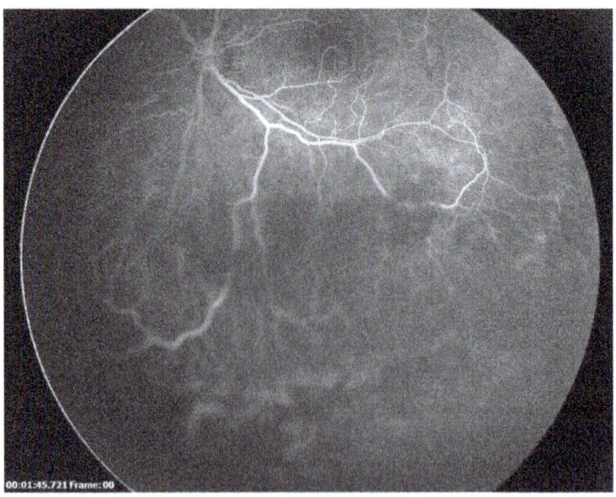

Fig. 27.78 Angiography reveals no proliferations at the inferior pole. The hypofluorescent structure at the inferior pole is blood

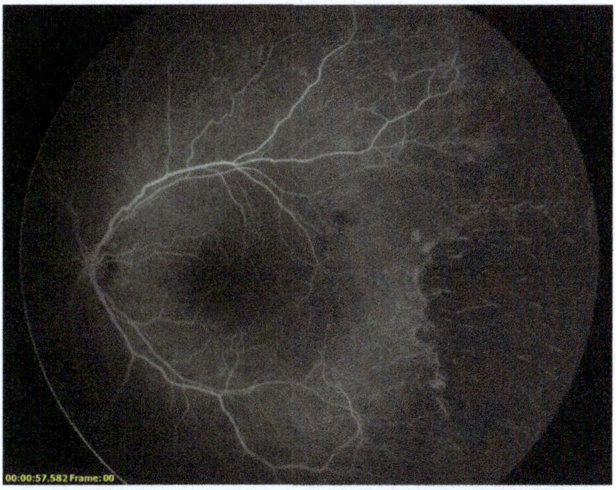

Fig. 27.79 LE: Three months later. Note the vessel malformations

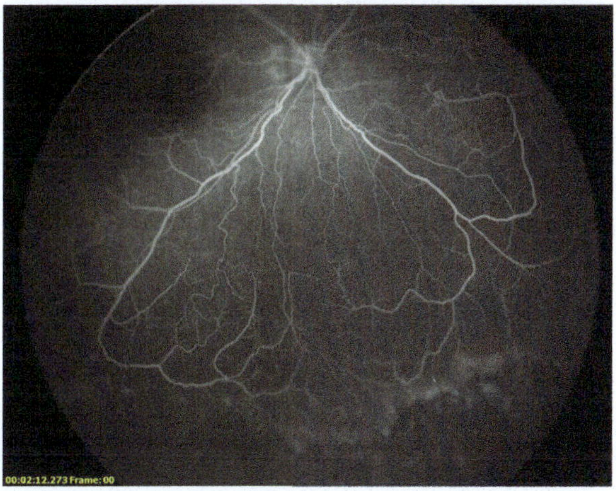

Fig. 27.80 RE: Three months later. Vessel malformation in the nasal periphery

- March 25th: **Laser photocoagulation** of retina

Seven years follow-up: Referral due to epiretinal hemorrhage in the left eye. ERG is performed and there are responses from both cones and rods, even though the response of the cones is somewhat low.

<u>Ocular examination:</u>

Retinoscopy and visual acuity:

- RE: + 2.5 / −2.0 / 5 = 0.4;
- LE: + 3.5 / −1.5 / 5 = 0.3

Regarding retinal status pathological vessels can be seen in FA, but no proliferations are present (Figs. 27.76, 27.77, and 27.78). On the left eye, preretinal bleeding is detected, but no proliferations are present. Therefore, there is no treatment indication at this time. A follow-up, 3 months later showed a complete resorption of the hemorrhage (Figs. 27.79 and 27.80).

Conclusion: This neonate was treated with two Avastin injections and finally with laser coagulation. Remark: It is very unusual that a neonate requires three Avastin injections [7]. Seven years after treatment with Avastin and delayed photo laser coagulation for ROP zone I a pathological angiography is present. Pathological vessels in retina and choroid have been described by [8]. Continued follow-ups are proposed at the place of residence.

27.17 Case Report No. 17: Delayed Treatment of ROP Plus Disease (Figs. 27.81, and 27.82)

General history:

Born 24 week GA with a weight of 695 g

Ocular history:

In week 38 ROP 3 plus was detected and no treatment was initiated (Fig. 27.81). In week 43 a ROP 3 with much activity at the temporal ridge was detected (Fig. 27.82).

Surgery:

- Week 43: Bilateral Lucentis injection

Follow-up:

- Week 54: Marked reduction of leakage.

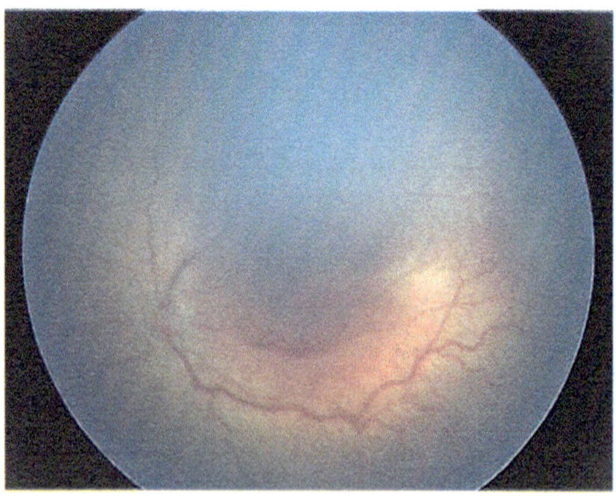

Fig. 27.81 A ROP with plus disease which was wrongly interpreted as preplus

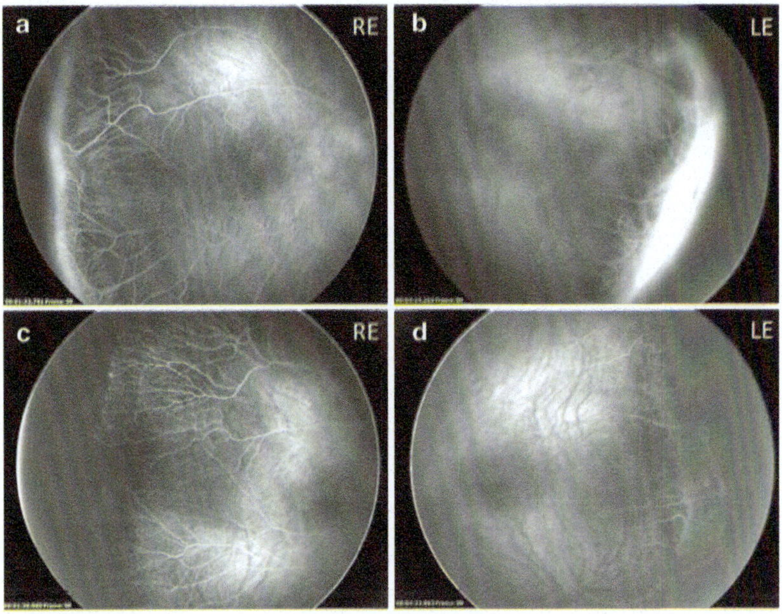

Fig. 27.82 The angiography pictures (**a**, **b**) were taken 4 weeks after the picture in Fig. 27.1. Both eyes were treated with intravitreal Lucentis. Note the strong leakage at the temporal ridge. The angiography pictures (**c**, **d**) were taken 11 weeks after the Lucentis injection. Observe the absent leakage

References

1. Nishina S, Suzuki Y, Yokoi T, Kobayashi Y, Noda E, Azuma N. Clinical features of congenital retinal folds. Am J Ophthalmol. 2012;153(1):81–7.
2. John VJ, McClintic JI, Hess DJ, Berrocal AM. Retinopathy of prematurity versus familial exudative Vitreoretinopathy: report on clinical and angiographic findings. Ophthalmic Surg Lasers Imaging Retina. 2016;47(1):14–9.
3. Chen CJ, Han IC, Goldberg MF. Variable expression of retinopathy in a pedigree of patients with Incontinentia Pigmenti. Retina. 2015;35(12):2627–32.
4. Swinney CC, Han DP, Karth PA. Incontinentia Pigmenti: A Comprehensive review and update. Ophthalmic Surg Lasers Imaging Retina. 2015;46(6):650–7.
5. Lytvynchuk LM, Glittenberg CG, Ansari-Shahrezaei S, Binder S. Intraoperative optical coherence tomography assisted analysis of pars Plana vitrectomy for retinal detachment in morning glory syndrome: a case report. BMC Ophthalmol. 2017;17:134.
6. Miranda HA 2nd, Costa MC, Frazão MAM, Simão N, Franchischini S, Moshfeghi DM. Expanded Spectrum of congenital ocular findings in microcephaly with presumed Zika infection. Ophthalmology 2016;123(8):1788–1794.
7. Jing Feng, Jing Qian, Yanrong Jiang, Mingwei Zhao, Jianhong Liang, Hong Yin, Yi Chen, Wenzhen Yu and Xiaoxin Li. Efficacy of primary Intravitreal Ranibizumab for retinopathy of prematurity in China Ophthalmology, 2017–124, 3, Pages 408–409.
8. Lepore D, Quinn GE, Molle F, Orazi L, Baldascino A, Ji MH, Sammartino M, Sbaraglia F, Ricci D, Mercuri E. Follow-up to age 4 years of treatment of type 1 retinopathy of prematurity Intravitreal Bevacizumab injection versus laser: fluorescein angiographic findings. Ophthalmology. 2018;125(2):218–26.

Chapter 28
Treatment Failures of ROP Disease

28.1 Case Report No. 18: 2× Recurrence After Laser Treatment for Zone I (Aggressive Posterior ROP) (Figs. 28.1 and 28.2)

This was the first ROP case in which we performed an intravitreal anti-VEGF (Avastin) treatment. The neonate had ROP 3 plus in zone I, we performed two times a laser treatment, but every time a recurrence occurred. Therefore, we injected intravitreal Avastin as rescue treatment.

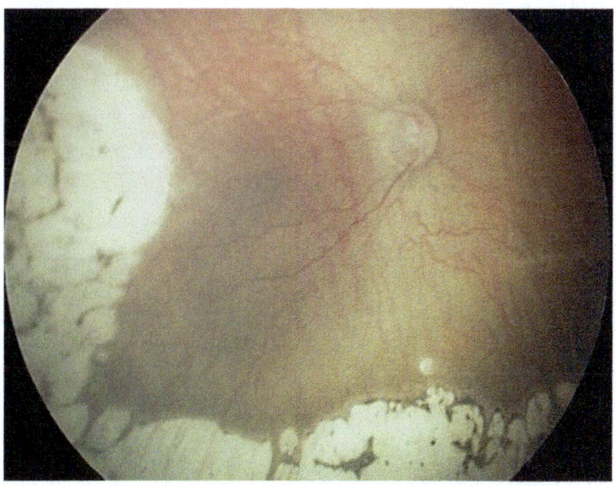

Fig. 28.1 Final postoperative image. Extensive laser coagulation

---

Electronic Supplementary Material The online version of this chapter (https://doi.org/10.1007/978-3-030-13701-4_28) contains supplementary material, which is available to authorized users.
The videos can be accessed under http://extras.springer.com/Search. Enter the ISBN number of your book and download the videos.

U. Spandau, S. J. Kim, *Pediatric Retinal Vascular Diseases*,
https://doi.org/10.1007/978-3-030-13701-4_28

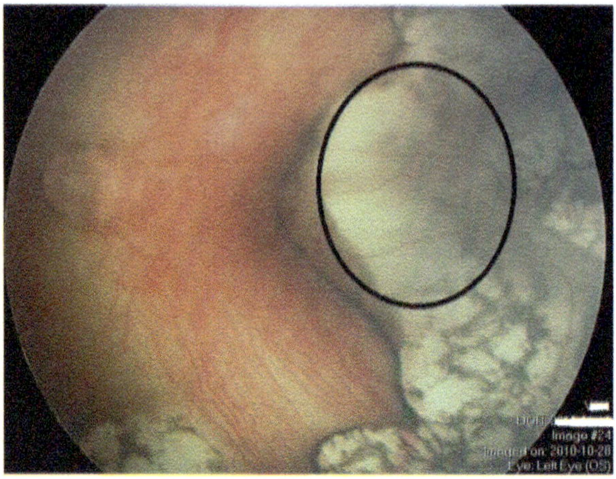

Fig. 28.2 Final postoperative image. Note the very central laser coagulation almost engaging the macula and the focal detachment (stage 4A) on the ridge (circle)

Before this case our primary treatment for ROP zone I was laser coagulation. After this difficult case we changed our treatment regime to anti-VEGF as primary treatment for zone I.

General history

A neonate born in week 24 with a birth weight of 716 g. Difficult necrotizing enterocolitis and short-bowel syndrome after bowel resections occurred.

Ocular history:

- Week 32: Diagnosed as ROP in zone I (Aggressive posterior ROP)
- Week 32: Laser treatment with 3118 effects (RE) and 2472 effects (LE).
- Week 34: A recurrence occurred. There were no skip lesions present but new ischemic tissue was present at the ridge. A completing laser treatment with 788 effects (RE) and 415 effects (LE) was performed.
- Week 36: A recurrence occurred. Iris rubeosis and plus disease developed although the complete ischemic retina was treated.
- Week 36: An intravitreal Avastin was performed as rescue therapy
- Week 36: 1 day postop: Marked improvement of the plus disease
- Week 40: Bilateral quiet eyes (Figs. 28.1 and 28.2). The right eye has an attached retina. The left eye has a focal detachment on the ridge causing a dragging on the macula.

8-year follow-up:

- Right eye: −5,25/− 2,5 cylinder 40°.
- Left eye: −4,25/−2 cylinder 150°.
- Visual acuity with both eyes was 0,25 with own glasses. It is likely that the left eye has a visual acuity below 0,1 due to the macular heterotopia.

Conclusion:

Despite a complete laser coagulation, a plus disease can reoccur in zone I. This phenomenon does not happen in zone II. The retina does not tolerate a too central laser coagulation. Consequently, we changed our treatment algorithm. For zone I an anti-VEGF treatment is the primary treatment (Fig. 28.3).

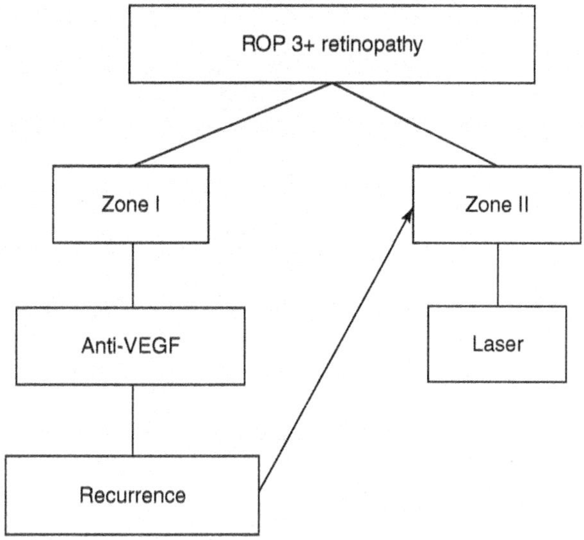

Fig. 28.3 Our treatment algorithm for ROP plus disease

28.2 Case Report No. 19: Vitrectomy for Stage 4A Retinal Detachment (Figs. 28.4, 28.5, 28.6, 28.7, 28.8, and 28.9)

General history:

A preterm born girl born in week GA 25 + 2 and a weight at birth of 743 g. Acute sectio due to B-streptococcus colonized placenta. After 2 days a lung bleeding occurred necessitating a stay of 3 weeks in a respirator. Congenital alfa-streptococcus and staphylococcus aureus sepsis during these 3 weeks.

Ocular history:

- Week 34: Laser photocoagulation (2677 effects (RE) and 2499 (LE)) for ROP 3+ in posterior zone II in a hospital elsewhere
- Week 36: Bilateral Lucentis injection due to deterioration to stage 4A
- Week 37: Bilateral cerclage due to persistent activity
- Week 41: Persistent activity; referral to our hospital
- Week 41: Examination with Retcam and Retcam angiography:
- Right eye: Detached temporal retina with subretinal exudates. Big skip lesion in the temporal periphery. 360 degrees cerclage (Figs. 28.4, 28.5, and 28.6).
- Left eye: Detached temporal retina with much subretinal exudates. Temporal proliferations. 360 degrees cerclage (Figs. 28.7, 28.8, and 28.9).
- *Angiography*: Very late effect.
- Right eye: Hypofluorescence at temporal pole, big skip lesion at the temporal ridge from 8 to 10 o'clock (Fig. 28.6).
- Left eye: 360 degrees proliferations, especially temporal, superior and at 6 o'clock (Figs. 28.8 and 28.9).

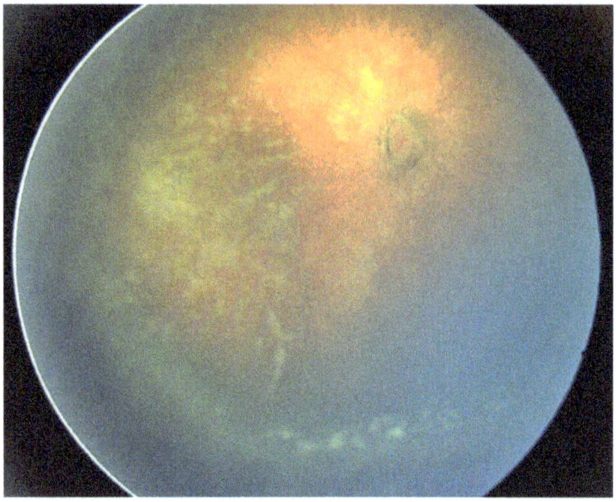

Fig. 28.4 Right eye: Colour picture: Increasing exudates from posterior pole to the periphery

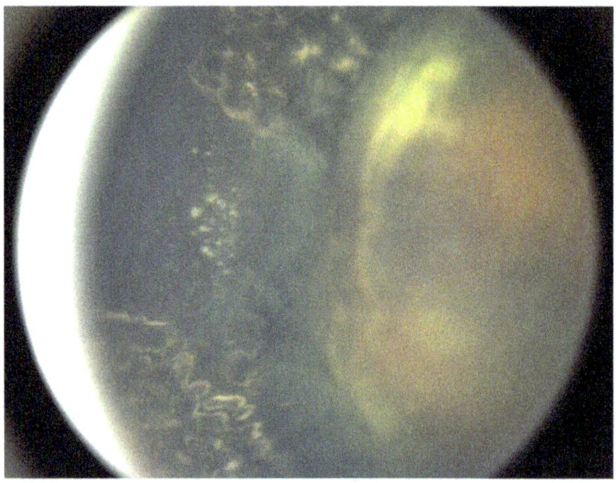

Fig. 28.5 Right eye: Colour picture: Big skip lesion at the temporal ridge from 8 to 10 o'clock and many exudates at the ridge

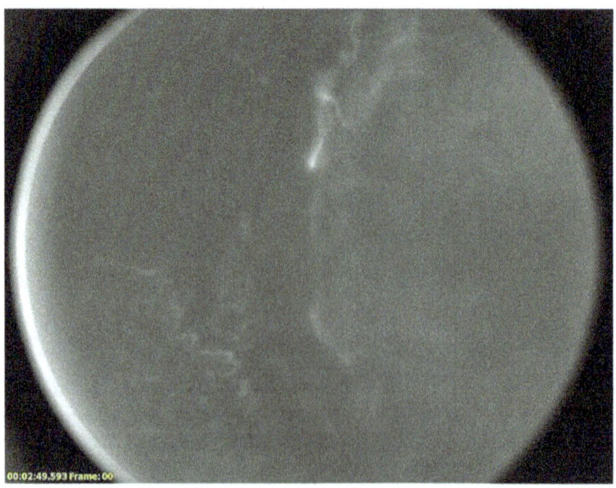

Fig. 28.6 Right eye. Angiography: Big skip lesion at the temporal retina from 8 to 10 o'clock

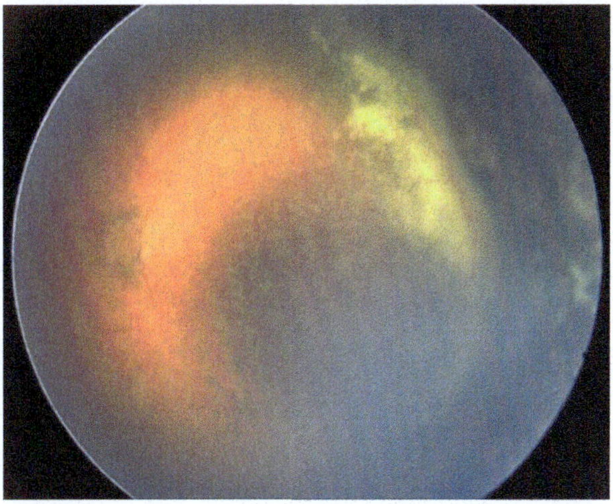

Fig. 28.7 Left eye. Colour picture: Many exudates and not treated ischemic retina at the temporal retina

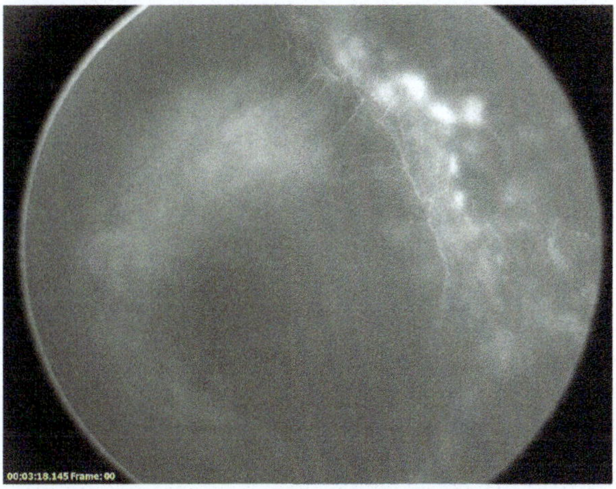

Fig. 28.8 Left eye. Angiography: Undertreated ischemic retina with leakage and pathologic vessels

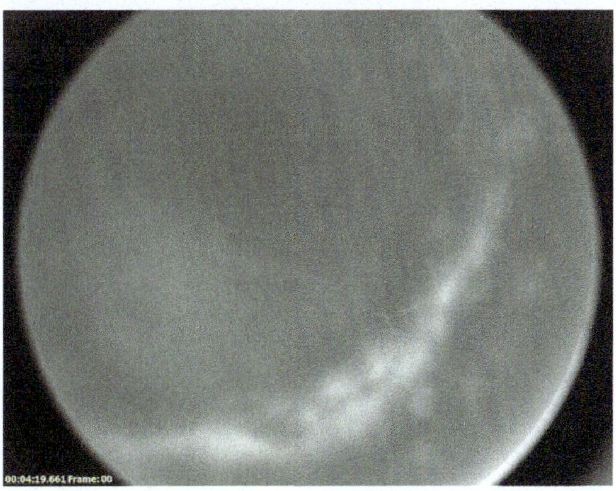

Fig. 28.9 Left eye. Angiography: Leakage and proliferations at the ridge

Surgery: Same day:

- Right eye: 27G lens sparing vitrectomy + endolaser + Lucentis (see video)
- Left eye: 27G lens sparing vitrectomy + endolaser + Lucentis (see video)

- 11 months follow-up: Fixates very badly, both eyes with much esotropia, bilateral −11 diopters
- 12 months after birth: Removal of encircling band.
- 16 months follow-up: Huge improvement of visual acuity after removal of encircling band. Fixates faces and toys with the left eye. Esotropia right eye. Right eye: −8 diopters; Left eye: −11 diopters. Examination of retina: Myopic fundus, attached retina, no exudates, no hemorrhages, laser effects in the periphery

Conclusion:

(1) The cause for the progression of the ROP disease was an incomplete treatment with laser coagulation (Figs. 28.5 and 28.6). (2) The encircling band caused a grave myopia (−12 diopters). The myopia reduced after removal of the encircling band from −12D to −9D in the right eye and −11D to −10D in the left eye.

28.3 Case Report No. 20: Bilateral Stage 4A and Stage 4B Detachment and Retinal Redetachment (Figs. 28.10, 28.11, 28.12, 28.13, 28.14, 28.15, 28.16, 28.17, 28.18, and 28.19)

General history: Born in week 22 with a weight of 525 g.

Ocular history:

- 03/2010: ROP 3+ in zone I; treated with intravitreal **Lucentis**
- 05/2010: Recurrence of ROP, treated with laser photocoagulation
- 08/2010: Nystagmus
- 09/2010: Retinal detachment stage 4B left eye and stage 4A right eye: Bilateral **lens sparing vitrectomy + Lucentis** (Figs. 28.10, 28.11, 28.12, 28.13, 28.14, and 28.15)
- **2 weeks after vitrectomy**: Redetachment in the right eye; left eye stable: Second **vitrectomy right eye + Lucentis** (Figs. 28.15, 28.16, 28.17, 28.18, and 28.19)

Final follow-up at 12/2010**:**

Attached retina right eye and stable status left eye.

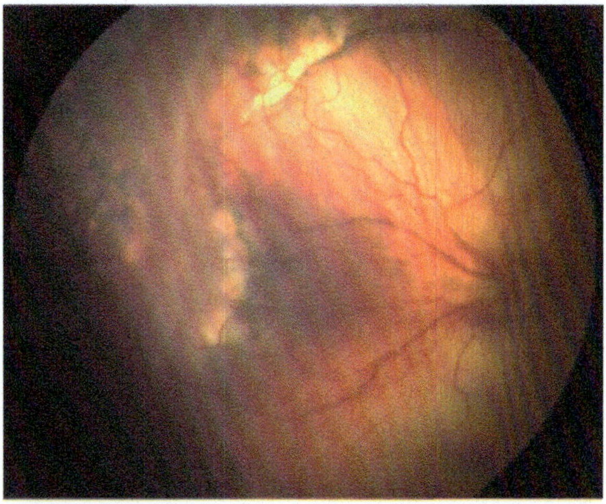

Fig. 28.10 RE: Colour photograph. Before first vitrectomy. Retinal detachment stage 4A

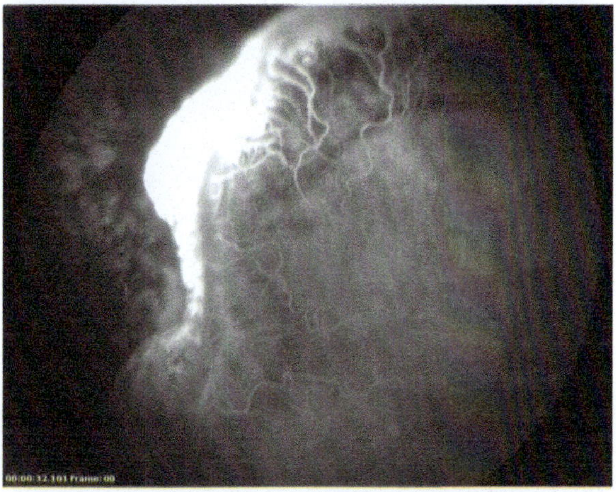

Fig. 28.11 RE: Angiography. Before first vitrectomy. Fibrovascular proliferations along the ridge

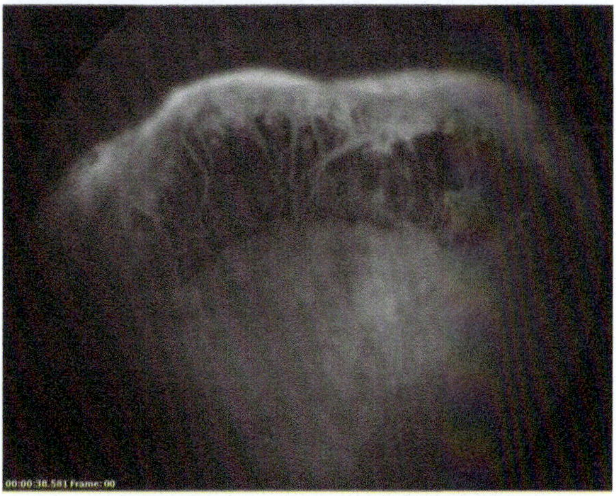

Fig. 28.12 RE: Angiography. Before first vitrectomy. Fibrovascular proliferations along the ridge

Fig. 28.13 LE: Colour photograph. Before first vitrectomy. Stage 4B with submacular hemorrhage

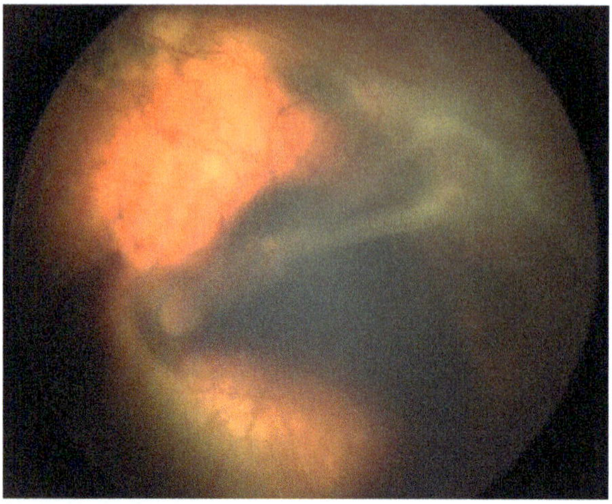

Fig. 28.14 LE: Angiography: Before first vitrectomy. Extensive leakage in the periphery

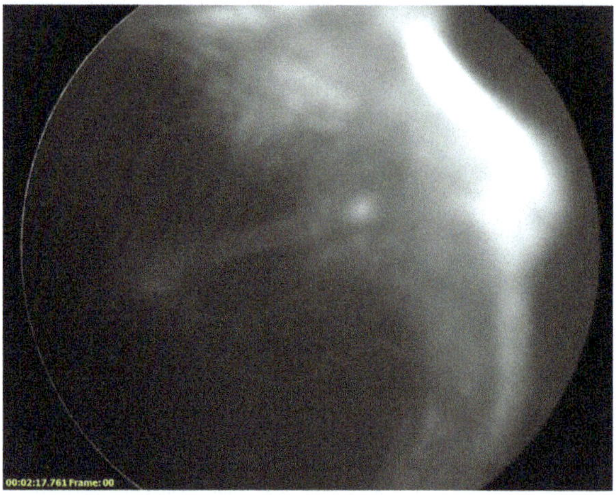

Fig. 28.15 RE: Colour photograph. Three weeks after first vitrectomy. Redetachment with submacular hemorrhage

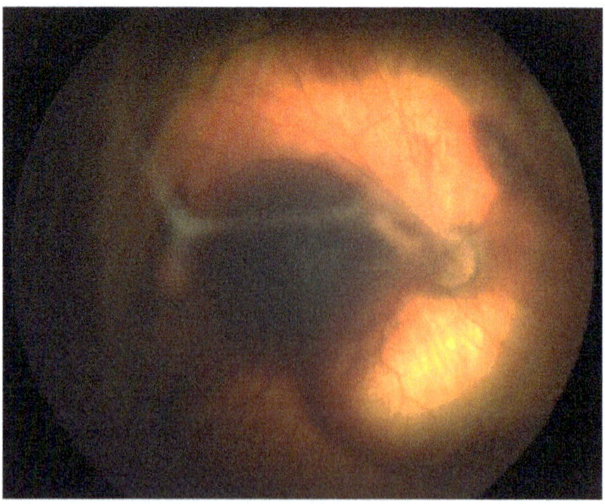

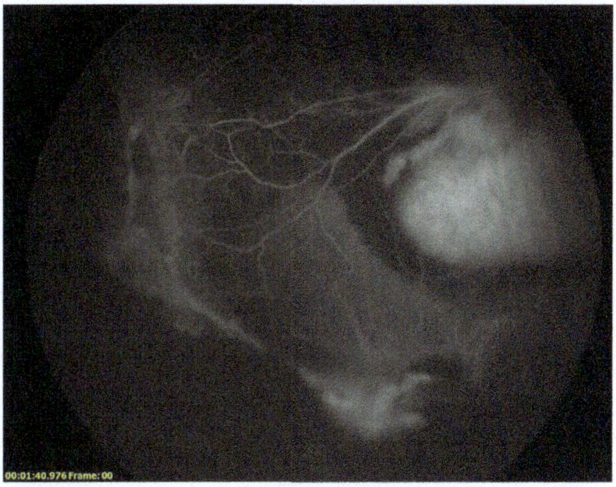

Fig. 28.16 RE: Angiography: Three weeks after first vitrectomy. Redetachment with submacular hemorrhage

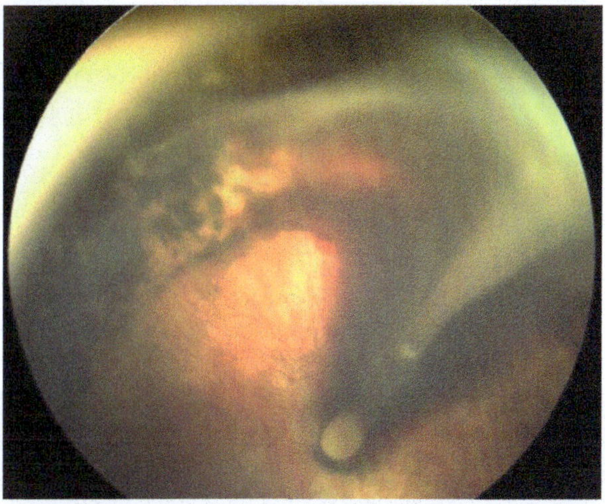

Fig. 28.17 LE: Colour photograph. Three weeks after first vitrectomy. Clear improvement

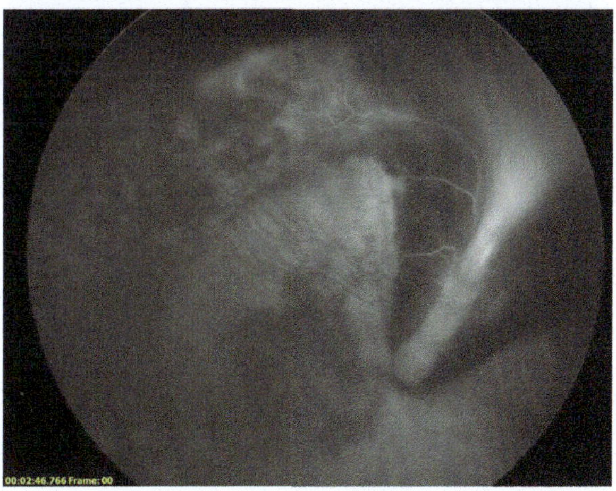

Figs. 28.18 and 28.19 LE: Angiography. Three weeks after first vitrectomy. Much leakage from the fold in the periphery

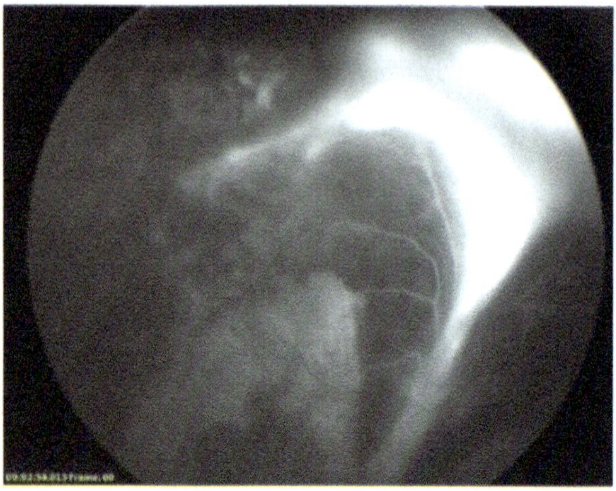

Figs. 28.18 and 28.19 (continued)

28.4 Case Report No. 21: Vitrectomy for ROP Stage 4b with Shallow Detachment and Exudates (Figs. 28.20, 28.21, 28.22, 28.23, and 28.24)

A premature born neonate in week 23 with a birth weight of 665 gram. Developed ROP 3+ in week 35 and received consequently a laser treatment with 1992 effects in the right eye and 1930 effects in the left eye. Both eyes progressed and were retreated 3 weeks later with laser treatment of 300 effects in both eyes. The right eye progressed and 3 weeks later the neonate was referred to our hospital. We scheduled immediately an examination in general anaesthesia and diagnosed a stage 4A detachment on the RE. Subretinal exudates were present around the optic disc and along the arcade (Figs. 28.20, 28.21, and 28.22). Skip lesions were found (Fig. 28.21) and a fibrovascular membrane had developed (Fig. 28.22). The left eye was normal (Fig. 28.23). A lens sparing vitrectomy with Lucentis injection was performed. The 1-week follow-up showed an attached retina and a marked reduction of exudates (Fig. 28.24).

Conclusion: The cause for the progression of the ROP disease was an under-treatment with laser coagulation. In this case, you can try to treat the eye first with anti-VEGF and completing laser and later with vitrectomy if necessary. We chose vitrectomy because the macula was detached.

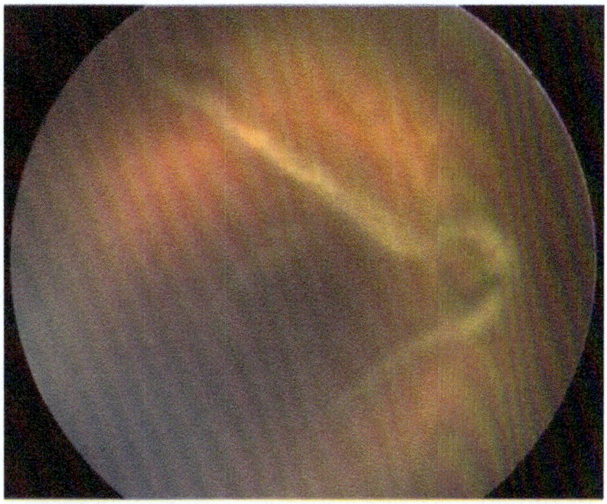

Fig. 28.20 RE: A stage 4B detachment with exudates around the optic disc and along the temporal arcade. The macula is detached. The reason for this detachment is an undertreatment with laser coagulation

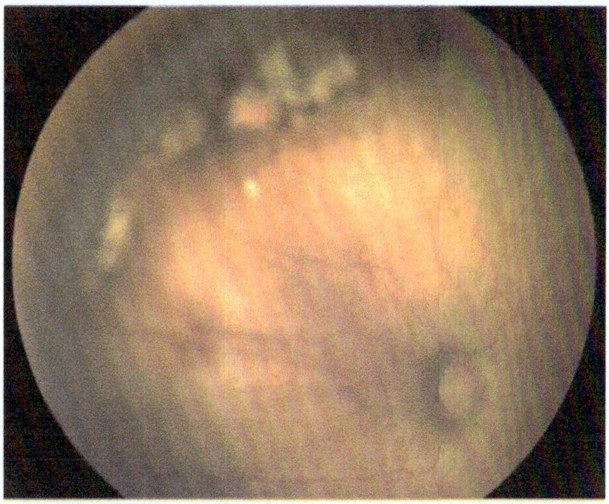

Fig. 28.21 RE: Note the non-treated ischemic retina in the periphery. Both eyes were treated again with laser. The left eye regressed but the right eye progressed

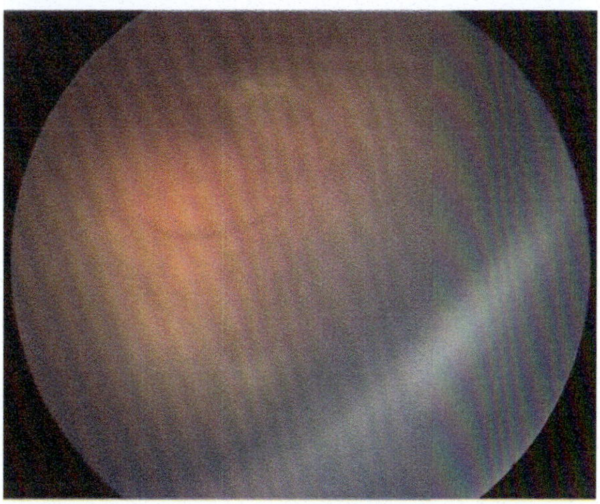

Fig. 28.22 A fibrovascular membrane developed from the ridge but did not reach the posterior lens

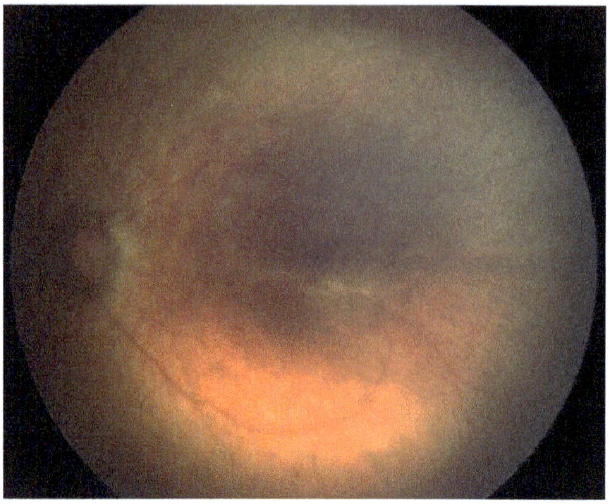

Fig. 28.23 The left eye was normal. The left eye regressed after the second laser coagulation

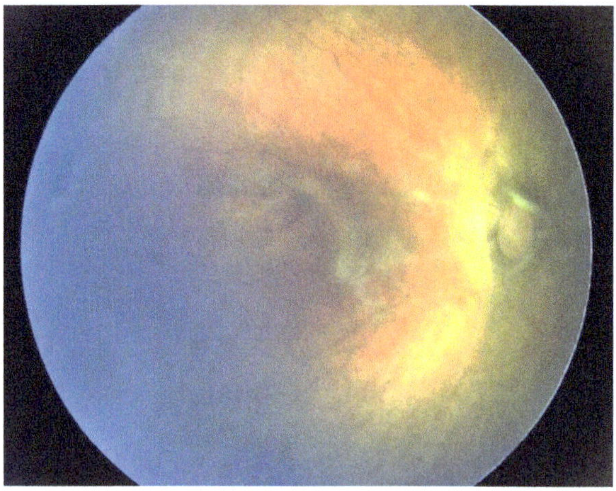

Fig. 28.24 RE: Follow-up 7 days after vitrectomy. The exudates are very much reduced, and the neonate could fixate much better

28.5 Case Report No. 22: Laser Coagulation and Lucentis for Stage 4A Detachment After Inadequate Laser Treatment (Figs. 28.25, 28.26, 28.27, 28.28, and 28.29)

This neonate was born in gestation week 24, the birth weight was 600 grams. This neonate was treated elsewhere with laser coagulation for ROP 3+. The disease persisted and a focal detachment temporal to the macula and a preretinal bleeding developed. Six weeks after the initial treatment the newborn was referred to us. We examined the newborn. The neonate is now 4 months old and weighs 4360 grams. Fundus examination revealed an overtreatment as well as an undertreatment of laser coagulation in both eyes (Figs. 28.25, 28.26, and 28.27). The right eye had a focal detachment at 3

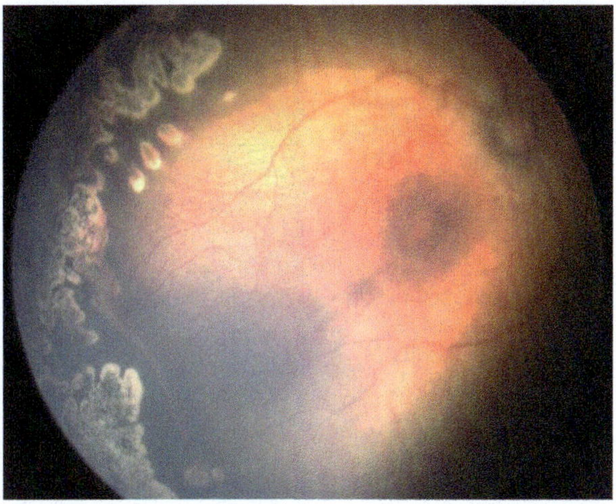

Fig. 28.25 RE: ROP 3 with plus disease. Note the undertreatment at the temporal ridge

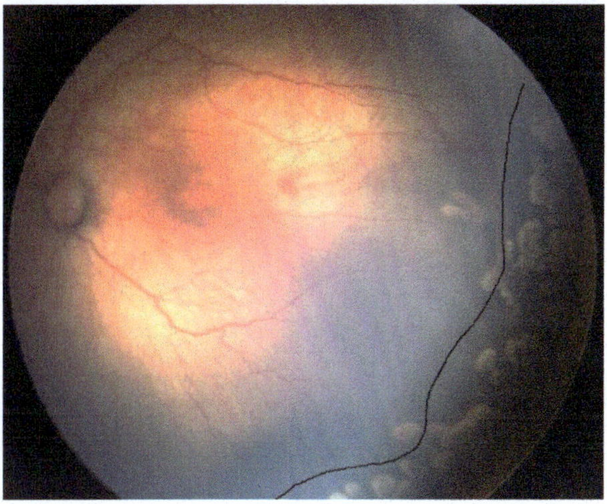

Fig. 28.26 LE: ROP 3 without plus. The laser effects are visible posterior to the ridge (overtreatment) and skip lesions can be seen anterior to the ridge (undertreatment)

and 9 o'clock with plus disease and the left eye had a focal detachment at 11 and 3 o'clock and no plus disease. The neonate was treated with completing laser coagulation (RE: 1157 effects, LE: 1364 effects) and an injection of Lucentis in the RE. The LE received no Lucentis injection because no plus disease was present.

One month later a central preretinal bleeding occurred on the left eye (Fig. 28.28). This eye was previously not treated with Lucentis. No treatment was initiated because the bleeding was central and not on the ridge, no focal detachment was observed and because laser coagulation was complete. At the three-month follow-up the hemorrhage had disappeared and the retina was completely attached (Fig. 28.29).

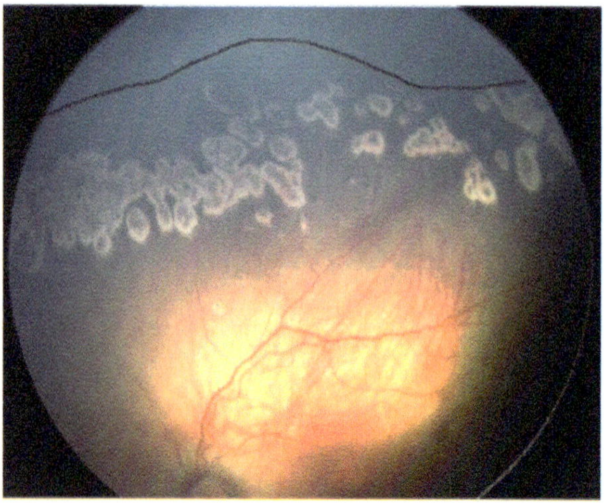

Fig. 28.27 LE The ischemic retina is not treated (undertreated) but the physiologic retina is treated (overtreated). Overtreatment should be avoided because physiologic retina is destroyed but it has no negative influence on the ROP activity. Undertreatment, however, is dangerous and must be avoided in any case because the ROP activity is not eliminated

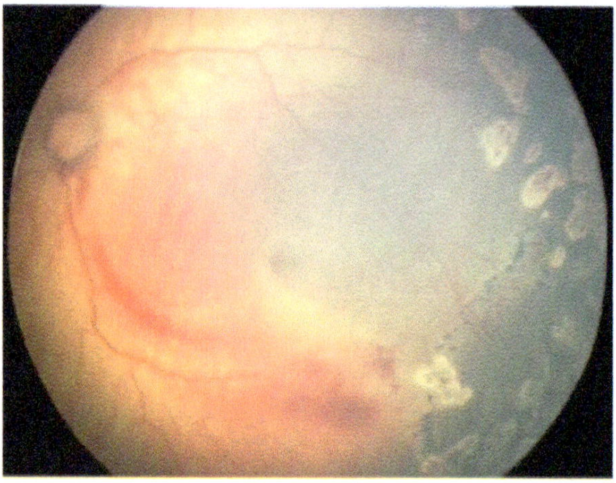

Fig. 28.28 **LE:** One-month follow-up: A preretinal bleeding occurred. No treatment was initiated

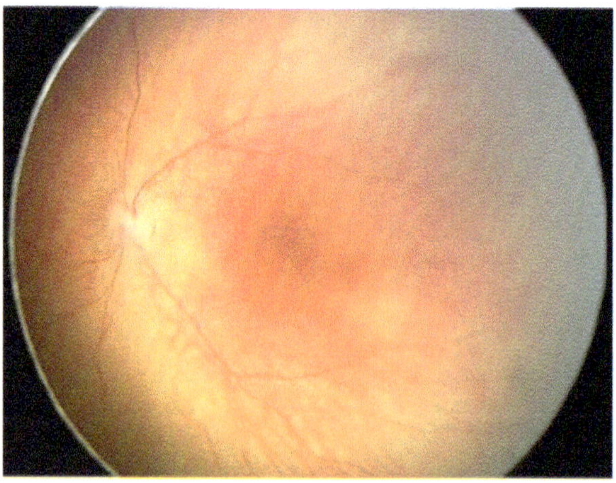

Fig. 28.29 **LE:** Three months follow-up: The preretinal bleeding disappeared

Conclusion: The cause for the progression of the ROP disease was an undertreatment with laser coagulation. If an undertreatment is present we recommend first a completing laser coagulation and an Lucentis injection. If the plus disease does not disappear after 2 weeks we recommend a lens sparing vitrectomy.

28.6 Case Report No. 23: Delayed Treatment in a 22-Week Newborn (Figs. 28.30, 28.31, 28.32, 28.33, and 28.34)

A 22 + 6-week newborn was diagnosed in week 39 with ROP 3+ in the right eye (Figs. 28.30 and 28.31). The left eye showed ROP stage 2. The neonate was referred to a treatment center but there she was diagnosed as ROP stage 2. No treatment

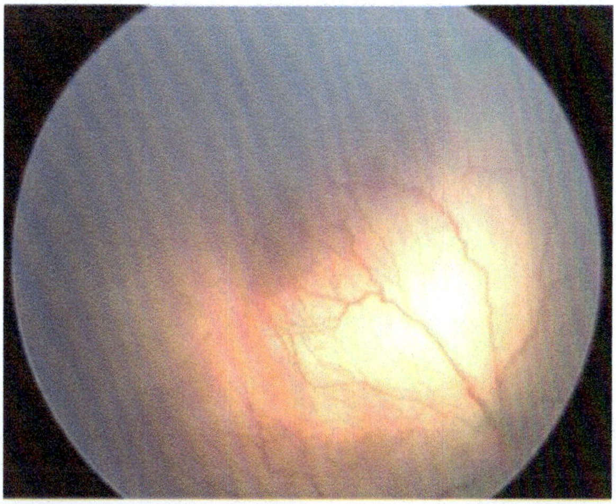

Fig. 28.30 **RE:** Week 39: A flat ridge on the temporal side is present. A posterior zone II is present

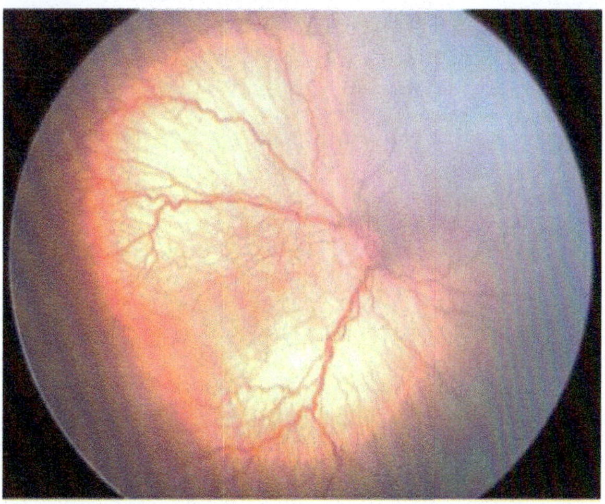

Fig. 28.31 **RE:** Week 39: The central vessels are tortuous and thick. A ROP plus disease is present

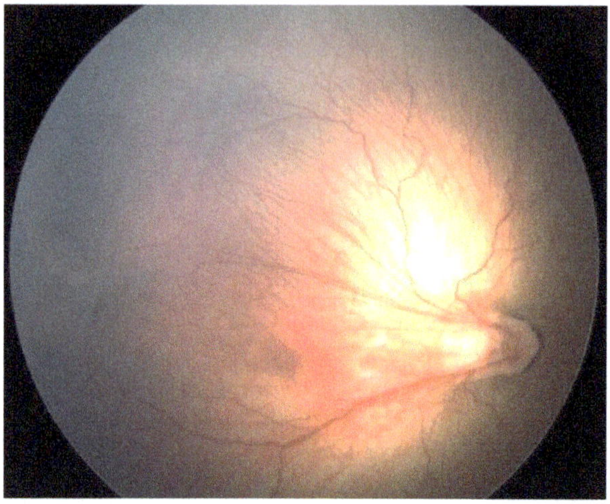

Fig. 28.32 RE: Two months later. A macular dragging is found

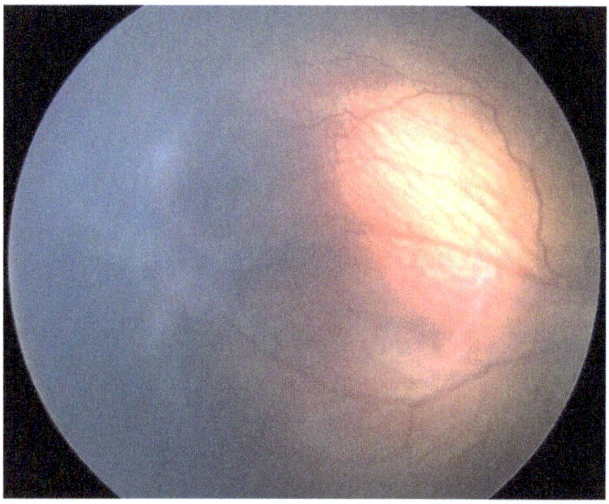

Fig. 28.33 RE: Two months later. An octopus formed retinal fibrosis is present on the ridge. A low retinal detachment was seen. Avastin was injected intravitreal

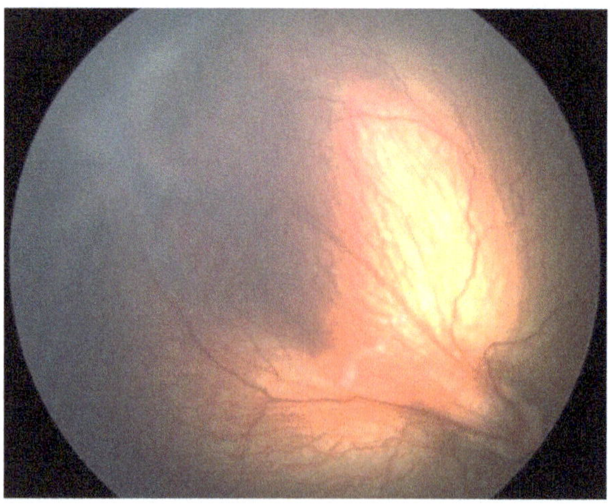

Fig. 28.34 RE: Two months later after Avastin injection. The macular dragging remains. A focal detachment cannot be detected. No further treatment is recommended. Note the tilted disc

was initiated. Two months later a macular dragging with focal detachment at the temporal ridge was observed (Fig. 28.33). An intravitreal treatment with Avastin was performed. A two-month follow-up showed an unchanged fundus (Fig. 28.34).

28.7 Case Report No. 24: Intravitreal Lucentis for ROP Stage 4A After Cryo and Laser Treatment (Figs. 28.35, 28.36, 28.37, and 28.38)

General history: A premature born boy in week 24 and a weight of 470 g and very slow gain of weight.

Ocular history:

- Week 32: Diagnosis of ROP 3+ In zone I.
- Week 32: Laser treatment

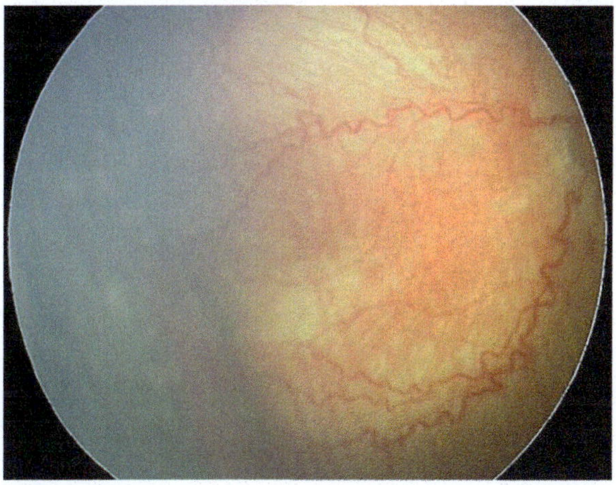

Fig. 28.35 RE: Central tortuous and thick vessels, temporal hemorrhage on the ridge. Attached retina. Calm on the nasal side

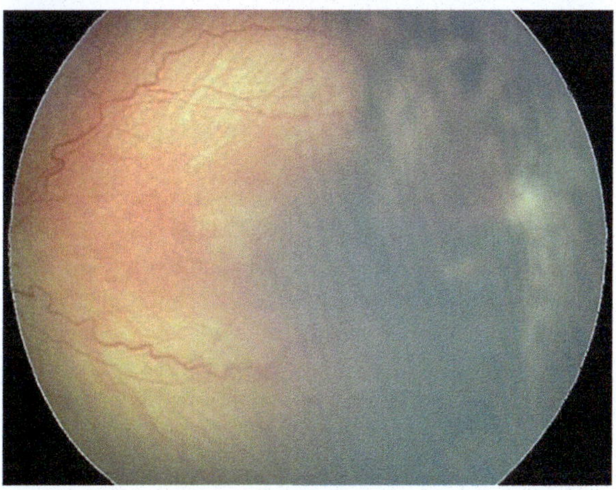

Fig. 28.36 LE: Rubeotic iris, centrally tortuous and thick vessels, temporal pigmented area with detached retina from 2 to 5o'clock, a nest of retinal proliferations on top of detached retina and the macula is attached

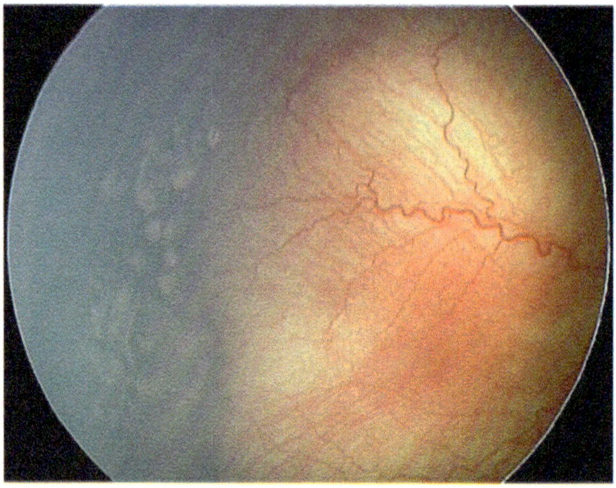

Fig. 28.37 RE: 1-month later: Resorbed hemorrhage and much less media opacities. The central vessels are still tortuous but less thick

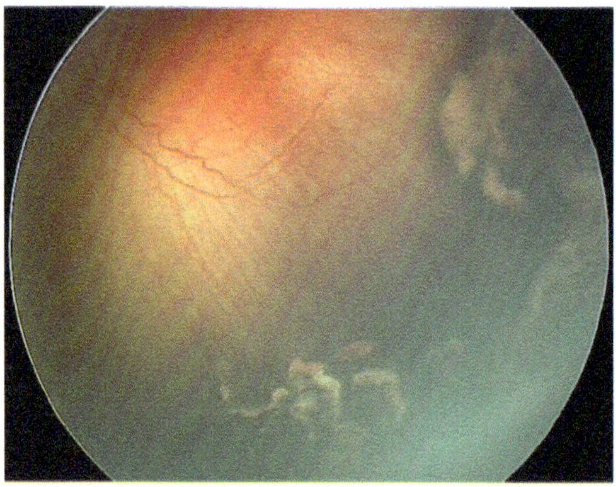

Fig. 28.38 LE: 1-month later: The hemorrhage has disappeared, the retina is reattached, and the vessels are almost normal

- In the follow-up a persistence of ROP disease and development of an iris rubeosis was detected. An undertreatment of laser was detected. Consequently, a repeated treatment was recommended.
- Week 37: Cryopexy treatment
- During the follow-up the iris rubeosis regressed but the morphology of the retinal vessels did not improve. In the left eye a ridge with proliferations and hemorrhage developed and in the left eye a thin retinal bleeding was found.
- Week 39: The patient was referred to our hospital.
- We scheduled immediately an examination in general anaesthesia. The examination with indirect ophthalmoscopy and Retcam showed:
- The *right eye* had no iris rubeosis. At the posterior pole tortuous and thick vessels were found and a temporal hemorrhage on the ridge was present. The retina was attached (Fig. 28.35). The *left eye* had an iris rubeosis. The central vessels were

tortuous and thick. Temporal a pigmented area with detached retina from 2 to 5 o'clock was seen and a nest of retinal proliferations on top of the detached retina. The macula was attached, and the nasal side was calm (Fig. 28.36).

- The *right eye* was diagnosed as ROP 3+. The *left eye* was diagnosed as ROP 4A.
- A bilateral intravitreal bevacizumab injection was performed.
- Week 44: The 1-month follow-up showed a resorption of the hemorrhages. The retina was attached in the left eye (Figs. 28.37 and 28.38).

Three-year follow-up: The 3y/o girl has a lot of worries. Her eyesight is relatively bad, she has nystagmus. She has grave myopia and astigmatism. The myopia is about 4 and 6 diopters with an astigmatism of 2–3 diopters.

Conclusion: The cause for the progression of the ROP disease was an under-treatment with laser coagulation. If ROP stage 4A develops, then an anti-VEGF injection may solve the problem. If no effect occurs 2 weeks after injection, we recommend a lens sparing vitrectomy.

28.8 Case Report No. 25: Vitrectomy for ROP Stage 4A

This neonate was born in week 24. In week 32 she was treated with bilateral Lucentis for ROP 3+ in zone I. In week 40 a recurrence in zone II occurred. A laser coagulation was performed. Within 2 weeks a retinal detachment developed in the left eye. A stage 4A detachment was diagnosed. The right eye regressed. Therefore, in week 42 an episcleral band was placed in the left eye. The detachment, however, persisted, and retinal exudates increased slowly. In week 46 the neonate was referred to our hospital for vitrectomy.

We performed an examination in general anaesthesia:

The right eye showed no active ROP disease. The left eye had a big preretinal hemorrhage at the temporal equator and many exudates at the posterior pole. A 360 deg impression of the encircling band was present. A light retinal elevation is seen at the temporal pole. The diagnosis was a stage 4A detachment and we decided to perform a lens sparing vitrectomy.

Surgery:

During the same session a 27G lens sparing vitrectomy with intravitreal Avastin injection was performed in the left eye. The surgery was without complications.

2 months follow-up: Visual function: Fixates light, left eye: esotropia. Retinoscopy: Right eye: +1,5 diopters; Left eye: −9 diopters.

4 months follow-up: Increase of myopia in the left eye from −9 diopters to −12 diopters.

Removal of cerclage 9 months after placement.

Ten months follow-up: Visually active, fixates well with the right eye, left eye: esotropia. Retinoscopy after removal of cerclage: Right eye: +1,5sph diopters; Left eye: -12sph diopters. Examination of retina: Right eye: Optic disc and macula normal, attached retina; left eye: Optic disc normal, macula with poor reflex, attached retina, no exudates.

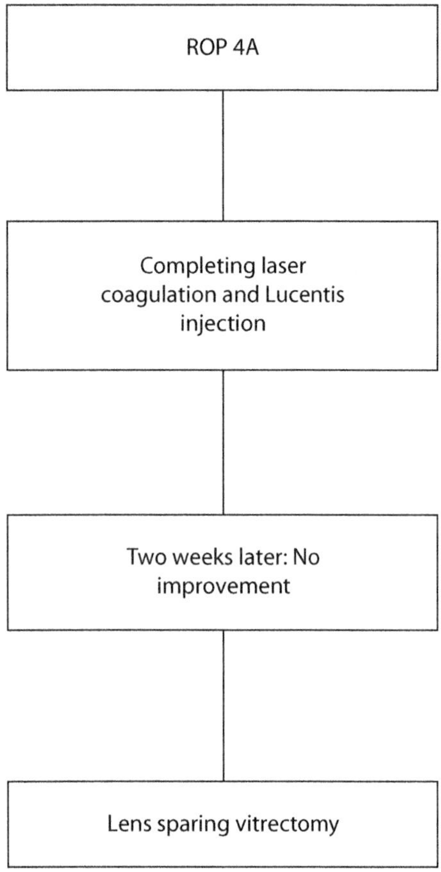

Fig. 28.39 Our treatment algorithm for ROP stage 4A

Conclusion: (1) The cause for the progression of the ROP disease is not really clear. The eye looked well laser treated. However, an undertreatment of the ridge cannot be excluded. Our treatment algorithm for ROP stage 4A is depicted in Fig. 28.39. (2) An encircling band causes a grave myopia. In this case a myopia of −12 diopters was induced. A one-sided encircling band causes a grave anisometropia and amblyopia.

28.9 Case Report No. 26: Failed Vitrectomy for ROP Stage 4B (Figs. 28.40, 28.41, 28.42, 28.43, 28.44, 28.45, and 28.46)

In week 23 born neonate. In week 35 treated with laser coagulation for ROP 3+. In week 39 treated with bilateral Lucentis and encircling band. In week 43 referral to our hospital for vitrectomy of a stage 4 detachment in the left eye. She was treated with chloramphenicol eye drops for an acute dacryocystitis in the left eye. The injection with Lucentis in the left eye was delayed for 2 days due to an increased risk for endophthalmitis due to the ongoing dacryocystitis.

An *examination* in general anaesthesia revealed the following findings:

- *Right eye*: Clear optical media. 360 deg cerclage impression. Big hemorrhage on the temporal ridge. Angiography shows much vascular activity at 9 o'clock and skip lesions 360 deg (Figs. 28.40, 28.41, and 28.42).
- *Left eye*: Hazy optical media. 360 deg cerclage impression. Retinal detachment nasal and inferior. Detached macula. Retcam angiography shows vascular activity temporal and skip lesion 360 deg (Figs. 28.43, 28.44, and 28.45).

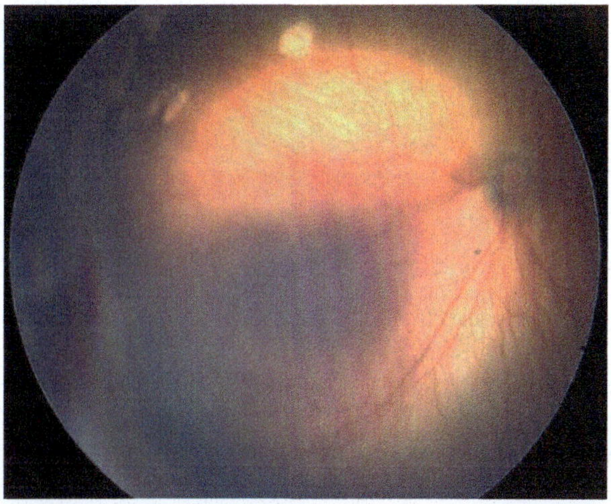

Fig. 28.40 RE: Hardly any plus, but a big hemorrhage on the ridge at 9 o'clock

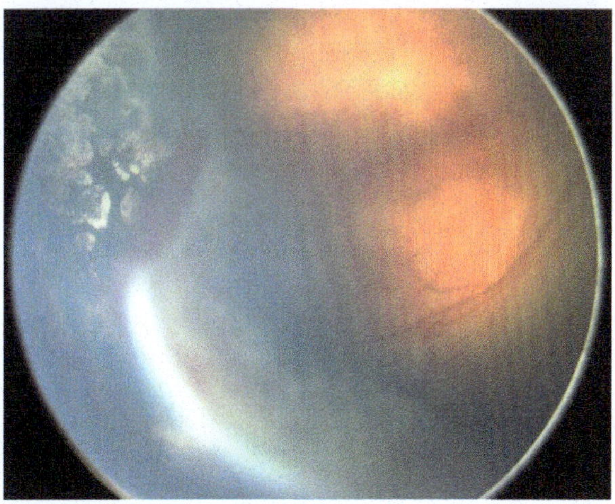

Fig. 28.41 RE: Skip lesions at the temporal ridge, a hemorrhage and a fibrovascular membrane from 6 to 9 o'clock

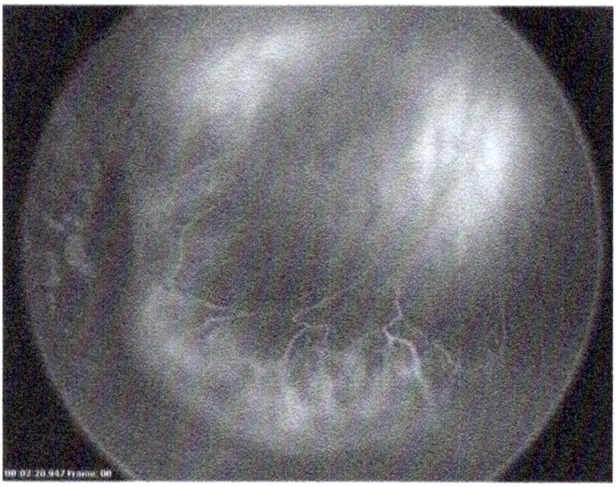

Fig. 28.42 RE: The angiography picture corresponds to Fig. 28.41. Leakage and proliferations from 6 to 8 o'clock

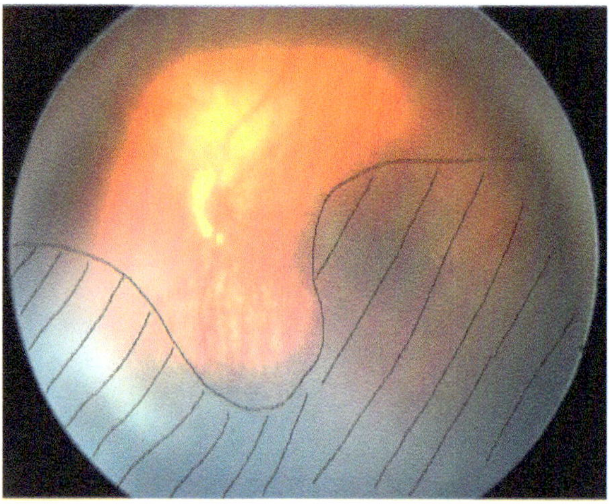

Fig. 28.43 LE: A stage 4B detachment. The macula is detached

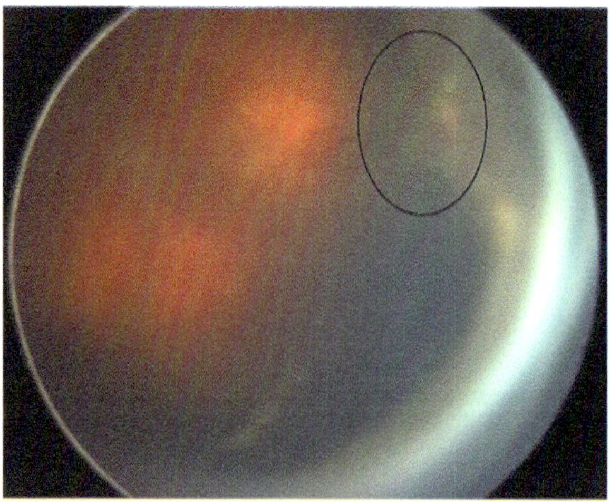

Fig. 28.44 LE: A contraction of retinal tissue at the ridge with focal detachment. Note also the white fibrovascular membrane in the temporal periphery

- The right eye is diagnosed as a persistence of ROP disease in zone II. Planned LIO and Lucentis injection. The left eye is diagnosed as stage 4B detachment. Planned lens sparing vitrectomy + Lucentis injection.
  Surgery:
- *Right eye*: Completing laser coagulation and Lucentis injection.
- *Left eye*: 27G lens sparing vitrectomy. It was very difficult to insert the trocars because the fibrovascular membranes were in the way. The lens was injured. The infusion was in the beginning not located inside the vitreous cavity and induced a retinal detachment. At the end of the surgery and 1 day postop the retina was attached. One week later, however, the retina detached (Fig. 28.46). We discussed with the parents the situation and informed them that in a next surgery a lensectomy would become necessary. The parents chose not to operate the eye.

Four months later the encircling band was cut in both eyes. An esotropia was present in both eyes and the neonate fixated light and started to play with toys.

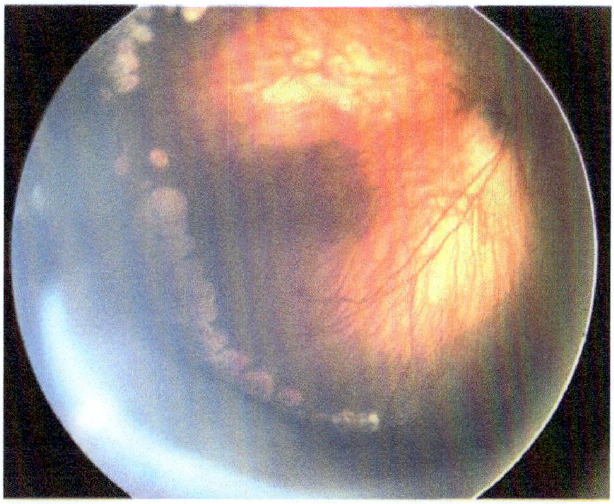

Fig. 28.45 RE: 4-month follow-up. Attached retina

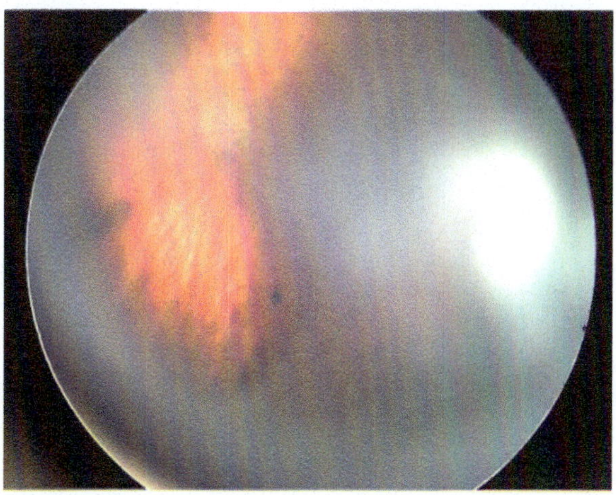

Fig. 28.46 LE: 4-month follow-up. The nasal retina is attached but the residual retina is detached. Note also the thick and white fibrovascular membrane at 3 o'clock

Chapter 29
Interesting Case Reports in ROP from the Literature

29.1 Very Late Reactivation of ROP After Intravitreal Bevacizumab Injection

Intravitreal anti-VEGF injection temporarily blocks the action of VEGF and can be followed by recurrence or reactivation of ischemic proliferative retinopathy. Therefore, eyes treated with intravitreal anti-VEGF usually show different clinical course from laser-treated eyes.

Recurrence or reactivation of ROP is one of the major concerns of anti-VEGF treatment for ROP. Blair and colleagues reported two cases of very late reactivation leading to retinal detachment after intravitreal bevacizumab.

Case 1

In 2016, Snyder et al. reported a case of late reactivation at the age of 2.5 years [1]. A summary of the case report is as follows. A female infant, whose BW was 630 g and GA was 24 weeks, developed aggressive posterior retinopathy of prematurity in zone I and intravitreal bevacizumab (0.625 mg) injection was done at 34 weeks PMA. At 51 weeks PMA, the baby showed reactivation of ROP (zone 2, stage 3 with plus disease) and 2nd injection of bevacizumab (0.625 mg) was done. At 80 weeks PMA, there was no recurrence of ROP and peripheral vascularization was deemed adequate. At 2.5 years, the right eye developed a vitreous hemorrhage and a tractional retinal detachment, and the left eye showed EFP (extraretinal fibrovascular proliferation) in zone II. The right eye underwent two vitrectomies and the left eye underwent peripheral laser ablation.

Case 2

In 2017, Hajrasouliha et al. reported a case of late reactivation of ROP resulting in bilateral tractional retinal detachment 3 years after intravitreal bevacizumab injection [2]. A female infant, whose BW was 739 g and GA was 24 weeks, developed bilateral posterior zone 2, stage 3+ ROP and intravitreal bevacizumab (0.625 mg) injection was done at 36 weeks PMA. Because the disease appeared quiescent at

U. Spandau, S. J. Kim, *Pediatric Retinal Vascular Diseases*,
https://doi.org/10.1007/978-3-030-13701-4_29

75 weeks PMA, the scheduled follow-up was increased to a 6-month interval. At 3 years of age, she developed bilateral peripheral retinal detachment with anterior fibrovascular proliferation and posterior exudates. Both eyes were treated with laser ablation to peripheral avascular retina, scleral buckle to support fibrovascular tissue, and intravitreal bevacizumab to reduce vascularity and exudation.

These two cases highlight different clinical course of anti-VEGF treated eyes compared to that of conventional laser treated eyes. Also, the cases raise questions on optimal follow-up protocol and the proper indications of laser treatment in eyes treated with anti-VEGF. Physicians should be aware of the possibility of very late reactivation of ROP and be cautious before increasing follow-up intervals. Shorter follow-up interval, peripheral retinal evaluation with fluorescein angiography and laser photocoagulation may be beneficial when peripheral avascular retina is persistent after anti-VEGF treatment.

29.2 Persistent ROP in Tetralogy of Fallot

There have been two case reports on atypical findings after ROP treatment in babies with tetralogy of Fallot (TOF). TOF refers to a combination of four cardiac anomalies including ventricular septal defect, pulmonary stenosis, right ventricular hypertrophy, and overriding aorta. TOF is one of the most common cyanotic congenital heart diseases and arterial oxygen saturation is low in patients with TOF, leading to tissue ischemia such as retinal ischemia.

In 2013, Paulus and Moshfeghi reported a case of persistent plus disease after laser treatment in a female infant [3]. A baby born at 29+ 2 weeks of gestation with a BW of 940 g was diagnosed as TOF and Di George syndrome. The baby showed type 1 ROP at 2 months after birth. Despite of regression of EFP after peripheral laser ablation, worsening plus disease developed. Although fluorescein angiography revealed no active ROP 2 months after laser treatment, plus disease was persistent for several months.

In 2016, Gunay et al. reported a case of persistent ROP in a female infant with TOF [4]. The baby was born at 35 weeks of gestation and BW was 1700 g. The baby developed zone II, stage 1 ROP with mild vascular dilatation and tortuosity at 39 weeks PMA. These findings were persistent even at 6 months of corrected age.

These cases imply that infants with a severe cardiovascular status may develop ROP.

29.3 Endophthalmitis After Intravitreal Injection for the Treatment of ROP

Although there are many studies on intravitreal anti-VEGF injection for ROP, only one case of infectious endophthalmitis after intravitreal injection, to the best of my knowledge, was reported (as of September, 2018).

In 2017, Wang and Xiang in Guangzhou, China, reported a case of bacterial endophthalmitis in a preterm infant after intravitreal bevacizumab injection [5]. A male infant with GA of 28 weeks and BW of 1.2 kg underwent intravitreal bevacizumab injection at 34 weeks PMA for the treatment of zone II, stage 2+ ROP. Povidone iodine solution was applied before injection and tobramycin/dexamethasone ointment was applied 3 times a day after injection. Four days after injection, fundus imaging revealed a whitish plaque in the left eye. After 3 days, fundus exam revealed enlarged plaque to a gray flocculent mass with vitreous haze and anterior segment exam showed conjunctival hyperemia and cornea edema. A diagnosis of bacterial endophthalmitis was made and a vitreous tap to collect vitreous sample and intravitreal vancomycin and ceftazidime injections were performed. Systemic antibiotics was not administered. After intravitreal antibiotics treatment, retinal findings and corneal edema improved and a favorable anatomic outcome was achieved 3 weeks after the intravitreal injection of antibiotics.

This case suggests that (1) frequent fundus exams may be necessary to detect infectious endophthalmitis early after intravitreal injection in patients with ROP, (2) intravitreal injection of broad-spectrum antibiotics may be effective without systemic administration of antibiotics, and (3) clinical characteristics of presumed bacterial endophthalmitis in a preterm infant after intravitreal injection was similar to that in adult patients. However, because information from a single case is very limited, physicians should be prudent in managing an unusual case of endophthalmitis after intravitreal injection for ROP.

29.4 Exudative Retinal Detachment After Laser Photocoagulation or Anti-VEGF Injection in ROP

Exudative retinal detachment has been reported after laser photocoagulation in ROP. In 2014, Ehmann and Greve reported two cases of bullous exudative retinal detachment after 10 and 7 days after laser photocoagulation, respectively [6]. In Case 1, subretinal fluid decreased after two intravitreal dexamethasone and three intravitreal bevacizumab injections. In Case 2, subretinal fluid almost disappeared after two intravitreal bevacizumab injections. However, the exact role of bevacizumab in these cases is not certain.

In 2018, Cabrera et al. reported a case of exudative retinal detachment after laser ablation [7]. A 469-g birth weight, 25-week GA female infant at 35-week PMA received a retinal laser photocoagulation for zone II, stage 3+ ROP. She developed a large macular exudative retinal detachment 5 days after the laser. On OCT, residual subretinal scar and outer retinal loss were detected with a later appearance of a dragged macula noted at 52-week PMA. The authors concluded that post-retinopathy of prematurity laser exudative retinal detachments can resolve without aggressive intervention but may cause permanent retinal sequelae.

A case of exudative retinal detachment after intravitreal bevacizumab injection has also been reported. Chhablani et al. reported a case of exudative retinal detachment with hypotony and patchy choroidal whitening [8]. A male preterm infant born at 28 weeks of gestation developed AP-ROP in zone I and treated with intravitreal bevacizumab. On the next day, hypotony and exudative retinal detachment with patches of choroidal whitening were detected and he was treated with topical steroids and cycloplegic eyedrops. The exudative retinal detachment resolved on the tenth day. The authors concluded that choroidal ischemia secondary to bevacizumab injection for the treatment of AP-ROP could be an unusual complication.

29.5 IOP Elevation After Intravitreal Anti-VEGF Injection

Although IOP elevation is theoretically possible after intravitreal injection in preterm infants, few studies dealt with this issue. A case series study in Switzerland showed that anterior chamber paracentesis was required to reduce IOP in 3 of 6 eyes treated with intravitreal ranibizumab (0.3 mg/0.03 ml) [9]. In these eyes, indirect ophthalmoscopic exams right after intravitreal injection showed poor central artery perfusion due to high IOP, which improved immediately after paracentesis. Although the definition of poor central artery perfusion is not clear in this report, physicians should be aware of possible IOP elevation after intravitreal injection in ROP and fundus exams should be done right after injection.

29.6 Other Unusual Responses After Intravitreal Anti-VEGF Injection in ROP

In a multicenter study in Taiwan, 2 of 49 eyes receiving intravitreal bevacizumab showed transient retinal vessel sheathing after injection [10]. The 2 eyes of 1 patient with bilateral stage 4A ROP developed transient retinal vessel sheathing in the inferior venous branch, which disappeared after vitrectomy. The authors of this study mentioned that although whether the vessel sheathing was due to increased IOP after injection or to the anti-VEGF agent remains unknown, it is more likely that transient sheathing was due to delayed effects of the injected agent rather than the immediate IOP elevation.

A case report in Thailand showed that two sites of choroidal rupture developed along the posterior edges of laser scars after laser photocoagulation and intravitreal bevacizumab for the treatment of AP-ROP in a preterm infant born at 28 weeks of gestation [11]. The authors speculated that the patients developed choroidal rupture because of the dual effects of laser ablation (resulting in chorioretinal scarring with loss of RPE and atrophy of choriocapillaris and larger vessels) and intravitreal bevacizumab (blocking VEGF which is essential for the development and maintenance of choriocapillaris).

References

1. Snyder LL, Garcia-Gonzalez JM, Shapiro MJ, Blair MP. Very late reactivation of retinopathy of prematurity after monotherapy with Intravitreal Bevacizumab. Ophthalmic Surg Lasers Imaging Retina. 2016;47:280–3.
2. Hajrasouliha AR, Garcia-Gonzales JM, Shapiro MJ, Yoon H, Blair MP. Reactivation of retinopathy of prematurity three years after treatment with Bevacizumab. Ophthalmic Surg Lasers Imaging Retina. 2017;48:255–9.
3. Paulus YM, Moshfeghi DM. Persistent plus disease after laser in retinopathy of prematurity with tetralogy of Fallot. Eur J Ophthalmol. 2013;23:764–6.
4. Gunay M, Yavuz T, Celik G, Uludag G. Persistence of retinopathy of prematurity in an infant with tetralogy of fallot. Case Rep Pediatr. 2016;2016:7070316.
5. Wang J, Xiang D. Early clinical characteristics of bacterial endophthalmitis in retinopathy of prematurity after intravitreal bevacizumab injection: a case report. Exp Ther Med. 2017;13:3563–6.
6. Ehmann D, Greve M. Intravitreal bevacizumab for exudative retinal detachment post laser therapy for retinopathy of prematurity. Can J Ophthalmol. 2014;49:228–31.
7. Cabrera MT, Brewer EM, Grant L, Tarczy-Hornoch K. Exudative retinal detachment documented by handheld spectral domain optical coherence tomography after retinal laser photocoagulation for retinopathy of prematurity. Retin Cases Brief Rep. 2018; https://doi.org/10.1097/ICB.0000000000000793.
8. Chhablani J, Rani PK, Balakrishnan D, Jalali S. Unusual adverse choroidal reaction to intravitreal bevacizumab in aggressive posterior retinopathy of prematurity: the Indian Twin Cities ROP screening (ITCROPS) data base report number 7. Semin Ophthalmol. 2014;29:222–5.
9. Menke MN, Framme C, Nelle M, Berger MR, Sturm V, Wolf S. Intravitreal ranibizumab monotherapy to treat retinopathy of prematurity zone II, stage 3 with plus disease. BMC Ophthalmol. 2015;15:20.
10. Wu WC, Yeh PT, Chen SN, Yang CM, Lai CC, Kuo HK. Effects and complications of bevacizumab use in patients with retinopathy of prematurity: a multicenter study in taiwan. Ophthalmology. 2011;118:176–83.
11. Atchaneeyasakul LO, Trinavarat A. Choroidal ruptures after adjuvant intravitreal injection of bevacizumab for aggressive posterior retinopathy of prematurity. J Perinatol. 2010;30:497–9.

Index

The videos for this book can be accessed under http://extras.springer.com/Search.

U. Spandau, S. J. Kim, *Pediatric Retinal Vascular Diseases*,
https://doi.org/10.1007/978-3-030-13701-4

The manufacturer's authorised representative in the EU is Springer Nature Customer Service Centre GmbH, Europaplatz 3, 69115 Heidelberg, Germany. If you have any concerns regarding our products, please contact ProductSafety@springernature.com

Printed and bound by CPI Group (UK) Ltd, Croydon, CR0 4YY
30/07/2026
02181675-0003